NEW DEVELOPMENTS IN MEDICINAL CHEMISTRY

Volume 1

EDITOR

Carlton Anthony Taft

Brazilian Center for Physics Research

Brazil

Co-Editor

Carlos Henrique Tomich de Paula da Silva

School of Pharmaceutical Sciences of Ribeirão Preto,

University of São Paulo

Brazil

eBooks End User License Agreement

CONTENTS

FOREWORD

Quantum mechanics (QM) plays an important role in Computational Medicinal Chemistry. In this book the current state-of-the-art for QM-based methods are discussed including density functional methods, bioisosterism and quantum chemical topology, free energy simulations, solvation thermodynamics, docking and scoring, weak interactions as well as selected applications to Cancer, Aids, Alzheimer, Parkinson and other diseases. QM-based methods are important in ligand-protein binding which is the essence of drug discovery and design. They can be also very useful for determining electronic descriptors which are necessary in bioisosterism, QSAR and other approaches.

Computational medicinal chemistry can predict energies, geometries and diverse physicochemical properties essential for novel drug discovery and optimization. Interactions between a ligand and a molecular target structure can be investigated using molecular interaction fields (MIFs). It is possible to identify regions where specific chemical groups of a ligand molecule can interact favorably with another target molecule, suggesting pharmacophore models or virtual receptor sites. The authors discuss the extensive use of molecular interaction fields in drug discovery including 3D-QSAR, virtual screening, and ADMET prediction.

QSAR has been applied to research and development of pharmaceutical chemistry for more than 40 years, maintaining the predictive ability of the approach as well as its receptiveness to mechanistic or diagnostic interpretations. The authors present and discuss the basis of the QSAR approach in a clear and intuitive way. Toxicology predictions in Medicinal chemistry is also discussed.

In Medicinal Chemistry, drug chirality is an important theme for design and development of new drugs. The authors bring forth a new understanding of the role of molecular recognition in pharmacologically relevant events. Three methods used for the production of a chiral drug are discussed, i.e the chiral pool, separation of racemates, and asymmetric synthesis. Although the use of chiral drugs predates modern medicine, only since the 1980's has there been a significant increase in the development of chiral drugs.

Since the choice of appropriate synthetic approaches are crucial for the efficiency of the drug discovery process, with the introduction of microwave-assisted organic synthesis in 1986, the efficiency of microwave flash-heating chemistry in dramatically reducing reaction times has recently fascinated many pharmaceutical companies, which are incorporating microwave chemistry into their drug development efforts. In this book, the authors extensively explore details of the high-speed medicinal chemistry using focused microwaves.

One of the classes of compounds with great interest in Medicinal Chemistry, which has been largely investigated and synthesized, is the carbohydrates family. The large number of these compounds in nature and their diverse roles in biological systems validate the increasing interest for their chemical and biological research. Blood groups determinants (ABH), tumor associated antigens and pathogen binding sites are some of the relevant glycoconjugates found in mammalian cells. The demand for glycans and glycoconjugates for various studies of targets involved in several serious diseases have been continuously growing. The authors discuss the importance of drug design based on carbohydrate structure for the treatment of parasitic diseases (*T. cruzi*) and virus infections (influenza and HIV), as well as the development of glycoconjugate antitumour vaccines related to the structure of human mucin-associated glycans.

The book also includes an important review and discussion about one of the most promising targets in the study of Alzheimer's disease (AD), the Glycogen Synthase Kinase-3β (GSK-3β), as well as the inhibitors that are being developed. This enzyme has been associated with the primary abnormalities found in AD, including hyperphosphorylation of the microtubule-associated protein tau, which contributes to the formation of neurofibrillary tangles, a second trademark of the disease, and its interactions with other Alzheimer's disease-associated proteins.

This book thus attempts to convey a few selected topics stimulating the fascination of working in all the multidisciplinary areas, which overlaps knowledge of chemistry, physics, biochemistry, biology and pharmacology, describing some of theoretical and experimental methods in Medicinal Chemistry. It is interesting to consider the information described in this book as the starting point to access available and diverse knowledge in this exciting Medicinal Chemistry field.

Prof. Dr. Ramaswamy Sarma
State University of New York
Albany, NY, USA

PREFACE

This book is aimed at, from students to advanced researchers, for anyone that is interested or works with medicinal chemistry, at experimental or theoretical levels for many therapeutic purposes. We attempt to convey a few selected topics stimulating the fascination of working in these multidisciplinary areas, which overlaps knowledge of chemistry, physics, biochemistry, biology and pharmacology. This book contains 7 chapters, of which 3 are related to theoretical methods in medicinal chemistry whereas the others deal with experimental/mixed methods.

In modern computational medicinal chemistry, quantum mechanics (QM) plays an important role since the associated methods can describe molecular energies, bond breaking or forming, charge transfer and polarization effects. Historically in drug design, QM ligand-based applications were devoted to investigations of electronic features, and they have also been routinely used in the development of quantum descriptors in quantitative structure-activity relationships (QSAR) approaches. Today, QM-based methods are crucial in ligand-protein binding which is the essence of drug discovery and design. In chapter 1, we present an overview of the state-of-the-art of QM-based methods currently used in medicinal chemistry. Bioisosterism, quantum chemical topology, free energy simulations, solvation thermodynamics, docking and scoring, weak interactions as well as selected applications to various diseases are discussed.

Glycogen Synthase Kinase-3β (GSK-3β), a serine/threonine kinase, has emerged as one of the most attractive therapeutic targets for the treatment of the Alzheimer's disease (AD). This enzyme has been linked to all the primary abnormalities associated with AD, including hyperphosphorylation of the microtubule-associated protein tau, which contribute to the formation of neurofibrillary tangles, and its interactions with others Alzheimer's disease-associated proteins. Thus, the significant role of GSK-3β in essential events in the pathogenesis of AD makes this kinase an attractive therapeutic target for neurological disorders. Chapter 2 explores the nature and the structure of this promising enzyme, focusing on the structure-based design of new GSK-3β inhibitors.

Computational chemistry can be used to predict physicochemical properties, energies, binding modes, interactions and a large amount of helpful data in lead discovery and optimization. Interactions between a ligand and a molecular target structure can be investigated using molecular interaction fields (MIF). Employing such approaches, it is possible to identify regions where specific chemical groups of a ligand molecule can interact favorably with another target molecule, suggesting pharmacore models or virtual receptor sites. In chapter 3, we discuss how molecular interaction fields have been extensively used in drug discovery projects including a variety of applications: 3D-QSAR, virtual screening, similarity of protein targets and specificity of ligands, prediction of pharmacokinetic properties and determination of ligand binding sites in biomolecular target structures.

The development of quantitative structure-activity relationships (QSARs or 2D QSARs) is a science that has developed without a defined framework, series of rules, or guidelines for methodology. It has been more than 40 years since the QSAR paradigm first found its way into the practice of agrochemistry, pharmaceutical chemistry, toxicology, and eventually most facets of chemistry. Its staying power may be attributed to the strength of its initial postulate that activity is a function of structure as described by electronic attributes, hydrophobicity, and steric properties as well as rapid and extensive development in methodologies and computational techniques that have ensued to delineate and refine the many variables and approaches that define the paradigm. The overall goals of QSAR retain their original essence and remain focused on the predictive ability of the approach and its receptiveness to mechanistic or diagnostic interpretations. Our intention with chapter 4 is to offer the basis of the QSAR approach in a clear and intuitive way, with maximum simplification and trying to close the gap that exists between maths and students of pharmacy. Moreover, the interpretation of the equations is even more important than statistically obtaining significant and robust relationships. We will show our results on Choline Kinase (ChoK) inhibitors as antiproliferative agents to demonstrate the possibilities of the Hansch model in the drug design process.

The issue of drug chirality is now a major theme in the design and development of new drugs, and our aim in chapter 5 is to discuss its importance in Medicinal Chemistry, underpinned by a new understanding of the role of molecular recognition in many pharmacologically relevant events. In general, three methods are utilized for the production of a chiral drug: the chiral pool, separation of racemates, and asymmetric synthesis. Although the use of chiral drugs predates modern medicine, only since the 1980's has there been a significant increase in the development of chiral pharmaceutical drugs. The thalidomide tragedy increased awareness of stereochemistry in the action of drugs, and as a result the number of drugs administered as racemic compounds has steadily decreased. In 2001, more than 70% of the new chiral drugs approved were single enantiomers. Approximately 1 in 4 therapeutic agents are marked as racemic mixtures, the individual enantiomers of which frequently differ in both their pharmacodynamic and pharmacokinetic profiles. The use of racemates has become the subject of considerable discussion in recent years, and an area of concern for both the pharmaceutical industry and regulatory authorities. Pharmaceutical companies are required to justify each decision to manufacture a racemic drug in preference to its homochiral version. Moreover, the use of single enantiomers has a number of potential clinical advantages, including an improved therapeutic/pharmacological profile, a reduction in complex drug interactions, and simplified pharmacokinetics. In a number of instances stereochemical considerations have contributed to an understanding of the pharmacological effects observed for a drug administered as a racemate. However, relatively little is known of the influence of patient factors (e.g. disease state, age, gender and genetics) on drug enantiomer disposition and action in man. Examples may also be cited where the use of a single enantiomer, non-racemic mixtures and racemates of currently used agents may offer clinical advantages. The issues associated with drug chirality are complex and depend upon the relative merits of the individual agent. In the future it is likely that a number of existing racemates will be re-marketed as single enantiomer products with potentially improved clinical profiles and possible novel therapeutic indications.

Microwaves are a powerful and reliable energy source that may be adapted to many applications. Since the introduction of microwave-assisted organic synthesis in 1986, the use of microwave irradiation has now introduced a completely new approach to drug discovery. The efficiency of microwave flash-heating chemistry in dramatically reducing reaction times has recently fascinated many pharmaceutical companies, which are incorporating microwave chemistry into their drug development efforts. Thus, the time saved by using focused microwaves is important either in traditional organic synthesis or in high-speed medicinal chemistry, which has been analyzed by us in chapter 6.

The high abundance of carbohydrates in nature and their diverse roles in biological systems validate the increasing interest for their chemical and biological research. Carbohydrates can be found as monomers or oligomers, or as glycoconjugates, which are formed by an oligosaccharide moiety joined to a protein (glycoproteins) or to a lipid moiety (glycolipids). Blood groups determinants (ABH), tumor associated antigens and pathogen binding sites are some of the relevant glycoconjugates found in mammalian cells. It is well known that carbohydrate and glycoconjugate molecules are implicated in many cellular processes, especially in biological recognition events, including cell adhesion, differentiation and growth, signal transduction, protozoa, bacterial and virus infection, and immune response. Therefore, the demand for glycans and glycoconjugates for various studies of targets involved in several serious diseases have been continuously growing. In chapter 7 we discuss the design of drugs based on carbohydrate structure for treatment of parasitic diseases (*T. cruzi*) and virus infections (influenza and HIV). Moreover, the development of glycoconjugate antitumor vaccines related to the structure of human mucin-associated glycans will also be outlined.

Some contents of this book also reflect some of our own ideas and personal experiences, which are presented in selected topics. It is interesting to consider the information described in this book as the starting point to access considerable available and varied knowledge in the Medicinal Chemistry field.

CONTRIBUTORS

Carlton A. Taft	Full Professor, Brazilian Center for Physics Research, Rio de Janeiro, Brazil
Carlos H. T. P. Silva	Associate Professor, School of Pharmaceutical Sciences of Ribeirão Preto, University of São Paulo, Ribeirão Preto, Brazil
Adriana M. Namba	Postdoctoral Researcher, School of Pharmaceutical Sciences of Ribeirão Preto, University of São Paulo, Ribeirão Preto, Brazil
Vinícius B. Silva	Fellow, School of Pharmaceutical Sciences of Ribeirão Preto, University of São Paulo, Ribeirão Preto, Brazil
Jonathan R. Almeida	Fellow, School of Pharmaceutical Sciences of Ribeirão Preto, University of São Paulo, Ribeirão Preto, Brazil
Ana C. García	Assistant Professor, Department of Pharmaceutical Chemistry, School of Pharmacy, Granada, Spain
Miguel A. Gallo	Full Professor, Department of Pharmaceutical Chemistry, School of Pharmacy, Granada, Spain
Joaquín M. Campos	Full Professor, Department of Pharmaceutical Chemistry, School of Pharmacy, Granada, Spain
María del C. Núñez	Assistant Professor, Department of Pharmaceutical Chemistry, School of Pharmacy, Granada, Spain
Antonio Espinosa	Full Professor, Department of Pharmaceutical Chemistry, School of Pharmacy, Granada, Spain
Peterson Andrade	Fellow, School of Pharmaceutical Sciences of Ribeirão Preto, University of São Paulo, Ribeirão Preto, Brazil
Lílian S. C. Bernardes	Assistant Professor, Federal University of Santa Catarina, Santa Catarina, Brazil
Ivone Carvalho	Full Professor, School of Pharmaceutical Sciences of Ribeirão Preto, University of São Paulo, Ribeirão Preto, Brazil
Vanessa L. Campo	Postdoctoral Researcher, School of Pharmaceutical Sciences of Ribeirão Preto, University of São Paulo, Ribeirão Preto, Brazil
Valquíria A. Leoneti	Postdoctoral Researcher, School of Pharmaceutical Sciences of Ribeirão Preto, University of São Paulo, Ribeirão Preto, Brazil
Maristela B. M. Teixeira	Fellow, School of Pharmaceutical Sciences of Ribeirão Preto, University of São Paulo, Ribeirão Preto, Brazil

CHAPTER 1

Current State-of-the-art for Quantum Mechanics-based Methods in Drug Design

Carlton Anthony Taft[1] and Carlos Henrique Tomich de Paula da Silva[2]

[1]*Brazilian Center for Physics Research, Rua Dr. Xavier Sigaud, 150, Urca, 22290-180, Rio de Janeiro, Brazil and* [2]*School of Pharmaceutical Sciences of Ribeirão Preto, University of São Paulo, Av. do Café, s/n, Monte Alegre, 14040-903, Ribeirão Preto, São Paulo, Brazil*

Abstract: We review the current state of the art for quantum mechanics-based methods in drug design and selected applications to various diseases. We present a brief introduction and give current trends for each section. We review bioisosterims and quantum chemical topology (shape, conformation, multipole moments, hydrogen bonding, fingerprint, charge distributions), free energy simulations (equilibrium, non-equilibrium), Molecular Interaction Fields (grids, hotspots, fingerprints), solvation (MD/MM-PBSA-GBSA, FEP/TI/LIE, COSMO, PCM/DFT), docking (algorithms, scoring, new approaches), summary of quantum mechanics approximations focusing on density functional methods (AM1, HF, Post-HF, MP, QM/MM), DFT(GGA, Meta-GGA, pure τ functionals, DHDF, MO6, vW-D, Hybrids)) and weak interactions (hydrogen, van der Waals, carbohydrate-aromatic, halogen, environmental electron densities). Using these models we present selected applications of our work during the last decade in which we proposed novel inhibitors for Cancer, Aids, Alzheimer, Parkinson and other diseases.

INTRODUCTION

With the tools of quantum mechanics and computational chemistry it is possible to characterize structure, energetics and dynamics of the interactions of atoms and molecules with their biological counterparts. The desired effect of drugs on humans is a result of the molecular recognition between drug and target (proteins). The type of binding, spatial arrangement and molecular electronic structure will determine the effectiveness and activity of the drug at its site of action. Although inexpensive approaches such as those based on molecular mechanics (MM) can aid in novel lead discoveries, QM-based approaches would be fundamental if quantum physical-chemistry effects are important, i.e charge transfer, polarization, forming/breaking, describing bonds, weak interactions, solvation and enthalpic/entropic effects.

In drug design, historically, QM-based tools were used for development of quantum descriptors for structure-activity correlations in QSAR experiments. Semi empirical level QM calculations have also been used for development of descriptors and structure-activity correlations. However, problems in which molecular mechanics (MM) and semi-emprical models have failed are nowadays solved by QM-based methods. Some of these problems involve ligand-binding affinities, transition metal complexes, charge transfer effects, weak interactions, bond forming/breaking, enzymatic reactions by biological systems of pharmacological relevance, transition state configurations, solvation effects and accurate determination of free energies. QM-based approaches can also be used in developing tools for other fields such as quantum chemical topology in drug design and force fields for molecular mechanics and dynamics.

We discuss bioisosterism and quantum chemical topology in drug design involving quantum chemical descriptors such as shape, conformation, charge, electronic distribution, fingerprints, multipole moments, polarity and hydrogen bonding. We present free energy simulations tools FEP / REFEP / TI / FDTI /RTI/LIE / OS / ADuMWHAM / PT / PTTI / λ-dynamics / non-equilibrium methods. Docking techniques are discussed. The effects of flexibility, water, large databases, efficiency of scoring algorithms, importance of benchmarking, multiple protein structures, hybrids involving molecular dynamics (MD), Monte Carlo (MC) and DFT are discussed. The emphasis is, however, on new approaches and current trends. Molecular Interaction Fields are discussed. Basic quantum mechanical tools are summarized, i.e semi empirical, Hartree-Fock and Post-Hartree-Fock approximations. We review density functions methods with a brief historical introduction and emphasis on new density functionals. We also discuss weak interactions (hydrogen bonds, van der Waals, carbohydrate interactions, halogen bonds and environmental electron density effects).

BIOISOSTERISM AND QUANTUM CHEMICAL TOPOLOGY IN DRUG DESIGN

Maintaining or enhancing the original bioactivity, the concept of bioisosterism is applied in medicinal chemistry to make modifications to potential new drug compounds. Properties such as toxicity and solubility can be altered without loss of potency. The quantum chemical basis for biososterism can be used to identify the quantifiable physical characteristics that lead to similarity in biological activity. Using *ab initio* data, we can find bioiosteric fragment replacements with original electronic, geometric and physical chemical properties which can be linked to broader chemical characteristics relevant to biological activity. Capping groups can also be used to represent different chemical environments based on transferability. Bond properties can be obtained from the electron density and surface properties can be defined by partitioning the molecular isodensity surface. Efficient algorithms can also allow us to use pharmacophores to compare the spatial distribution of molecular features allowing rapid alignment into chemically significant orientations. Gaussian overlay fingerprints as well as force field and *ab-intio* calculations of 3d structures can be used for shape comparisons to indicate fragment replacements. Saddle points of the electron density between bonded nuclei also yields useful information. Quantum chemical descriptors with information on biological activity for known drugs can be obtained from isolated molecular wave functions and stored [1-26].

Among the quantum chemical descriptors we have shape, conformation, size, charge and property distribution fingerprints, electronic distribution, atomic multipole moments, polarity, surface properties and hydrogen bonding among others [1-4].

Some of the important factors to fit a ligand into the binding site are size and shape. Formation of binding conformations can be influenced by stable conformations of linkers whose groups are defined as fragments with two connection points to a parent compound. Detailed *ab initio* calculations of conformational and steric properties can be stored in databases. In addition it is possible to evaluate linker conformation using geometric measures. For comparison of volume overlap for prealigned structures there are 3D fingerprints as well as linker dimensions and volume [1-5].

Directional properties such as dipole moments may be influenced by fragment conformations. A molecular conformation bound to a target can be related to the stable conformers linkers can adopt. For each linker, electronic and structural properties for low energy conformations can be calculated by full optimization using *ab-intio* methods and stored in databases.

In general, conformers with unique back-bones and the most diverse set of side chains should be included. By aligning the linkers we can determine the similarity in linker conformation. The global conformation of a molecule is determined by the relative orientation of two linker connection points. Geometric orientation and separation of the second linker relative to the first can describe the conformation of the linker. Atomic Cartesian coordinates for bonds and atoms inside linkers can be compared once the linkers are prealigned in a reference axis system. However, different torsional rotations can be obtained with identical backbone conformations and it is not possible to guarantee always identical molecular geometries in a parent compound by closely matching linker geometric parameters. Obtaining similar impacts on global conformation of parent compounds should be the main usage of linker geometric parameters [1-15].

The spatial dimension of each linker in its standard orientation can be used to compare the linker size. Capping by an isodensity surface the atomic volumes of all atoms inside the linker, yields the linker volumes. The binding site of a target can also be influenced by steric interactions due to shape fingerprints. It is of interest to use linker isosters with similar shapes. In order to gain a measure of linker volume overlap, fingerprints can be compared with the spatial distribution of chemical physical properties of stored linkers. In addition, spatial distribution of H-bond atoms can also yield linker replacements via fingerprint identification whereas, in contrast with shape fingerprints, only the requested physical properties are used [1-25].

The electrostatic interaction with other moieties can be determined by the distribution of charges and is important for ligand-protein binding. The charge density can be obtained with high details using *ab initio* calculations.

Multipole moments can be described using spherical harmonics and stored up to the quadrupole moment whereas directionality can also be included yielding a measure of similarity in charge distribution.

In cases, such as for example, when part of a linker's isodensity surface is relatively more important, an additional, nondirectional descriptor such as polarity can be stored. This polarity can be defined in a linker as an average of the mean value of the electrostatic potential across each atom's surface grid.

Both the ionization energy and the electrostatic potential can be stored across atomic grids on the isodensity surfaces whereas the energy required to remove electron n from point r is given by the ionization energy. Regions most susceptible for charge transfer to electrophiles are correlated with regions of lowest ionization energies on a molecular surface.

Although it is not easy to directly calculate H-bond acceptor and donor strengths, it is possible to store *ab initio* descriptors. These can be correlated with the electrostatic potential and ionization energies on the isodensity surface of H-bond acceptor atoms and the electrostatic potential energy at the nuclear position of an H-bond acidic proton. Using shape fingerprints to compare the positions and strengths of donor and acceptor atoms it is then possible to count the number of donor and acceptors [1-25].

It is also possible to use *ab initio* bond lengths and quantum chemistry descriptors to predict lipid and solubility parameters. Fitting of nonlinear or linear expressions to *ab initio* quantum chemistry descriptors is the basic approach used in the development of QSPR and QSAR models. Consequently, storing a wide range of theoretical parameters in databases is important for future development of models. Among the basic properties generally stored and used are volume, charge, dipole moment, quadrupole moment, Laplacian, Lagrangian kinetic energy, force exerted on nucleus by atomic density, attractive energy of atomic density to nucleus, electron-electron repulsion and total potential energy.

The delocalization index of a pair of bonded atoms, derived from the electron pair density, gives an intuitive measure of bond order. This model, at the RHF level, yields results in agreement with the classical conceptual `Lewis model`. Based on the degree of electron pair overlap between A and B, the delocalization index yields a quantitative and intuitive method of comparing bond orders as well as quantifying charge delocalization throughout an entire structure. A similar property called the localization index describes the extent to which electrons are localized on a single atom. Using volume integrals of the pair densities, the atomic overlap matrix can be evaluated, charge delocalization throughout an entire structure can be investigated and delocalization between atoms and ring positions can be compared.

Using the fragmentation approach, the linkers groups stored in databases can be found yielding drug like molecules. The data from fragmentation to be stored in database can be classified using simple architectures emphasizing atomic as well as whole linker properties. The database can often be accessed via Web interfaces, allowing interactive construction of database search queries without need to install new softwares. Weighted Euclidean distances from linkers in property space can be used for scoring hits whereas search tolerance in the property value can be used to normalize distances.

The 'Quantum Isostere Database' (QID) [1] is a Web based tool designed to find bioisosteric fragment replacements for lead optimization using *ab initio* data. QID stores a range of novel quantum chemical descriptors for fragments of known drug compounds taken from the World Drug Index (WDI) [26]. Physical descriptors with clear meaning are chosen such as electrostatic energy, surface and geometric parameters. Further fundamental physical properties are linked to broader chemical characteristics relevant to biological activity. Conformational dependence is explicitly dealt with and capping groups are used to represent different chemical environments based on background research into transferability of electronic descriptors. The resulting database has a Web interface that allows medicinal chemists to enter a query fragment, select important chemical features and retrieve a list of suggested replacements with similar chemical characteristics [1-26].

FREE ENERGY SIMULATIONS

The thermodynamic quantity, free energy, defines binding affinity. The binding pose is the orientation of a ligand in a protein binding pocket whereas the enthalpy is the energy of interaction for a singly such pose. Entropy represents the sum over all possible poses since not only the optimum poses, but also multiple poses are possible. The entropy will be high when multiple low enthalpy poses are possible and low if a single pose is favored. It is a very demanding problem to determine entropy by summing over the enthalpies of multiple poses [27-76].

At constant pressure and temperature a system will spontaneously evolve in the direction of decreasing Gibbs free energy until equilibrium is reached ($\Delta G=0$; $\Delta G=\Delta H - T\Delta S$). ΔS and ΔG are changes in entropy and enthalpy respectively. This equation reflects the tendency for the thermal motion to disrupt association and bond formation and the natural preference for lower potential energies, i.e the enthalpy-entropy compensation phenomenon whereas various combinations of unfavorable/favorable entropy/enthalpy components can lead to protein-ligand binding (ΔH reduces to the change in internal energy).

The equilibrium between a ligand A and its receptor B can be witten as a dissociation/association phenomenon, whereas at temperature T=298 K and P = 1 atm with reactants and products at a concentration of 1 M, $\Delta G`$ (free energy change in a hypothetical standard reference state) can be written as a function of the concentrations of the species using the law of mass action, leading to $\Delta G`= RTln([A]_{eq}[B]_{eq}/(AB]_{eq}) = RT \ln K$. The exponential relationship between the free energy and equilibrium constant (K_d) indicates that even small changes in free energy have considerable effects on the equilibrium constant.

The calculated values of ΔG needs to be accurate to be helpful. The quality of the potential used to represent molecular energies as well as conformational sampling is important. At least the most populated states needs to be probed for free energy calculations and it is necessary to sample the various configurations as extensively as possible. Since at physiological temperatures proteins populate many conformational states, the notion of molecular simulations to obtain thermodynamic ensembles of conformations is intricately associated with that of free energy calculations.

In order to calculate affinity differences, initial efforts focused on approaches whereas one ligand is transformed incrementally into another via a series of *in-silico* non-physical states. Any path between the two states is legitimate (state function). Physical-chemistry determines the transformation. Firmly rooted in statistical mechanics, these protocols are Thermodynamics Integration (TI) and free energy perturbation (FEP). Each state along the transformation has to be coupled to the chemical topologies of both end points. The methods can be computationally expensive.

The increase in reference experimental results has been very important for improvement of theoretical predictions of affinities, receptor-ligand structures and empirical scoring functions. Although effects such as hydrogen bonding and apolar contacts may not be accurately incorporated, the chemically intuitive nature of the empirical scoring functions is important for computing and ranking quickly, large libraries of diverse compound docked to a target`s active site.

Fundamental to understanding the thermodynamic properties of many biologically important systems and phenomena, are the free energy simulation methods which are used to estimate protein stability, protein-ligand binding affinities as well as hydration free energies. From the difference in the free energies associated with the chemical transformation of one ligand into the other, in the solvent and bound environments, it is possible to determine the binding affinities of ligands. Effectively, the free energy of binding is the force behind ligand binding with target-protein in biomolecular systems.

The subtle balance between entropic and energetic effects yields the free energy originating from loss of conformations, translational, orientational degrees of freedom, direct ligand-protein interactions as well as (de) solvation effects of both ligand and host. Different specificities arise mainly from differing entropies and enthalpies. There is thus a need for methods that focus on entropy and binding energy accurately in order to reliably predict and reproduce novel drug activities. Consequently, computational techniques that estimate binding free energies play a very important role in understanding experimental structure-activity relations and affinities as well as screening and design of novel putative ligands. In this regards we focus in this chapter on some of the recent current trends for binding free energy calculations [27 -76].

In traditional thermodynamic integration (TI) and free energy perturbation (FEP) the vertical `arms` of the thermodynamic cycle are evaluated by alchemically morphing one ligand into the other in order to determine their free energy changes. At discrete points along the transformation pathway, between the end-states, multiple simulations are performed. The Hamiltonian for these simulations are defined as $H = T_x + (1 - \lambda)V_0 + \lambda V_1$ where λ indicates the distance along the transformational pathway and the potential energy contributions associated with the two end-points are given by V_0 and V_1 [28, 31, 47-48].

Many calculations of protein ligand binding have been made using full statistical thermodynamic treatment of protein-ligand binding. One of these methods is free energy perturbation (FEP) which represents a baseline capability whereas the free energy change is computed from the ensemble averages generated at discrete λ values. This method calculates the relative free energy of two systems A and B, via the Zwanzig equation [51] where the difference in free energy between systems A and B is given as the ensemble average of the exponential of the difference in energy of the two systems, divided by the Bolzmann's constant multiplied by the temperature [44]. The average is formed over the ensemble generated by system A, which is known as the reference state whereas system B is known as the perturbed state.

The average formed will only converge satisfactorily if the reference and perturbed states are similar with a good overlap between them. To ensure that this is the case, the two systems are connected by a reaction coordinate, λ which does not need to be a scaling coordinate, i.e could be an intermolecular distance, dihedral angle or reaction coordinate. This method has evolved and has been used for drug design purposes. However, the computational demands are significant since for each pair of ligands that are investigated, simulations at multiple λ values must be made. For the FEP method, the main limitation is the pre-selected binding site of the protein for a pre-selected pose. The ligand cannot easily cross the local energy barriers to explore different poses, which is an important issue, due to the fact that with the number of rotable bonds in the molecule there is a dramatical increase in the possible conformations to explore [33, 46-48].

Thermodynamic integration (TI) is a well-established rigorous free energy method based on the coupling parameter λ, described for FEP, whereas simulations are made with λ values, allowing good phase space overlap from systems A to B. The free energy gradient is the property accumulated by each simulation, which can be found by integrating over the measured gradients. Effectively, TI uses the gradient of the free energy, with respect to λ to construct the potential of mean force (PMF) across λ by calculating the gradient at various points along λ and then numerically integrating them to obtain the complete PMF [33, 42-49].

Alternatively the free-energy gradients may be calculated numerically by approximating the gradient by finite difference. In order to verify the accuracy of the approximation, both the forward and backward gradient may be calculated. If $\Delta\lambda$ is small enough the forward gradient should equal the negative of the backward gradient which would be a good estimate of the analytic gradient (FDTI) [33, 46-47]

The benefit of FDTI over FEP is that the overlap between the reference and perturbed states is significantly improved through the use of small values of $\Delta\lambda$ and the Zwanzig equation is expected to converge well. The advantage of FDTI over TI is that it may be performed in any FEP-capable simulation package. The disadvantage of TI and FDTI is that the final numerical integration can magnify any random errors in the gradients leading to a loss of precision in the results [33, 46-47].

Replica exchange TI (RTI) incorporates Hamiltonian replica exchange moves between adjacent λ simulations whereas λ moves are made periodically in such a way that each configuration is exchanged with a neighbor. In order that these moves adhere to a detailed balance, they are accepted or rejected with the equivalence of two metropolis tests. RTI increases sampling, especially of the solvent, by providing the possibility of ensembles making large jumps in phase space. In addition, as simulations are able to move freely, configurations which are more favorable to a particular area of λ, may migrate there [46]. A similar technique may be used to combine replica-exchange with FEP, resulting in replica-exchange FEP (REFEP) [31, 46-48].

Adaptive umbrella sampling and the related adaptive umbrella weighted histogram analysis method (ADuMWHAM) treats λ as a dynamic coordinate and perform moves in λ throughout the simulation. An umbrella potential is iteratively refined to encourage even sampling of the λ coordinate. After this is achieved, the umbrella equals the negative of the potential of mean force along λ from which the relative free energy may be obtained. AdUmWHAM is a modification of adaptive umbrella sampling that uses the weighted histogram analysis method (WHAM) to combine the statistics of all previous iterations efficiently when refining the umbrella. The disadvantages of these methods is that the moves along λ are driven by the umbrella potential and cannot progress too quickly for the rest of the system to respond, leading to `Hamiltonian lag` [47].

Parallel tempering (PT) enhances sampling through the use of multiple replica of the system, each running at a different temperature whereas neighboring temperatures are tested according to a PT Monte Carlo (MC) test. If this test is passed, the coordinates of the system at these temperatures are exchanged and at the end of the simulation the set of trajectories at each temperature form a correct ensemble distribution. Parallel tempering thermodynamic integration (PTTI) enhances sampling through the use of multiple replicas of the system, each running at a different temperature [47].

The linear interaction method (LIE) is based on linear response theory and estimates the binding free energy of a compound from the ensemble average of the potential interaction energy. It can be used as a semi empirical scoring function, calculating binding free energies between the protein and ligands. Molecular dynamics simulations of both bound and unbound states of a ligand can be performed and the simulation averages of the interaction energies between the ligand and its environment used to determine binding free energies. It can address the electrostatic contribution to the binding free energy as the difference of adding a charge distribution to an uncharged compound, free, when bound to the protein, and in solution. By assuming for both charged and uncharged states a quadratic form of the free energy landscape, linear response theory can estimate the free energy difference between them. The calculation is simplified by the observation that the electrostatic interactions will average to zero if applied to a simulation of the uncharged species. This holds if without a net charge, the neutral form of molecules are placed in a homogeneous medium or if extensive orientational sampling in polarized environments are indicated. For the nonpolar part, the free energy of cavity formation is estimated by using the empirical observation that both the free energy and the Van der Waals potential energy of nonpolar compounds, correlate linearly with the size of the molecule [31,48].

Another method is the one-step (OS) perturbation method, in which a possible unphysical reference molecule, which shows similarity to a range of relevant ligands, is simulated and free energies for all these ligands are obtained from a single simulation. Unlike TI or FEP, the OS method uses the thermodynamics cycle rather than connecting two states A and B by simulations at many intermediate states. This method relies on the definition of a single reference state or compound S, which samples the relevant degrees of freedom for both states A and B. The Zhanzig`s equation [51] can be applied, when a state S has been found to calculate ΔA_{AS} whereas because free energy is a state function, the difference between states B and A can be calculated as $\Delta A_{BA} = \Delta A_{BS} - \Delta A_{AS}$. One way of constructing S is by using soft atoms whereas the interactions are modified in such a way that the singularity has been removed for overlapping particles. A tremendous gain in efficiency of OS over TI or FEP is possible if one state S can be chosen, which may be used to calculate free energies for a series of endstates A, B, C......whereas only a single simulation at state S is required and the Zwanzig equation can be applied *a posteriori* because only the less computationally demanding calculation of determining the differences $H_A - H_S$ is required [31].

Both OS and LIE methods have their weaknesses and strengths. For prediction of nonpolar compounds the LIE results are reportedly rather poor whereas the OS methods performs better. The apolar art of the LIE equation is more empirical in nature whereas the OS method can be derived from statistical mechanics. The OS method with a neutral reference state performs poorly when electrostatic interactions are involved whereas the LIE method is better for these interactions [31,50-55].

Since a combination of LIE and OS (LIE/OS) can lead to an increase in accuracy, a new combination was proposed taking into consideration the best of both methods. The apolar contribution to the free energy can be calculated by the OS approach improving the LIE estimate of polar contribution to the binding free energies, where the OS approach performs particularly poorly. The combined approach is reportedly more accurate than any of the two separate methods, is computationally slightly more demanding than LIE, has the advantage that most of the computational effort goes into simulations of physically relevant states with only a slight loss in precision. The usage of empirical parameters, other than the force-field description of the molecular system, is no longer necessary when calculating relative free energies of binding [31].

In the λ-dynamics simulation method the λ parameter is propagated along with the atomic coordinates during a simulation and treated as a dynamic variable with a fictitious mass. This simulation can simultaneously evaluate multiple ligands establishing a constraint whereas the sum of λ^2 over all the ligands is equal to 1. All ligands compete for a common receptor based on their relative free energies using multiple copy simultaneous search methods, similar to those of binding experiments and structure-based design [28,60-62].

The extended Hamiltonian for a λ-dynamics system can be written as the sum of kinetic and potential energy terms. The kinetic energies are the sum of energies derived from atomic coordinates and λ variables whereas the hybrid function for L ligands and a protein is constructed from x and x_i coordinates for the environment and the ligand i respectively as well as the biasing potential F and the coupling parameter λ^2. The use of λ^2 ensures that λ values are in the range [0,1] throughout the simulation trajectory. Given two ligands i and j, with biasing potentials F_i and F_j, the difference in free energy can be determined from the simulation [28,60-63].

An alternate method obtains relative free energies from a single λ-dynamics simulation. This is effectively a generalized ensemble TI method whereas snapshots from a λ-dynamics trajectory are sorted into bins according to their λ value and the traditional TI equation can be used to compute the change in free energy associated with each individual bin [63].

In λ-dynamics, biasing potentials can be used as a reference free energy or can be the free energies associated with the corresponding ligand transformations in the solvent environment. They can also serve for biasing potentials focusing the sampling in a particular region of phase space. For a given simulation, biasing potentials can be chosen to reduce the barrier height between different states along the reaction coordinates. The estimated free energies of each ligand from a simulation can also be selected as the biasing potentials for the corresponding ligands in the subsequent simulation. Data from multiple simulation trajectories can be combined to obtain more accurate estimates of the free energy [64,68].

In multiple topology representations for λ-dynamic, multiple ligands are represented explicitly in a simulation although they do not interact with each other directly, i.e the ligands sample independent conformations within the binding pocket. Restraining potentials can be added to the hybrid potential so that ligands that are only weakly coupled to the environment do not wander outside the vicinity of the binding pocket. The restraining potential depends on λ_i and the atomic coordinates of ligand i as well as the average coordinates of the environment atoms, x_o and ensures that the ligands remain in low-energy regions of conformational space and can also prevent high-energy states that cause instability [28,33,46-47,60-65].

λ-dynamics has been incorporated into some modeling software packages whereas the system is partitioned into the environment and the individual ligands. Initial values of the parameters are specified for each partition of the system and additional restraining potentials can be applied to a specific partition. Some workers treat λ as a dynamic variable that is varied via Monte Carlo schemes after every molecular dynamics step in which the atomic coordinates are propagated [66,67].

One of the advantages of λ-dynamics over TI and FEP methods can be attributed to its ability to assess the thermodynamic properties, in a single simulation, of multiple chemical moieties which can include multiple substituents attached to a common ligand as well as individual ligands. λ-dynamics has also demonstrated its ability to rapidly and reliably differentiate between good and poor binders whereas for most drug design problems it is sufficient to identify the poor binders. Variation of λ-dynamics include constant pHMD (CPHMD) in which fictitious λ particles are used to propagate titration degrees of freedom and the end-states represent the deprotonated (λ=0) and protonated (λ =1) states [73].

Recently a dynamic λ parameter was incorporated into the adiabatic free energy dynamics (AFED) method for generating free energy profiles along reaction paths by choosing switching functions that generate a high barrier between the endpoints and by carefully assigning the temperature and mass of λ [74]. Another approach use λ as a self-regulating sampling variable to efficiently traverse high-energy barriers and to thoroughly explore low-energy biasing. By using multiple copies of a subset of the system and intermittently varying their associated λ values a copy in a high-energy region will adopt a small λ value and will sample more broadly until it finds a low-energy region [75]. However, λ-dynamics have focused on simulating differences at single sites in a given system including explicitly represented ligands to amino acid side chains within peptides as well as chemical moieties attached to a specific substituent site on a common core compound [28,62,64,76].

The theoretical foundation of binding free energy predictions based on atomistic representations of the protein-ligand complex is based on statistical thermodynamics whereas at equilibrium we can write the biomolecular reaction for the standard free energy of association as -RTln($1/K_i$). Classical statistical thermodynamics relationships connect the macroscopic thermodynamic properties to microscopic properties via molecular, canonical ensemble partition functions of the complex, the individual species and the solvent. Although the partition functions, in principle, enumerate all the possible microscopic states of the molecules, the direct calculation of the partition function, in practice, for complex systems such as solvated proteins, is unfeasible due to the configurational integral. Although there have been ingenious efforts to decompose the free energy into numerous components in order to approximate the calculations, the difficulties persist mainly due to the error in the calculations of the free energy components which is larger than the actual absolute value of the binding strength [28-55].

It is necessary to sometimes inject empirically derived corrections or simplifying assumptions. In the path-integral method for predicting relative binding affinities of protein-ligand complexes a different approach is presented based on a stochastic kinetic formalism. Inspired by Feynman's path integral formulation there was an extension of the theory to classical interacting systems whereas the ligand is modeled as a Brownian particle subjected to the effective nonbonding interaction potential of the receptor which allows the calculation of the relative binding affinities of interacting biomolecules in water to be computed as a function of the ligand's diffusivity and the curvature of the potential surface in the vicinity of the binding minimum. These calculations are reportedly exceedingly rapid and in test cases, the correlation coefficient between actual and computed free energies > 0.93 for accurate data sets [30].

In rational drug design the lack of sufficient computational resources remains one of the factors preventing the general application of free energy methods. In recent years many nonequilibrium (NE) free energy methods have been made parallel and more accessible regarding computational resources [33, 36, 45, 71]. The nonequilibrium methods do not use the potential energy differences used in FEP calculations, instead, λ is incremented n times (where n is a constant for the calculation) from 0 to 1, with simulation sampling allowed between increments and the work performed, as a consequence of each λ increment, is summed. Estimating the free energy difference through the work, determined from the potential energy differences, invariably produces a systematic error due to the nonequilibrium nature of the perturbation process. The Hamiltonian lag, i.e the simulation lags behind the changing potential, contributes positively yielding the dissipated work, whose average is positive and is associated with the increase of entropy during an irreversible process [33,72].

Various NE free energy methods use a basic rule of thermodynamics which states that over the course of an isothermal, reversible process linking two equilibrium states, the work performed on the system is equal to the free energy difference between the two states. However, for a process linking two states (switch) to be truly reversible it must in principle be infinitely long, thus switches cannot be truly reversible and the NE free energy calculations depend on the closeness between switch and reversible limit. There are a number of switching methodologies. In practice, the number of switches needed to produce an accurate estimate of the free energy difference depends on the nature of the distribution of work values produced by the nonequilibrium calculation [33, 49, 72].

The Bennett's acceptance ratio (BAR) is an interesting development of the switching methodology, with switches in both forward and backward directions used to calculate the free energy differences. This is estimated from the lower bound found through the average work and slowly increased iteratively until the difference is satisfied. The free energy with the lowest variance for a given set of forward and backward work values is produced by BAR and may be one of the efficient nonequilibrium work estimators [33,71].

Another interesting set of methods use weights for the size and position of increments to improve the sampling of the switches. Particular areas of a switch may be more or less prone to producing large work values. It is possible to reduce the amount of work through the use of favorable system configurations or very small λ increments [33].

Configuration bias sampling uses the idea of sampling to bias the configurations, which are used to increment λ, producing switches with a lower work distribution. Due to the possible presence of a nonsymmetric bias in Jarzynski equality (JAR) calculations, it may become necessary to make a choice between JAR estimates in the forward and backward directions [33, 36].

The harmonic oscillator (HO) systems for NE sampling considers the systems A and B, with the same number of oscillating particles N but with differing Hamiltonians, in terms of x_i the reference coordinate for particle i and ω_A and ω_B for the force constant of the two systems, which control the size of oscillations the particles will undergo as well as the size of phase space each system explores. The HO model is very simple and many of its properties can be calculated analytically, including free energy differences. This is very useful as the results from this protocol can be compared to the correct answer rather than an answer found using an exhaustive free energy protocol [33].

DOCKING

Today, for drug discovery programs, simulation and computational modeling have become important components, whereas for modeling of protein-ligand binding, a well established technique is molecular docking, with numerous applications ranging from industrial drug research to pure fundamental studies. However, today's molecular docking programs still fail to satisfy the expectations of researchers, despite two decades of significant investments in developing docking softwares, leading to limited *in silico* ligand screening in the drug discovery process. For many workers, the search for improving molecular docking is focused on the search for a better representation of intermolecular interactions energies, scoring functions and docking algorithms that perform global optimizations on multidimensional potential energy surfaces. Free energy calculations focus on the main forces contributing to ligand-protein binding (hydrogen bonds, electrostatics, hydrophobic, van der Waals, etc) [77-483].

In general, the problem of finding the low-energy binding modes of a ligand is based on 'the lock and key mechanism' within the active site of a known receptor and is what defines the molecular docking problem. A vast literature is devoted to these methods. An important objective is to search large sets of compounds for new lead structures from protein-ligand docking and drug optimization. However, the design space grows combinatorialy with the number of degrees of freedom of the interacting molecules and all possible docking configurations cannot be completed. As an example, for a protein receptor that occupies a volume of 60 Å^3, with a translational resolution of 1 Å, rotational resolution of 20^0 in each axis, potential ligands and protein receptor with 35 and 3,500 atoms respectively, it would be necessary to make on the order of ~ 10^{14} pairwise nonbonding evaluations, in order to take into consideration all possible docking configurations. Computational power thus becomes a limiting factor [443].

Numerous protein-ligand docking programs have been developed to efficiently discover lead compounds for a target protein from large compound databases. Docking programs can be assessed if the pose or binding mode of a crystal structure can be reproduced or whether the predicted score can be correlated with experimentally measured binding affinity. In general docking algorithms are highly successful at generating good binding modes whereas scoring functions are less successful at correctly identifying binding modes. In comparing docking programs, some of which can generate conformations very close to crystal binding structures, it is generally not known which conformation created by which program is close to the true structure. It is thus of interest to further improve scoring methods to rerank conformations generated.

Although docking of small molecules to protein binding sites, i.e key structure-base drug design (SB) methods was pioneered during the early 1980s, with the treatment of the protein and ligand as rigid bodies, various problems still continue to afflict docking. Issues, such as flexibility in the receptor and ligand, covalent interactions, handling water molecules, metals and scoring are problems that still continue to afflict docking. In this chapter we will review some of the recent trends regarding docking and scoring methods.

The consensus scoring (CS) method for example, generally provides stable results, since it combines multiple scoring functions (sf) in order to supplement the weakness of a single sf. For blind trials, CS has been suggested to be a reliable method that improves false or positive hit rates. Among the consensus scoring (CS) methods, bootstrap-based consensus scoring (BBCS), derived from the idea of bootstrap aggregating (bagging) and based on ensemble learning, combines multiple scorings, each of which has the same functional form but different energy-parameter sets [78]. One of the objectives of BBCS is to circumvent the problem that it is not easy to uniquely determine the energy-parameter set that provides the global minimum of binding free energy over all complexes when the number of data in a training set is not enough. Two steps are used to generate the multiple energy-parameter sets, i.e generation of training sets by a bootstrap method and optimization of the energy-parameter set by a Z-score approach, based on energy landscape theory [128, 132].

One of the various scoring functions is given as a function of the protein and ligand coordinates, sum of the energy contributions from each hydrogen bond, metal contacts and specific aromatic interactions where each contribution is multiplied by linear penalty functions. A measure of hydrophobic contact is also provided as a function of protein-ligand atom pairs and parameters involving pairs of nonpolar and polar atoms. Among the various options, multiple predictors can be combined by rank-by-number as well as by rank-by-wcs (weighted consensus score). In the first method an average score is calculated for every docking and the consensus rank of each structure is obtained by sorting in ascending order. In the wcs method the protein-ligand docking structures, including decoys, are ranked according to the ascending order of scores calculated by each predictor. A matrix rank is obtained and a weighted consensus score is defined. Finally, the consensus rank of each docking structure is obtained by sorting in descending order. However since all complexes cannot be used as a training set, there will be some error between a semi-complete and actual constructed scoring function. The idea of the BCS method is to reduce this error [283].

The entire surface of a protein molecule in solution is covered by water molecules yielding properties which are different from those in the bulk. Experimental results indicate the existence of large networks of water molecules in the vicinity of the surface which remain mobile, are loosely bound to surface with short interaction times whereas others are well bound to ligand binding sites where they can mediate the interactions between the ligand and the protein, stabilizing the complex in solution via hydrogen-bonded networks, participating in selectivity, specificity, recognition and stabilization processes of the active sites. Water molecules have also served to improve the performance of virtual screening, providing a structural rationale for ligand-derived pharmacophore models of binding sites and improving the predictive ability and rationalization of three-dimensional quantitative structure-activity relationship (QSAR) models [90,140-228].

There is often thermodynamically favorable release of water molecules during the binding of a ligand to a protein receptor. The retention of bound water molecules may be also associated with an entropic penalty outweighed enthalpically via favorable hydrogen-bonding interactions. Computer simulations can determine the displacement of tightly bound water molecules and predict hydration sites. Targeting, mimicking, displacement of water molecules can be performed in structure-based drug design in order to improve the binding affinity of ligand molecules. In some cases, the recruitment of tightly bound water molecules can bridge the interactions between the ligands and the protein resulting in decrease of binding affinity of ligands.

In de novo drug design, tightly bound water molecules can play an important role in modulating the binding modes and chemical diversity of designed ligands by imposing steric and hydrogen-bonding constraints. However, diverse studies with small as well as large datasets of ligand-protein complexes could not produce conclusive, non-contradictory evidence that the inclusion of tightly bound water molecules improves docking accuracy. Determining the ideal scoring function, in general and for this type of research in particular, is not a straightforward task since they must return free energy of protein-ligand binding and account for multiparticle changes associated with ligands, proteins and the surrounding aqueous medium upon binding [79].

The docking algorithm is related to the mathematical problem of global optimization yielding diverse approaches such as incremental construction of an optimal ligand pose (DOCK [246], FlexX [247], Surflex [111]), Monte Carlo algorithms (GlamCock [241], ICM [240]), genetic algorithms (Autodock [105,417], Gold [104], MolDock [245]), hierarchical scoring functions for crude shape fitting and linear optimization of ligand pose (QXP [251], LigandFit [252], Glide [112]) and systematic analysis of possible minima using graph searches (eHits [250].

Docking methods are often characterized by docking success rates which specifies the percentage of correctly predicted ligand positions as well as virtual screening studies in which ligands known to be active for a particular target protein are mixed with inactive ones (decoys) and rank-ordered according to their predicted scores. It is important to make standard benchmarking properties which include test sets of protein-ligand complexes, data sharing, preparation of protein ligand structures for modeling sets of active and decoy ligands for virtual screening experiments. Although programs like AutoDock and Glide estimate the free energy of protein-ligand binding it is believed that binding energy prediction is a post-docking procedure and therefore more computationally demanding methods such as linear interaction energy approximations and free energy perturbation methods are required. We note that one of the objectives is still to improve speed and quality of binding energies calculated from docking programs [105,417, 112].

Three specialized high accuracy scoring functions and an innovative molecular docking algorithm were recently introduced in the Lead Finder docking software [79]. This algorithm combines the classical genetic algorithm with various local optimization procedures and resourceful exploitation of the knowledge generated during the docking process. The scoring functions are based on a molecular mechanics functional which explicitly accounts for different types of energy contributions scaled with empirical coefficients to produce three scoring functions tailored for 1) accurate binding energy predictions 2) correct energy-ranking of docked ligands poses and 3) correct rank-ordering of active and inactive compounds in virtual screening experiments.

The purpose of the first function is to accurately estimate the free energy of ligand binding for a particular structure of a protein-protein complex. The purpose of the second scoring function is to give the highest score to the correct experimental ligand pose. Finally, another set of scaling coefficients was designed to yield maximum efficiency in virtual screening experiments. The local pose optimization is viewed as a valuable component of genetic algorithm which facilitates faster evolution of individuals in addition to usual genetic operations such as recombination and mutation. The pseudo Solis-Wets (PSW) optimization is based on a random displacement in each degree of freedom, following the chosen direction when the energy of a new ligand pose is lower. Before the start of a docking process, the conformation of a ligand in solution is optimized, its energy is then used as a reference in energy calculations and its structure used as a source for generating the initial pool of individuals by randomizing the translational and orientation coordinates of a molecule. The genetic algorithm uses the notion of a niche to cluster individuals with similar genotypes and to restrict their expansion [79, 105].

The protein structure, in an aqueous environment for a living organism, can differ from the monocrystal structure. 3D structures determined by NMR spectroscopy are not completely sensitive to the conformational state of the molecules and are less reliable than X-ray results, which does not always yield the structural determination of some fragments due to the partial disorder in crystals. In addition, in order to reduce the time to obtain X-ray results, the resolution is often chosen to be lower than necessary for reliable localization of the hydrogen atoms, yielding imprecise determination of which tautomeric forms of ligand and proteins are interacting [98, 298].

In addition to the unreliability of some 3D structures of proteins used in docking programs, the scoring functions are also not always examined for macroscopic physicochemical properties and consist in general of discrete values dependent of the types of interactions, i.e hydrophobic, hydrophobic, H-acceptor, H-donor, *etc.* Some scoring functions characterize Gibbs free energy or the potential energy to determine the thermodynamics of ligand-receptor interactions. The question arises however, if this criteria is correct. Does ligand and receptor know whether their interaction is stable or unstable, with low or high free energies respectively, or does the kinetic factors play a more important role in the interaction? Is there a strong dependence on the interaction of some active centers of the molecules and not on the total interaction energy, leading to the sometimes observed poor relation between scoring functions? What about Gibbs free energies and other parameters describing the biological activities of the compounds?

Another important issue is insufficient consideration of the receptor and ligand flexibilities. In some methods a ligand is decomposed into small rigid fragments, which are reassembled to fit the binding site. The problem may not have an unambiguous solution since the ligand decomposition may have subjective errors, there may be many variants of adjustment of the fragments to each other and it may be necessary to estimate the conformational flexibility of the whole system. Some authors propose that the reasons for the low predictivity of the docking, with rms deviations above 2 Å may be attributed to the experimental data and the weaknesses of the docking methods [303].

A new methodology to describe the interactions in 'receptor-ligand' complexes was introduced in order to address some of the above-mentioned problems, i.e the 3D/4D QSAR algorithm BiS/Multiconformational (BiS/MC) and CoCon algorithms [98]. The first algorithm performs the restricted docking of compounds to receptor pockets. The other algorithm determines the relationships between the bioactivity and the parameters of interactions in the 'receptor-ligand' complexes, including a new formalism for estimating hydrogen bond energies. 3D structures of the ligand-receptor complexes are used and the receptor geometry in the complexes is prepared for the interaction with a ligand changing, to a lesser degree, as it receives different ligands.

The method aligns molecules onto each other by considering their Coulomb and van der Waals potentials at points on the molecular surface. The algorithm reconstructs the model receptor as being complementary to the field of the generalized molecular set whereas the receptor is represented as a set of pseudoatoms whose parameters can be calculated from the complementarity formalism. The molecules are oriented in the complementary receptor model and the maximum total probability of the interactions of a molecule with the model receptor is optimized. The use of probability increases the influence of the most important 'receptor atom-ligand atom' interactions on the molecular orientation. The model receptor is flexible and every ligand is represented as a set of conformers, found with the algorithm, interfaced with the MM3 force field which allows taking into account the flexibilities of both the receptor and ligands. The reconstruction of the complementary model receptor is performed by means of an algorithm which gets additional information on the molecular orientation in the receptor cavity.

The BiS/MC method uses the MERA (Model of Effective Radii of atoms) force field which is a nonparametric model for simulating the effective atomic radii whereas each atom fills the space allowed by other atoms such that the atom is represented by an expanding balloon. Other expanding spheres limit the expansion of the atomic spheres such that the expansion of the balloon ceases when the external pressure provided by the other atoms is equal to the internal pressure of the balloon. The internal density of the atom i is proportional to its inverse volume such that the external density equals the sum of the inverse volumes of spheres with radii equal to the distances between atoms i and j. It is possible to calculate the zero-order approximation volume of each atom whereas the sum of the atomic volumes must be equal to the molecular volume allowing the calculation of the density of the compound [309].

A new approach (CoCon) for determination of mechanisms of biological action of compounds as well as search for active centers of ligands and receptors was reported [98]. The basic idea of the CoCon algorithm is that biological activity of a compound depends mostly on the interaction ability of the active centers of the receptor and ligand sites whereas relationships are created between the biological activity and the parameters of interactions in the 'receptor-ligand' complexes. The interaction depends on the atom-atomic potentials of van der Waals and Coulomb interactions which permit the decomposition of the interaction energies in search of the best linear relationship between the biological activity and the parameters of the interaction. In CoCon the parameters that determine biological activity belong to the receptor and ligand atoms that are supposed to be active centers. Forward and backward stepwise procedures of the regression analysis can be used for the decomposition with this algorithm. The leave-one-out cross validation technique can be used to estimate the quality of the relationships [98].

There is still considerable debate regarding whether the conformation of the protein in the ligand-bound state was induced by the ligand or whether this state already existed before binding by the ligand and was selected from an ensemble of different conformations. Certainly, for the determination of the conformation of the protein to which it is bound, the ligand plays a central role. For half a century the existence of ligand-induced flexibility was considered inconsequential or rare whereas today it is known that a large number of proteins contain as much as three flexible residues in the active site and thus single rigid dockings predict incorrect binding pose for most ligands. Major domain rearrangements, simpler backbone-loop and side-chain movements are often observed in flexible residues leading in general to an unclear picture of protein changes induced by ligands. Simultaneous ligand effects on protein conformation, separating the amount of protein effects on ligand conformation, inadequate understanding of receptor flexibility, due to paucity of experimental data, are some of the issues that need to be addressed in theoretical-computational techniques [336].

If we start by assuming that any holo form of the protein would be adequate, we note that even a slight change in the protein conformation can have a significant effect on docking results. At the next step, one can accept small changes in receptor conformation using soft scoring functions to evaluate the binding to a rigid protein, i.e soft functions (sf) that accepts overlap between ligands and protein and accounts for some plasticity of the receptor as well as being computationally efficient since only the scoring function parameters needs to be changed. The disadvantage is that sf cannot handle major structural rearrangements such as back-bone movements [177].

Rotamer exploration and multiple protein structures (MPS), i.e survey methods, are similar to simulating ligand flexibility by exploring multiple ligand conformations offering an alternative way to model receptor flexibility. One method consists of simulating side-chain movements by exploration of rotamer libraries. Another method, which can be computationally expensive as the number of conformations increase, consists of docking ligands to multiple receptor structures which allows a wide range of conformational flexibility, being restricted however to the MPS set being used. Another disadvantage is the ambiguity caused by multiple equally good docked poses and of false positive results [339].

The rotamer exploration approach may fail if desired rotamer is not included in library and may be biased by rotamer library whereas only side-chain conformational changes are allowed and multiple solutions may lead to ambiguity in interpretation. The MPS multiple dockings approach can have a high computational cost and novel conformation cannot be found with ambiguity in interpretation of multiple equally good solutions. There are no quantification of conformational changes for specific ligands and the calculations are biased by the input set of conformations. The approach may also fail if specific ligand induces novel conformations not included in the MPS set.

We can significantly reduce the cost of multiple dockings by using average receptor grids generated from MPSs taking into account the range of flexibility with ensemble docking methods which has however the difficulties of including significant structural diversity in the average grid as well as the danger of obtaining artificial ligand poses that match only the artificial average grid structure and not any real conformation of the protein.

The quantitative characterization of ligand-induced receptor movements was first reported using classical molecular interaction potentials (cMIP) and volumes to quantify the binding sites of proteins without the usage of ligand properties. A knowledge-based approach for handling receptor flexibility was proposed interfacing biology (protein structure using data analysis and modeling techniques) with chemistry (small molecule properties), i.e quantitative structure-induced conformation relationship (QSiCR) analysis, whose difference with QSAR is that the former predicts the effect of ligands on the structural conformation of key residues in the active site of the protein instead of the concentration or biological activity of the ligand. In the QSiCR approach we first identify the observable conformational differences in the active site of mainly ligand-bound forms of crystal structures of proteins. It is then possible to identify suitable position-invariant residues in the active site from the same set of structures in order to define a frame of reference. Conformational changes are defined in terms of geometrical quantities such as distances of variable residues from invariant residues, which are modeled as functions of ligand properties using statistical-computational methods [336,339].

A multiple protein structure (MPS) can be obtained by experimental methods or computational techniques such as rotamer libraries, molecular dynamics simulations (MDS), normal mode analysis (NMA) and Monte Carlo sampling. MDS- the time-dependent behavior of a molecular system is calculated and is considered to be the method that most rigorously attempts to study receptor flexibility for docking). In MDS the equations of Newton's second law of motion yields a trajectory that describes the positions of the atoms as they vary with time. Insights into protein folding and flexibility were the early objectives of MDS whereas recent applications has been more devoted to exploring receptor flexibility before docking, to simulate induced-fit, to include solvent effects, to refine docked complexes and calculate binding free energies. Multiple low-energy states of proteins are generated by MDS at the pico- and nano- second levels of theory whereas minor readjustments in the active-site atoms are included and a set of MPS for docking a ligand is obtained. However, major hindrances in running a MDS is the large computational power required as well as the incomplete knowledge and understanding of the forces determining protein flexibility. In addition, large structural changes may be missed as the computational feasible times of simulation are often unrealistically short as compared to the known real timescales of protein folding/unfolding events [336].

In order to identify flexible regions of the receptor at low computational cost, normal mode analysis (NMA) is an alternative to MD. The NM are defined by the eigenvectors of the Hessian matrix of the potential energy and the protein movement is represented as a superposition of normal modes, fluctuating around a minimum energy conformation. After the introduction of coarse-grained representations of the protein, NMA gained widespread usage. The space defined by the first most relevant NMA eigenvectors provides a correct picture of the flexibility of proteins in aqueous solution at a low computational cost.

Some of the approaches to incorporate protein flexibility in docking include the use of soft potentials, rotamer exploration, multiple protein structures (MPS) multiple dockings, multiple protein structures (MPS) ensemble docking, hybrid methods and MD simulations after docking. Some approaches permit pilot docking of ligands allowing small clashes with protein residues and subsequently *in silico* generation of the protein conformations that have adjusted themselves to the ligands [337,338]. Other hybrid approaches use rotamer exploration, a combination of soft potentials and/or active-site mutation to simulate induced-fit effects. Hybrids methods can use a combination of multiple ligand pose generation with soft potentials and complex-relaxation to allow receptors to adjust to ligands, with multiple dockings of each ligand to selected receptor conformations with the best-docked structures and further refinement of the complexes [339-340].

At a high computational simulation cost, MDS can be used after docking to examine the stability of the docked conformation and the strength of binding, allowing also for receptor and ligand rearrangements in order to obtain lower energy conformations of the docked complex. A drawback of this approach is that the conformations explored by MDS are dependent on the starting solution provided to the simulator as well as the initial velocity.

Using docking with soft potentials, completely novel conformations cannot be found, there is a low level of ligand effects, no quantification of conformational changes and bias by input conformation. Only subtle side-chain changes are detected. It is easy to interpret and has low computational cost. It can also detect subtle changes than other methods overlook.

In the MPS ensemble docking there is a small chance of finding novel conformations. Average protein structure may not give a real conformation. There is no quantification of conformational changes and may fail if ensemble is biased. However there are multiple ways of generating multiple structures and ligand effects are included to moderate level. There are side-chain and backbone changes but restricted by the ensemble set used.

In the MDS after docking methods there is an analysis of huge output effort-intensive. It has a high computational cost, is biased by starting structures and initial velocities and my fail owing to short simulation times and miss the best solution. On the other hand it can find novel conformations to a limited extent with moderate to high level of ligand effects. It has side-chain and backbone movements but is restricted by simulation time. There is quantification of conformational changes and solvent effects and membrane-bound proteins can be handled.

Hybrid methods, although requiring more computational time an effort than rigid body docking, have the advantage of considering all types of conformational changes. Side-chain and backbone movements and novel conformations can be found to some extent. However, if multiple equally good solutions are found interpretation may be difficult and it may miss large conformational changes.

Cross-docking, or using a protein structure from a complex containing a different ligand, provides a good assessment of a docking program's ability to reproduce X-ray results. Cross docking [318] was performed with various softwares. Using the protein structure from the complex that contains the bound ligand most similar to the docked ligand increases docking accuracy for all methods ('similarity selection'). Identifying the most successful protein conformer ('best selection') and similarity selection substantially reduce the difference between self-docking and average cross-docking accuracy. There is an identification of universal predictors of docking accuracy. There is consistent behavior across most protein-method combinations. Models for predicting docking accuracy built using these parameters can be helpful in selecting the most appropriate docking methods.

With increasing x-ray structures available researchers often use molecular docking programs to find novel ligands via virtual screening of compound libraries. With docking programs being upgraded with new technology and new programs being developed there has been a growing need for appropriate evaluations of these programs focused on virtual screening, pose prediction or various combinations. Metrics, standardized data sets and statistical analysis can be useful for evaluating real performance differences between docking programs.

In recent work, PhDOCK, ICM, GLIDE, FlexX, DOCK and SURFLEX were evaluated by comparing their utility in selecting active compounds from a database of decoys as well as generating and identifying docking poses which are close to the X-ray conformation [77]. Despite its limitations the Directory of Useful Decoys (DUD) can be used to evaluate the performance of docking programs in virtual screening and remains a valuable virtual screening benchmark available to the entire chemistry community [263].

Among the docking methods used by the workers, the flexible anchor-and-grow algorithm was used in DOCK 6.1, base fragment placement and incremental construction was used in FlexX V2.03, an algorithm with precomputed grids occurring in a hierarchical fashion was used in GLIDE v4.5, optimization of flexible ligands by internal coordinates in a grid-based receptor field was used by ICM v3.5-1, 3D pharmacophores simultaneously docked into the target binding site and then scored using the contact scoring function was used in PhDOCK, and empirical Hammerhead scoring function using an idealized active site ligand to generate ligand poses by incremental construction and a crossover procedure that combines pieces from distinct poses was used in the Surflex algorithm. The ability of a docking program to reproduce a ligand pose close to that found in an X-ray complex is often a critical determinant of the program's effectiveness for structure-guided design. Analysis of the softwares indicated general trends in accuracy that are specific for particular protein families. Modifying basic parameters in the software was shown to have a significant effect on docking and virtual screening results, suggesting that expert knowledge is critical for optimizing the accuracy of these methods [77].

There was recently [404] reported an assessment of some programs for ligand binding affinity prediction. FLEXX, X-Score, AutoDock and BLEEP were examined for their performance in binding free energy prediction in various situations including co-crystallized complex structures, cross docking of ligands to their non-cocrysallized receptors, docking of thermally unfolded receptor decoys to their ligands, and complex structures with 'randomized' ligand decoys. There was not found a satisfactory correlation between the experimental estimated binding free energies over all the datasets tested. A strong correlation between ligand molecular weight-binding affinity correlation and experimental predicted binding affinity correlation was found.

In order to identify receptor-ligand interactions through an *ab inito* approach workers have recently demonstrated a qualitative relation between the electric characteristics and binding affinity of a complex-receptor-ligand; a large binding affinity correlates with a large charge transfer which allows analysis of binding interactions of complexes using small computational resources with acceptable reliability of the results [402].

Largescale applications of high-throughput molecular mechanics with Poisson-Boltzmann surface area (PBSA) for routine physics-based scoring of protein-ligand complexes were made [403]. Statistically significant correlation was observed with experimentally measured potencies. The calculations illustrate the feasibility of procedural automation of physics-based scoring calculations to produce ordered binding-potency estimates for protein-ligand complexes with sufficient throughput for realization of practical implementation into scientist workflows in an industrial drug discovery research setting.

A new alternative method for the evaluation of docking performance was recently reported: RSR vs RMSD, i.e an assessment criterion for docking poses in which experimental electron density is taken into account when evaluating the ability of docking programs to reproduce experimentally observed binding modes. Three docking programs (Gold, Glide, and Fred) were used to generate poses for a set of protein-ligand complexes for which the crystal structure is known. The new criterion is based on the real space R-factor (RSR) which measures how well the ligand fits the experimental electron density by comparing that density to the expected density, calculated from the predicted ligand pose. The RSR-based measure is compared to the traditional criterion, the root-mean-square distance (RMSD) between the docking pose and the binding configuration in the crystallographic model. The results highlight several shortcomings of the RMSD criterion that do not affect the RSR-based measure. The RSR-derived approach allows a more meaningful *a posteriori* assessment of docking methods and results [405-410].

There was recently reported [411] a research work on binding estimation after refinement, a new automated procedure for the refinement and rescoring of docked ligands in virtual screening. BEAR (Binding estimation after refinement) is reportedly a novel automated computational procedure suitable for correcting and overcoming limitations of docking procedures, such as the generation of unreasonable ligand conformations and poor scoring function, which uses molecular dynamics simulation followed by MM-PBSA and MM-GBSA binding free energy estimates as tools to refine and rescore the structures obtained from docking virtual screenings. As binding estimation after refinement relies on molecular dynamics, the procedure can be adjusted to the needs of the end-user in terms of computational time and the desired accuracy. Binding estimation after refinement and re-scoring, in a validation test, resulted in a significant enrichment of known ligands among top scoring compounds compared with the original docking results. After refinement, binding estimation has direct and straightforward application in virtual screening for correcting both false-positive and false-negative hits, which should facilitate more reliable selection of biologically active molecules [411-419].

An investigation of flexible protein-ligand docking [420] was recently reported. The new simulated annealing protocol termed disrupted velocity simulated annealing (DIVE-SA) outperformed the replica-exchange method and the traditional simulated annealing method in identifying correct docking poses. Atomic velocities were reassigned periodically to encourage the system to sample a large conformational space. Scaling potential energy surfaces reduces structural transition barriers which could further facilitate docking. The DIVE-SA method was evaluated on its ability to perform flexible ligand-flexible protein docking. To reduce computational time and to avoid possible unphysical structural changes resulting from the use of nonoptimal force fields, a soft restraint was applied to keep the root-mean-square-deviation (RMSD) between instantaneous protein structures and a chosen reference structure small. Their work demonstrates the important role that flexibility plays in accepting different ligands and should profitably not be restrained in molecular docking so that more diverse ligands can be studied [94,420-426].

A novel visualization tool for the analysis and comparison of molecular docking (PosDock) [427] which processes a docking results database and displays an interactive pseudo-3D snapshot of multiple ligand docking poses such that their docking energies and docking poses are visually encoded for rapid assessment. The docking energies are represented by a transparency scale whereas the docking poses are visually encoded by a color scale[427-429].

A study of assessment of scaffold hopping efficiency by use of molecular interaction fingerprints was recently reported [97] whereas a novel scoring algorithm based on molecular interaction fingerprints (IFPs) was comparatively evaluated in its scaffold hopping efficiency against four virtual screening standards (Glide, XP, Gold, ROCS and a Bayesian classifier). Decoy databases for the targets under examination were obtained from the Directory of Useful Decoys and were further enriched with approximately 5% of active ligands. Structure and ligand-based methods were used to generate the ligand poses and a Tanimoto metric was chosen for the calculation of the similarity interaction fingerprint between the reference ligand and the screening database whose enrichments were found to depend on the pose generator algorithm. In spite of these dependencies enrichments using molecular IFPs were reportedly comparable to those obtained with GlideXP, Gold, ROCS and the Bayesian classifier [97, 430-441].

Recent work have emphasized the importance of rescoring docking hit lists for model cavity sites. The strategy is to rescore top-ranked docked molecules using a better but slower method such as molecular mechanics-generalized Born surface area (MM-GBSA) techniques. These more physically realistic methods have improved models for solvation, electrostatic interactions and conformational changes [442]

Recent work reports a computation methodology, which leads to the ability to partition the Gibb's free energy for the complexation reaction of aromatic drug molecules with DNA. Using this approach, it is now possible to calculate the absolute values of the energy contributions of various physical factors to the DNA binding process, whose summation gives a value that is reasonably close to the experimentally measured Gibb's free energy of binding. Application of the methodology to binding of various aromatic drugs with DNA can provide answers regarding the main contributors to the stabilization of aromatic ligand-DNA complexes [443].

A recent work introduces CONFIRM (connecting fragments found in receptor molecules whereas a pre-prepared library of bridges is searched to extract those which match a search criterion derived from known experimental or computational binding information about fragment molecules within a target binding site. The resulting bridge 'hits' are then connected, to the fragments and docked into the target receptor. Docking poses are assessed in terms of root mean squared deviation from the known positions of the fragment molecules as well as docking scores, should known inhibitors be available [96].

A recent work was presented assessing the role of polarization in docking. The strategy for including ligand and protein polarization in docking is based on the conversion of induced dipoles to induced charges. These have a distinct advantage in that they are readily implemented into a number of different computer programs, including many docking programs and hybrid QM/MM programs. Induced changes are also more readily interpreted. In this study the ligand was treated quantum mechanically to avoid parameterization issues and was polarized by the target protein, which was treated as a set of point charges. The induced dipole at a given target atom, due to polarization by the ligand and neighboring residues, was reformulated as induced charges at the given atom and its bonded neighbors and these were allowed to repolarize the ligand in an iterative manner. The final set of polarized charges was evaluated against the default empirical Gasteier charges, and against nonpolarized and partially polarized potential-derived charges. Inclusion of polarization does not always lead to the lowest energy pose having a lower RMSD. However, whenever an improvement in methodology, corresponding to a more thorough treatment of polarization, resulted in an increased cluster size, then there was also a corresponding decrease in the RMSD. The options for implementing polarization within a purely classical docking framework are discussed [91].

A Bayesian model averaging for ligand discovery was recently reported [100]. The Bayesian analysis of high-dimensional descriptor data using Markov chain Monte Carlo (MCMC) simulations for learning classification trees is a novel method for pharmacophore and ligand discovery. Experimentally determined binding affinity data is used to assess model averaging algorithms and then applied to large databases. The main Bayesian algorithm, in addition to achieving high specificity and sensitivity, also lends itself naturally to classifying test sets with missing data and providing a ranking for the classified compounds. The approach has been used to select and rank potential biologically active compound and could provide a powerful tool in compound testing.

A study was presented regarding identifying receptor-ligand interactions through an ab initio approach. A qualitative relation was demonstrated between the electric characteristics and binding affinity of a complex receptor-ligand; a large binding affinity correlates with a large charge transfer. This allows the analysis of binding interactions of any complex using small computational resources with acceptable reliability of the results [402].

A novel scheme was proposed in which a panel of plausible pharmacophore hypothesis candidates were assembled to construct a pharmacophore ensemble (PhE) which in turn was treated as input for regression analysis via support vector machines (SVM). Each pharmacophore member in the PHE represents a protein conformation or a number of protein conformations with closed spatial arrangements. Unlike any other analog-based modeling methods, this PhE/SVM scheme can take into account protein plasticity, which is of critical importance to be addressed when the target protein can adopt significantly various conformations to interact structurally with diverse ligands, by using PhE in place of protein conformation ensemble [234].

MOLECULAR INTERACTION FIELDS

 For characterizing the ability of a molecule to interact with other molecules, Molecular Interaction Fields (MIF) are extremely useful. The Molecular Electrostatic Potentials can represent the energy of interaction of a molecule with a positive charge located at the cartesian coordinates of the molecule neighborhood. A more complex chemical probe representing any kind of functional group can be used to replace the positive charge, which can highlight graphically areas of space with energetically favorable interactions produced by molecules holding a probelike group [444-451].

The Grid-inDEPENDENT Descriptors (GRIND) represent [444] a class of alignment-independent three-dimensional molecular descriptors derived in such a way as to be highly relevant for describing biological properties of compounds. Chemically interpretable and easy to compute GRIND was obtained starting from a set of molecular interaction fields, computed by the first step, in which the fields are simplified, and a second step, in which the results are encoded into alignment-independent variables using a particular type of autocorrelation transform. The molecular descriptors so obtained can be used to obtain graphical diagrams called 'correlograms' and can be used in different chemometric analyses, such as principal component analyses or partial least-squares. An important feature of GRIND is that the molecular interaction fields can be regenerated from the autocorrelation transform and the results of the analysis represented graphically together with the original molecular structures, in 3D plots. ALMOND is a software package for the computation, analysis and interpretation of GRIND yielding highly predictive and interpretable models [444-447]

For identifying regions of strong interactions between biological receptors and ligands, the MIF`s can be extremely useful yielding important applications in drug discovery. Using analytic expressions, the MIF can be sampled at regular intervals over the space surrounding the molecules at certain `grid modes` yielding thousands or hundreds of thousands of data points for regular size molecules. Of particular interest are the `hot spots`, i.e regions of space holding the most negative (favorable) energy values representing potential locations where a ligand can place a functional group similar to the probe. These hot spots, which can be identified by visual inspection of graphical representations, can also represent groups of the receptor binding site with which the molecule could establish favorable binding interactions.

Hot spots can also be extracted by computational methods summarizing the most relevant information contained in hundreds of thousands of MIF nodes. Although in principle, not simple, the development of computational algorithms to extract these regions has potential applications in docking simulations, molecular superposition algorithms and other areas. Various methods have been proposed for obtaining hot spots from MIF as well as from grid MIF. Most of the methods proposed have drawbacks and different limitations that hamper their general application in the field of drug design [444-449].

Among these methods, AMANDA [448] is a simple but efficient algorithm which can be used to extract a set of hot spots from any MIF which can be applied to small molecule design. This algorithm requires that the starting MIF nodes are tagged by the atom contributing most to the field energy. A node prefiltering is first carried out by applying a energy cutoff in order to discriminate between relevant nodes and those representing weak or nonspecific interactions, which are removed. A list of remaining m_i nodes assigned to every atom (i) in the molecule is then built. A nonlinear fraction of the total number of nodes is determined, containing a few nodes for small regions and more nodes for larger regions.

First, the node with the lowest energy value is selected. Then the Euclidean distances between the chosen node and the rest of the members of the list is computed and added to their field energy values to yield a simple scoring for every mode and algorithm step. The node with the best scores is selected and the procedure is repeated. The algorithm guarantees selection of at least one node for every atom of the molecule for which the list of prefiltered nodes is not empty. The total number of nodes selected for a whole molecule depends on the number of atoms and groups able to produce relevant interactions. In order to be useful for drug design, the hot spots must depict the regions around a ligand which are more likely to participate in noncovalent bonding interactions with its receptor. Consequently, the quality of a hot spot extraction algorithm depends on how complete and accurate this picture is. In order to validate the method, hot spots for a collection of ligands were generated for comparison with experimental data for a collection of ligand-receptor complexes [448].

There was recently reported [449] a high-throughput virtual screening of proteins using grid molecular interaction fields. This new computational algorithm for protein binding sites characterization and comparison uses a common reference framework of the projected ligand-space four-point pharmacophore fingerprints, includes cavit shape and can be used with diverse proteins as no structural alignment is required. Protein binding sites are first described using GRID molecular interaction fields (GRID-MIFs) and the FLAP (fingerprints for ligands and poteins) method is then used to encode and compare this information. The discriminating power of the algorithm and its applicability for large-scale protein analysis was validated by analyzing various scenarios: clustering of protein families in a relevant manner, predicting ligand activity across related targets, and protein-protein virtual screening. In all cases, the results showed the effectiveness of the GRID-FLAP method and its potential use in applications such as identifying selectivity targets and tools/hits for new targets via identification of other proteins with pharmacophorically similar binding sites [449-450].

EasyMIFs and SiteHound; a toolkit for the identification of ligand-binding sites in protein structures was recently reported [451] whereas SiteHound uses molecular interaction fields (MIFs) produced by EasyMifs identify protein structure regions that show a high propensity for interaction with ligands. The type of binding site identified depends on the probe atom used in the MIF calculationl. [451].

SOLVATION

The need for predictive thermodynamic models is high enough that engineers are willing to accept inaccuracies in order to improve cost and time saving. Solvents are used in manufacturing and pharmaceutical drug development and researchers spend considerable time after synthesis to identify appropriate solvents and scale up to high-volume manufacturing [452-454]. In diverse areas, industrial as well as biomedical and chemical research, the determination of solvation free energies is important whereas their evaluation is a long-standing evolving challenge in computational chemistry. Upon formation of a ligand and receptor bound complex, the desolvation penalty is important in drug design. The partitioning between various solvents, i.e acid-base equilibrium (log P) is useful in pharmacokinetics. The molecular mechanical force field parameters (well depth, Lennard-Jones and atomic partial charges) are sensitive parameters for determination of solvation free energies.

A direct comparison between experimental and calculated free energy values can be often made since the absolute solvation free energies have been experimentally determined for several small molecules. The success of drug development and manufacture can be significantly increased with good predictive properties of which solvent selection is one of the important potential applications for predictive models. Although one of fast ways of obtaining necessary phase-equilibrium data is via predictive thermodynamic models. These methods, however, require regressed parameters from experimental data. An approach used to account for liquid-phase nonidealities as well as characterization of molecular interactions is solvation thermodynamics [48, 335, 452-462].

When the simulation describes ligand and receptor solutes immersed in a structureless continuum representation of the solvent, we have a family of methods for the estimation of binding affinities whereas continuum solvent models can address apolar as well as polar effects. The favorable interaction energy between a polar solvent like water and a charge can represent the electrostatic solvation energy which can be obtained by solving the Poisson-Boltzmann (PB) equation. This contribution is also called the reaction field arising from the solvent in response to the charge. The Born energy refers to the initial analytical expression derived by Born to calculate this energy for simple spherical ions. The approximate but fast generalized Born (GB) method can also address polar solvation. Combination of solvent accessibility (SA), molecular mechanics (MM), PB and GB yields the MM-PBSA and MM-GBSA methods [460].

Continuum solvation models (CSMs) such as the polarizable continuum model (PCM), the polarizable conductor model (CPCM), the solvation models (SMx), the conductor like screening model (COSMO) have efficiently incorporated solvation effects into quantum chemical calculations. These methods have in common that a cavity is constructed around the solute molecule outside of which a dielectric continuum (solvent) is assumed. The electric field arising from nuclei and electron distribution is screened by the polarization of this continuum whereas the effect of polarization can be represented by the surface charge density which it produces on its boundary, i.e the interface to the solute and thus the whole effect of the dielectric polarization can be described by the screening charges arising on the interface. The problem can then be described by a local system, i.e the solute together with a cavity surface. The CSMs indicate that cavity sizes about 20% larger than the vdW surfaces yields the best results. The COSMO-RS which starts from CSM going beyond the dielectric assumption using local ensembles of ideally screened molecules contacting on the vdW surface with pairwise interactions [179, 452].

The full MM-PBSA method also takes into account non-polar contributions to binding related to the solvent accessible surface area (SASA) buried with binding, which is usually interpreted as the hydrophobic effect. Solvation may also contribute to van der Waals interactions between receptor and ligand. The conformation reorganization energy (strain energy) is also included. Single static structures or conformational ensembles can be used to determine the changes in solute entropy upon binding. The system is partitioned into solvent and solute regions and different values of the dielectric constant assigned to each region whereas the aqueous solution is typically represented with a dielectric constant close to 78 (water). It is difficult to find an optimal general effective dielectric constant for proteins. Lower values means, stronger desolvation penalty for charges which become more buried with complexation, and weaker screening of the ligand-receptor Coulomb interactions. The dependence on the exact value is dampened since the magnitude of both effects will respond in an opposite and compensatory fashion.

What is the best way to map the dielectric boundary between solute and solvent? What is physically the most relevant surface to define this boundary which could be located at the solvent accessible van der Waals or the molecular surfaces? Partitioning of the dielectric regions is sensitive to discretization which could be, in principle, addressed by continuous dielectric functions. Using the van der Waals surface as a dielectric boundary results in buried regions with high dielectrics which artificially stabilizes the electrostatic solvation energies which are however, less severe than when the molecular surface is chosen to delineate the dielectric boundary The solvent accessible surface avoids the problem of interstitial high dielectric cavities. The PB method can also take into account the screening effects of counterions via the ionic strength. Dielectric constants, atomic charges and ionic strengths are mapped on grids. Finer grids thus represent more realistically the system, improving the calculations. Focusing techniques are necessary to retain acceptable boundary conditions with fine enough grids.

Apolar groups in water tend to self-associate in an effort to minimize their exposure to water which needs to be accounted for in binding free energy calculations. Non polar contributions favoring association include van der Waals and hydrophobic effects. Free energy of transfer of pure hydrocarbons from their neat liquid state to water is one of the manifestations of the positive unfavorable hydrophobic effects. It is in general assumed that non-polar free energies of binding of a ligand to a receptor should contain a term proportional to the amount of SASA buried upon complexation which is, however, somewhat empirical and phenomenological, although a term treating hydrophobic effects needs to be included in the nonpolar contribution. In general continuum models emphasize the important role of non-polar effects as a main driver of association which can overcome the expected decrease in configurational entropy with binding.

Although the entropic effects can oppose association or not, there are various contributions involved, whereas the difficulties in dissecting these entropic contributions have made difficult the development and testing of theoretical entropic contribution models. Nonetheless, the change in solvent entropy upon binding is implicitly included in the MM-PBSA method. Regarding solute entropy a pragmatic approach assumes that for similar mass ligands binding to the same protein yields similar entropic contributions which can be ignored for relative ranking of ligand affinities. This can lead to calculated absolute free energies which are too favorable consistent with the neglect of relatively large entropies of translation and rotation opposing binding. MD simulations can also be combined with MM-PBSA whereas the solute entropy is calculated from normal mode analysis for several snapshots and then averaged over the snapshots (MD/MM-PBSA) [461]. Overall, it seems that theoretical accounts for the various solute entropic contributions remains challenging.

Continuum solvent models can be used with single point calculations (SP/MM-PBSA) or an ensemble of configurations. Although the SP model is a simplification since free energies reflect all configuration states populated by the system at a given temperature, this method can be conveniently applied to structural models obtained from cruder scoring schemes including large number of docked compounds. A common strategy to combine conformational sampling with continuum solvent approach is to first generate structural models and explicit solvent with MD simulation which should produce a thermodynamic relevant ensemble of solute structures. After removal of the explicit solvent the continuum solvent model can then be applied to snapshots of these solute structures.

It is also possible to generate conformational ensembles directly with continuum solvation models. In realistic virtual screening experiments with hundreds of thousands of compounds the docking poses can be initially generated with fast empirical scoring functions. Efficient energy minimization algorithm can allow tens of thousands of docking poses to be rescored. On the other hand, solute entropies may be added when a relatively small number of poses is rescored. In general, the physics-based free energy scores can, in principle, be productively applied to the reranking of large number of docking poses of diverse ligands in virtual screening.

The LIE approach, similar to continuum solvation models, only needs to consider the free and bound configurations of the ligand, i.e only the end points needs to be simulated and no unphysical transformation from one ligand to another is required. The method considers the van der Waals and electrostatics interaction energies between the environment and the ligand. The free energy of binding is expressed as a linear combination of these interactions energies using MD or MC ensemble averages, either with the ligand bound to a solvated receptor or with the free solvated ligand. It is argued that intramolecular conformational energies, entropies and receptor desolvation are embedded in the linear response approximation and the adjustable parameters of the model. The treatment of long-range electrostatic interactions can be a complicating factor which is a well known limitation for simulations with explicit solvent [462].

There are also many unanswered questions regarding the empirical parametrization of the LIE method. The fact that LIE is computationally less costly and can perform well with truly diverse scaffolds is an advantage over FEP/TI methods. In addition large savings in calculation time can be obtained by replacing explicit hydration by a continuum solvent model such as generalized Born or PB. The continuum model can also be used in combination with MD, MC or MD/MC (HMC) protocols as well as energy minimization only. In addition to electrostatic and van der Waals terms, LIE can also include the number of hydrogen bonds between ligand and its surroundings, accepted or donated, apolar, aromatic or polar ligand SASA, receptor SASA and ligand or receptor intramolecular energy. The presence or absence of a chemical functionality in the ligand as well as the number of ligand rotable bonds can also be used. As in traditional QSAR, LIE/ELR models may be derived from a training set and used in prediction modes. In general, at a cheaper computational cost, LIE can rival the accuracy of FEP/TI when a suitable training set is available.

A general consensus indicates that polar desolvation which opposes binding in aqueous solution should not be neglected. In continuum solvent models the hydrophobic effect is accounted for by a non-polar solvation SASA-dependent term which favors binding. Its contribution provides in many cases a main driving force for binding. Of course, the addition of apolar groups only favors binding if it does not introduce steric clashes or conformational strain in the bound ligand and if the apolar groups do not further desolvate polar groups.

Among the a priori models which predict intermolecular interaction based on a few adjustable parameters and molecular structure are COSMO-RS and COSMO-SAC which are extensions of a dielectric continuum-solvation model to liquid-phase thermodynamics, i.e models which predict liquid-phase activity coefficients. COSMO-based models require input in the form of a molecule-specific distribution of the surface-charge density, a sigma profile which can be generated from single structures by performing computational expensive quantum-mechanical calculations [452].

Conceptually, COSMO-based models create a cavity with the exact size of a molecule within a homogeneous medium, or solvent, of a dielectric constant and then place the molecule inside the cavity. The solvation free energy represents the change in Gibbs free energy associated with moving a molecule from a fixed position in an ideal gas to a fixed position in a solution. The cavity-formation free energy represents the change in Gibbs free energy required to form a cavity within a solution S of the exact size of the molecule. The charging free energy represents the Gibbs free energy required to remove the screening charges from the surface of the molecular cavity. We determine the solvation free energy from the sum of the cavity-formation free energy and the charging free energy.

A sigma profile is a probability distribution of the surface-charge density of a molecule or a mixture. COSMO-based models construct the molecular shaped cavity within the perfect conductor according to a specific set of rules and atom-specific dimensions. The molecule's dipole and higher moments withdraw charges from the surrounding medium to the surface of the cavity in order to screen or cancel the electric field both inside the conductor and tangential to the surface, allowing the molecule to move freely within the system without altering the system's overall energy. The induced charges are calculated on the solute surface in discretized space from Poisson's equation and the zero total potential boundary condition [452].

The average of the segment surface-charge densities from COSMO calculations yields new surface-charge densities. The sigma profile for a molecule can be defined as the probability of finding a segment with a surface-charge density. One assumption of a sigma-profile generation procedure is that the optimization geometry from the calculation in the vapor phase is identical to the optimal geometry in the condensed phase which can save large amounts of computational time for calculations on larger molecules. Factors such as solvent polarity, molecular size and solvent-solute interactions could affect a solute molecule's structural conformation leading to different structures in a condensed phase than in an ideal gas.

Another assumption requires that the molecule be in the lowest-energy conformation once optimized although several low-energy structural conformations may exist because of the freedom in choosing dihedral angles whereas each conformation results in a slightly different sigma profile and therefore may affect property predictions. Consequently, in essence thermodynamics methods based on COSMO are a priori prediction methods based on molecular structures and a few parameters that are fixed for all of the compounds requiring no experimental data and rely on sigma profiles specific to each molecule as their only input.

One of the methods used to address this challenge involves the explicit simulation of a large number of solvent molecules with periodic boundary conditions. In other approaches the effect of solvation can be incorporated implicitly via continuum approximations. With computational cost limitations, the molecular dynamics free energy perturbation (FEP/MD) method with explicit solvent molecules provides an arguable realistic treatment of solvation. There are many methods with varying accuracy, computational cost and sophistication using a wide range of available implicit solvent methods.

A recently developed massively parallel hybrid DFT/DFT method treats at an *ab initio* DFT level the chemically active part of the system, i.e first solvation shells. For the remainder of the solvent an approximate orbital free DFT is used such that thousands of solvent molecules can be included in the calculations. The computational cost is low since the solvent molecules in the orbital-free region have fixed internal structures and frozen electron densities. In this method the flow of molecules across the DFT/orbital-free-DFT interface is allowed and all interactions in the system are treated at the DFT level preserving the fidelity of the simulations for the reactive part of the system. The DFT equations in the chemically active *ab initio* part of the system are solved with highly parallel real-space multigrids methods (RMG). A grid spacing of 0.32 bohr is used in the calculations, corresponding to a kinetic energy cutoff of 48 Ry. Ultrasoft pseudopotentials as well as the generalized gradient approximations are also used. This method was applied to investigate functional implications of multistage copper binding to the prion protein [459].

Computation of absolute solvation free energies of small molecules using explicit and implicit solvent model was recently reported. The absolute hydration free energy for a set of neutral ligands spanning diverse chemical functional groups commonly found in drug-like candidates was calculated using the molecular dynamics free energy perturbation method (FEP/MD) with explicit water molecules and compared to experimental data as well as its counterparts obtained using implicit solvent models. The hydration free energies are calculated from explicit solvent simulations using a staged FEP procedure permitting a separation of the total free energy into polar and nonpolar contributions. The nonpolar component is further decomposed into attractive (dispersive) and repulsive (cavity) components using the Weeks-Chandler-Anderson (WCA) separation scheme [454].

In order to increase the computational efficiency, all of the FEP/MD simulations are generated using a mixed explicit/implicit solvent scheme with a relatively small number of explicit water molecules in which the influence of the remaining bulk is incorporated via the spherical solvent boundary potential (SSBP). The performances of two fixed-charge force fields designed for small organic molecules, the General Amber force field (GAFF) and the all-atom CHARMm-MSI are compared. Because of the crucial role of electrostatics in solvation free energy, the results from various commonly used charge generation models based on the semiempirical (AM1-BCC) and QM calculations (CHelpG and RESP) are compared. The solvation free energies of the test set were also calculated using Poisson-Bolzmann(PB) and Generalized Born model of solvation (GB).

The quantum mechanics (QM)-based FEP method was used for the calculation of solvation free energy differences. The method used molecular mechanics (MM) for treating the solvent and QM for treating the ligand. Results generated using this method were consistent with those generated using a conventional FEP method [455]

Calculations using conventional and QM/MD-based FEP methods were performed with the λ-coupling method used for transforming inhibitor A into inhibitor B as well as the thread technique for mapping structurally dissimilar molecules [456].

Computation of binding free energy with molecular dynamics and grand canonical Monte Carlo simulations (GCMC) were recently reported. In order to address the many problems associated with solvent simulation MD was coupled with GCMC simulations to allow the number of water to fluctuate during an alchemical FEP calculation. The atoms in a spherical inner region around the binding pocket are treated explicitly while the influence of the outer region is approximated using the generalized solvent boundary potential (GSBP). At each step during thermodynamic integration, the number of water in the inner region is equilibrated with GCMC and energy data generated with MD. It was concluded that solvation free energy calculations with the GCMC/MD method can greatly improve the accuracy of the computed binding free energy compared to simulations with fixed number of water [457].

Researchers often create a reciprocal map of a protein surface in an effort to understand protein binding and function. In order to define complementary maps multiple-copy methods (MCM) use probe molecules to define these complementary maps flooding the protein surface with hundreds of small molecule probes (MP) which are simultaneously and independently minimized to the protein's potential energy surface. The MPs map out hydrophobic regions, ion pairing, hydrogen-bonding interactions, etc, such that clusters of probes on the protein surface can define the most important among these interactions. (MCSS) Multiple copy simultaneous search is a MCM method which tends to remove probes throughout the minimization process. Root-mean-square difference (RMSD)-based clustering is used at each step and only the lowest-energy member of each cluster is retained. Additionally, an energy cutoff is used so that high-energy probes are removed throughout the minimization [458].

The prediction of potency of protease inhibitors using free energy simulations with polarizable quantum mechanics-based ligand charges and a hybrid water model was recently reported. The binding interactions and free energy of binding of the inhibitors and proteins were obtained by performing GBSA simulations in which the inhibitor partial charge accounts for the polarization induced by the protein environment. A hybrid solvation models was employed that retains selected explicit wear molecules in the protein with surface-generalized Born (SGB) implicit solvent. The data suggest that the presence of selected explicit water in protein and protein polarization-induced quantum charges for the inhibitor compared to lack of explicit water and a static force-field based charge model can serve as an improved lead optimization tool and warrants further exploration [335].

An interesting work was recently reported regarding dissecting ligand structures through solvent environment occupancy for which MD simulations in explicit water solvent is a very promising approach. Using statistical mechanics analysis combined with MD simulations, thermodynamics properties of water molecules can be computed and analyzed in a comparative view. Using this idea a set of analysis tools was developed to link solvation with ligand binding in a key carbohydrate binding protein. Water sites (WS) were defined in terms of the thermodynamic properties of water molecules strongly bound to protein surfaces. The results indicated that the probability of finding water molecules inside the WS with respect to the bulk density is directly correlated to the likeliness of finding an hydroxyl group of the ligand in the protein-ligand complex. This information can be used to analyze in detail the solvation structure of the carbohydrate recognition domain (CRD) and its relation to the possible protein ligand complexes and suggests addition of OH-containing functional groups to displace water from high WS to enhance drugs, protein affinity and/or specificity [166].

There was recently reported a universal approach to solvation modeling. It is a continuum mean-field model designed to address various electrostatic and non electrostatic interactions that develops between a molecule and a surrounding medium. The SM8 model may be combined with density functional theory or Hartree-Fock theory to describe a solute's electronic structure and its self-consistent-field polarization by a solvent. It uses class IV charge models to obtain accurate charge distributions in the vapor phase or in solution, even when using small basis sets that are affordable for large systems. Nonelectrostatic effects due to cavity formation, dispersion interactions and changes in solvent structure are included. An analytic surface area algorithm provides stable energy gradients that allow geometry optimization in solution. Computation of free energies of solvation are discussed [179]. Recent work (2010) investigates the cooperative effect of solvent using an ab initio hybrid cluster/continuum model [231].

SUMMARY OF QM METHODS

We address two main categories of QM methods, i.e computationally inexpensive semi-empirical for systems with experimental information and first principles methods without the usage of experimental data. Semi empirical, *ab initio* and DFT are among the most used QM methods whereas the fastest but least accurate are the semi empirical methods. The accurate *ab initio* methods are more computationally expensive [463-521].

The semi-empirical methods can treat valence electrons explicitly and use simplified versions of equations from *ab initio* methods, including parameters fitted to experimental data. They can handle however larger systems. Despite the fact that it is sometimes difficult to determine the quality of the results, since the calculations may require large parameter sets and input from experiments or *ab initio* calculations, semiempirical AM1 binding enthalpies sometimes show a good correlation with those computed at the MP2 level of theory. Nonetheless, although computationally demanding, first-principles methods, due to their enormous structural diversity, are in general better suited for dealing with drugs.

The level of sophistication used determines the number of atoms or electrons which can be included in the simulation. At the lower level we have the empirical potentials (10^1 to 10^6 atoms), Tight-binding calculations, Slater-Koster approximations on the order of 10^4 atoms. Higher level methods include density functional theory (DFT), i.e DFT based calculations with basis sets (GTO, plane waves) and correlations (LDA+corrections), Self consistent field (SCF) Hartree-Fock calculations using basis sets (STO, GTO, planes waves) and correlations (MP perturbation theory, CI, CC, CCSD, etc) are used. The SCF and DFT covers the range up to 10^2 atoms [519].

Empirical or ab initio derived force fields and semi-classical statistical mechanics are used for the atomistic methods to determine thermodynamic and transport properties. The quality of the force fields may have a strong influence on the results. Molecular mechanics energy functions which relates the total potential energy of the system to its atomic coordinates can be used for large systems. The potential energy contribution to the internal energy is expressed as a sum of terms including typically electrostatics, bonds, angles, torsion and van der Waals effects. The real differences in the various models are not apparent from their functional form, but contained in their embedded parameters.

The total potential energy is differentiable with respect to atomic coordinates allowing calculation of the force exerted on every atom, yielding the 'force field' which can be used to propagate simulations using molecular dynamics (MD). The various force-fields are known by their acronyms to the practioners, eg OPLS (Optimized Potentials for Liqid Simulations) [464], AMBER (Assisted model building with energy refinement) [465], CHARMM (Chemistry at Harvard Molecular Mechanics) [466].

Using *ab initio* methods the QM Schrodinger (or Dirac) equation can be numerically solved to calculate drugs as well as ligand-protein properties from first principles. However, in addition to being numerically expensive they can only study fast processes and relatively small systems. Nonetheless, they can yield essentially exact properties using only the atomic coordinates and species as input offering ways to systematically improve the results, assess the quality and handle processes that involve bond breaking/formation as well as chemical reactions.

The calculations can for example be upscaled by calculating diffusivities, elastic tensors, viscosities from atomistic simulations for later use in continuum models. Force-fields can be determined for later use in MD simulations. The calculations can be downscaled by fitting two-electron integrals in semi-empirical electronic structure methods to electron affinities and ionization energies and empirical force fields can be fitted to reproduce experimental thermodynamics properties.

The high computational demands on first-principles-based calculations placed a strong limitation on scientific research projects. Density functional theory radically changed this scenario opening the way for accurate descriptions of the electronic structure in various fields at yet a more computationally affordable cost. DFT-based applications in drug design have since appeared in the literature at an increasing pace. Electron correlation effects, neglected in the Hartree-Fock theory, are included in gradient-corrected DFT at a similar computational cost. Difficulties may be encountered in describing London dispersion forces which may be important for interactions involving drug-target complexes [469].

MD simulations can be of considerable interest for simulating biological systems since most living organisms work at about 310 K. The addition of QM methods to MD, within the DFT framework, i.e first principles MD was originally developed in 1985 in the Car-Parrinello molecular dynamics (CPMD) approach, in which MD simulations can be made with the potential energy of the systems being computed at the DFT level of theory [468].

The scope of DFT formalism in particular and QM methods in general has expanded considerable, with the advent of QM/MM schemes, which can take into account tens of thousands of atoms enabling the study of a protein active site at the QM level whereas the rest of the protein and the solvent is treated by means of classical MM force fields. The implementation of the CPMD and other modification of the QM/MM mixed codes provides a very interesting and stimulating way of investigating at the QM level, macromolecular systems of pharmacological interest.

In a QM/MM approach the computational effort is concentrated in the part of the system where it is most needed. The effects of the surroundings are taken into account with a more expedient model. The intricacies of QM/MM lies in finding an appropriate treatment for the coupling between QM and MM regions. Electrostatic, van der Waals and bonded interactions can be included between the QM and MM regions. Hydrogen link atoms are often introduced to saturate the shell of QM-atoms covalently bonded to MM-atoms. The QM region can be treated at levels of theory spanning from semiempirical to ab initio and DFT Hamiltonians [467].

For a Hamiltonian with M nuclei and N electrons, in the Born-Oppenheimer approximation, the electronic motion can be decoupled since the mass of the nuclei is much larger than the electron mass. The nuclei moves in a potential given by electronic ground state energy and the electrons can be relaxed to the ground state for a given ionic configuration. The total energy is the expectation value of the Hamiltonian and the many-electron wavefunction is in 3N dimensional space. The ground state wavefunction has the lowest energy and obeys the conservation laws and the symmetries of the particles.

Early approaches to solve the Schrodinger equations concentrated in improving the wavefunctions using Slater determinants in an HF approach. However, correlation is not included and configuration interaction (CI) had to be considered whereas the wavefunction is a linear combination of Slater determinants. The growth is factorial with the increase of the number of electrons and difficulties lies in exact solutions of these equations. *Ab initio* methods aim at the solution of the Schrodinger equation, which cannot be solved exactly for polyelectronic systems resorting to approximations.

Hartre-Fock (HF) is one of the simplest approximations whereas the probability of finding an electron is assumed independent of the probability of finding other electrons. Each electron feels the average potential of all the other electrons. This method only includes the quantum mechanical exchange term but does not include electron-correlation which may be computed in various ways. In the Moller-Plesset (MP) many perturbation theory it is treated as a perturbation and corrections can be made at any order of energy and wave function, of which MP is one the most common. The HF approximation can also be extended to several electron configurations leading to the so-called multiconfigurational methods, which although very computationally demanding can reach a very high level of accuracy.

For a molecule, solid or atom, i.e an N-electron system, the time-independent Schrodinger equation depends only on the potential yielding minimization or direct solution strategies. Effectively, we can obtain the ground state energy by minimizing the expectation value of the energy using the variational method. However, it was noted that it should be possible to use the density as key variable, as in condensed matter physics, providing thus a viable, versatile alternative. Systems differ only by their potential energy.

A prescription can be provided, which deals with the kinetic energy and the electron-electron interaction, mapping the many-body problem into a single–body problem. Although the charge density and electrostatic potential were not reproduced in the early 1920s, it was recognized that the kinetic energy density in a uniform electron gas approximation could lead to ground state minimization of the energy functional via constraints. With the developments of Green and correlation functions, the chain of correlation is broken and only in 1964 did Hohenberg and Kohn show that all properties of the many-body system could be determined and are a function of the ground state density

[470]. DFT has become since one of the most popular tools in electronic structure theory due to its excellent performance to-cost ratio as compared with correlated wave function theory (WFT). The accuracy of DFT depends on the quality of the exchange-correlation functional.

DENSITY FUNCTIONAL THEORY

Kohn and Hohenberg introduced Density functional theory (DFT) in the 1960's. This theory allows us to approximately solve the electron correlation problem with resource efficiency similar to that of Hartree-Fock (HF). The correlation effect in the formal DFT theory is included in the exchange-correlation potential for which the exact formula is unknown yielding various approaches for the implementation [468-521].

The Hohenberg-Kohn theorem states that for any system of electrons in an external potential the potential is determined uniquely, except for a constant, by the ground state density whereas the full many-body wavefunction and all other properties of the system are also completely determined. They indicated in a second theorem that a universal functional for the energy of the density could be defined for all electron systems whereas the exact ground state energy is the global minima for a given external potential. The density which minimizes the functional is the exact ground state density. Using a contradiction argument they proved that in principle one can find all properties which are functionals of the electron density. For all many body wavefunctions with the same density, we first minimize for a given density and then minimize to find the density with the lowest energy.

The idea seems simple. The genius of the work was to realize that this provides a new way to approach the many-body problem. The original many-body problem was replaced with an independent electron problem which can be solved by requiring the ground state density to be the same as the exact density. The Kohn-Sham equations can be divided into the exchange-correlation functional, for which we have an exact theory but unknown functionals and independent particles. The energy can be minimized with constraints once a form is assumed for the exchange correlation whereas the eigenvalues are approximations to the energies, to add or substract electrons. The practical DFT does not provide however a guide of how to construct the energy functionals for systems with homogeneous and non-homogeneous densities. We can see DFT as an effective single-body problem using the Kohn-Sham equations and we can rewrite the ground state energy functional in terms of functions including a non-interacting kinetic energy part as well as an exchange-correlation part that depends on the density [470].

Usage by early workers of real spatially inhomogeneous systems led to gradient-expansion approximation (GEA). The inclusion of more general density functionals and their derivatives in the early eighties, led to the generalized gradient approximations (GGA) which however does not describe very well weak interactions such as van der Waals interactions. Incorporation of the kinetic-energy density in addition to GGA led to early Meta GGAs [519]. Addition of the density and its derivatives led to beyond-GGA developments, i.e Meta-GGAs in order to address issues such as self-interactions, fourth order gradient expansions and finite exchange potential at the nucleus. Time-dependent DFT (TD-DFT) can be used to study excited states and spin-DFT (SDFT) employs one density for each spin. Indirect orbital approaches to minimize the energies include optimized-potential model (OPM) and the self-interaction correction (SIC) [484].

Summarizing, the last two decades have seen important progress in the development and validation of density functionals. The LSDA which yields good predictions for solid-state physics is not as useful for chemistry due to overbinding of chemical bonds and underestimation of barrier heights. The GGA functional yields more accurate predictions for thermochemistry than LSDA although they still underestimate barrier heights. In the third generation functionals the spin kinetic energy densities are included yielding the meta-GGAs whereas all these are local functionals.

Mixing with nonlocal HF exchange yields the hybrid functionals which are more accurate than local functionals for main-group thermochemistry. Much of the more recent focus is now on including noncovalent interactions.

Extensive applications of DFT methods in chemistry started with the introduction by Becke in 1993 of the B3LYP functional which largely replaced MP2 in theoretical energy evaluations [470,482]. The B3LYP functional combines

Hartree Fock, Slater, B88 exchange functional of Becke as well as the Lee-Yang-Parr (LYP) and Vosko-Wilk-Nusair (VWN) correlation potentials.

Although B3LYP has often replaced MP2 in theoretical energy evaluations it has been unable, for example, to predict the correct isomerization energy for simple alkanes yielding an increasing error with the size of the alkane systems [497].

Effectively, although widely used in the computational chemistry community, the most popular functional B3LYP reportedly has some shortcoming, i.e it systematically underestimates reaction barrier heights, it is better for main-group chemistry than for transiton metals and it is inaccurate for interactions dominated by medium-range correlation energy, such as van der Waals attraction, alkane isomerization energies and aromatic-aromatic stacking.

Many new DFT functionals have been proposed in order to determine which functional should be used when B3LYP fails. In addition, in drug discovery the geometrical optimization is important and to do this appropriately efficient energy gradient techniques are required for the DFT methods.

There is controversy regarding the dispersion problem. Some workers prefer to avoid hybrid functionals entirely. Others attribute DFT problems to the improper treatment of medium range correlation. It has also been concluded that the inclusion of dispersion correction in B3LYP will significantly reduce the maximum absolute errors although 2.0 kcal/mol seems to be an accuracy limit in predicting isomerization energies and heats of formation [497].

Some well-known challenges of the DFT methods are the electron density and the self interaction error, conventionally defined as inexactness for one-electron densities. Since the HF has a long range property and does not suffer from self-interaction it has been included in the hybrid functionals to compensate for the DFT short-comings. The HF and DFT exchange contributions are mixed in the half-and-half functional (BHandHLYP) in a 1:1 ratio [472,494].

Various popular functional have been proposed to improve the DFT functional exchange potential. The OPTX functional includes left-right correlation in addition to exchange. Another approach designed to treat biological systems, i.e H-bonding, adopts Gaussian-like behavior at long-range for an exact exchange energy density at long-range [485-486]. We thus have the B3lyp variants, O3LYP and X3LYP [519].

Considerable effort have been placed in recent years to obtain optimum generalized gradient approximation (GGA) functionals to solve the local limitation of DFT methods. Among these new functionals we have the PBEPBE and THCTH. PBE exchange is a simplified GGA functional whereas all of the parameters are fundamental constants with no empirical parameters. HCTH on the other hand contains 15 adjustable parameters [484, 519].

Early studies have shown that although other properties are seriously degraded, the accuracy of reaction barrier heights can be dramatically improved by increasing the percentage of 'exact' exchange in the 40 – 50% region. Other workers have indicated that in order to correct excess exchange mixing for the ground state it is necessary to include the kinetic energy density yielding BMK with 42% exact exchange [489].

Another method, the CAM-B3LYP (Coulomb-attenuating method-B3LYP) combines the features of hybrid functional with the long-range corrected functional. The exchange functional is a mixture of exact, i.e. Hartree-Fock and DFT exchange whereas the ratio of exact to DFT exchange varies in different regions of the molecule. This method appears to handle well charge transfer. Other approaches use empirical fits to calibrate new designed functionals. Some functionals such as MO52X, use for refinement of their parameters databases sets which include thermochemistry, diverse barrier heights, transition-metal reaction energies and noncovalent interaction energies. This method has been successful for investigating the isomerization energies of alkanes [520].

The M06 family of functionals seems promising for application to larger systems having been constructed to account for effects of noncovalent interaction and including variable amounts of HF exchange. Each individual functional has been designed for a particular application and together shows a good across the board performance. The M06-class functionals depend on spin densities, spin density gradients, spin kinetic energy densities and for nonlocal, Hartree-Fock exchange. The M06, a hybrid meta functional, is reportedly a functional with good accuracy 'across-the-board' for transition metals, main group thermochemisry, medium-range correlation energy, and barrier heights. M06-2X, another hybrid meta functional is not good for transition metals but has excellent performance for main group chemistry, predicts accurate valence and Rydberg elecronic excitation energies and is an excellent functional for aromatic-aromatic stacking interactions. M06-L is not as accurate as MO6 for barrier heights but is accurate functional for transition metals and is the only local functional with better across-the-board average performance than B3LYP. Note that for large systems only local functionals can be more affordable. The M06-HF has a good performance for valence, Rydberg and charge transfer excited states with minimal sacrifice of ground-state accuracy [496,500].

The vdW-D collaboration bridges the gap between the speed of DFT and the quality of QC calculations. This functional seamlessly augments the standard exchange-correlation functional used in DFT to include a fully nonlocal correlation term which appropriately describes dispersion interactions within these systems [521]. Nonlocal correlation effects may also be included using wave function methods based on the Kohn-Sham (KS) self-consistent field fields (SCF) solution, as for example in the double-hybrid density functionals (DHDF) where a perturbation second-order correction has been shown to include in particular midrange correlation effects [521].

By including also long-range effects through the above-mentioned empirical correction, the resulting method (B2PLYLP-D and mPW2PLYP-D) show excellent performance in a range of tests where standard DFT fails. An empirical term for long-range dispersion was included (DFT-D) improving the prediction of molecular structure and bond energies of noncovalently bound complexes, intermolecular interaction energies in DNA phases pairs, amino acid pairs and reaction energies in organometallic chemistry [499,500].

For the double-hybrid density functionals (DHDF), non local effects were included whereas a perturbation second-order correction is made to include in particular midrange correlation effects. Effectively, with the idea that not only exchange but also the correlation part in KS-DFT has nonlocal orbital-dependent components, semi-empirical hybrid functional with correction from perturbation theory termed B2PLYP was proposed. First a standard hybrid-functional containing common semi-local generalized gradient approximations (GGA) for exchange (X) and correlation (C) is defined. A normal SCF calculation is carried out with this hybrid-GGA. The resultant KS orbitals and eigenvalues are then used as input for a standard second-order Moller-lesset type perturbation theory correction that replaces part of the semi-local GGA correlation leading to the double-hybrid density functionals (DHDF). One of the shortcomings of these functionals is underestimation of the long-range dispersion (van der Waals) interactions. To correct this deficiency a empirical dispersion term (DFT-D, i.e a damped atom-pairwise potential) is added to the expression leaving the electronic part of the functional untouched [479].

The inclusion of long-range effects through empirical corrections yields the B2PLY-D and mPW2PLYP-D methods [237,312]. DFT calculations approaches for the vdW energy have been proposed such as adding correction terms to the standard DFT energy and perturbation methods in the DFT (DFT-SAPT) where the dispersion energy is included as a second-order energy as well as adding correction terms to the standard DFT energy [333].

A classification scheme for DFT functionals was recently reported, i.e pure GGA functionals including PBEPBE and HCTH, pure τ functionals including VSXC and TPSSTPSS as well as hybrid functionals including MO52X, B3LYP, BMK, BHandH, BHandHHYH and CAM-B3LYP) [501].

Since DFT methods may encounter problems in the excited states, due to the fact that long-range properties such as charge transfer are common in the excited states, TDDFT (a time-dependent procedure) can be used to study excited states. It is an exact quantum mechanical theory in which the time-dependent density is the fundamental variable and the exchange-correlation (XC) potential describes the many-body interactions. For small changes in the time-dependent XC potential, the linear response approach can be applied to solve the equations making it possible to obtain the excitation energies as poles of the frequency dependent ground state linear response functions. TDDFT has replaced HF-based single-excitation theories (CIS) for calculation of valence excitation energies. Inclusion of solvation leads to TDDFT/PCM and IEFPCM-TDDFT methods [490, 493, 501].

In addition to the relatively modest computational expense, a major boost for the advancement of the method has been the assurance that it is a formally exact theory [493]. However, in practice, there is need to use approximate xc potentials which may lead to errors in the computational results. There have been problems such as description of Rydberg excitations, treatment of extended π systems, absence of double and higher excitations and the 1/R dependence of charge-transfer (CT) excitation energies. Although there is belief that any problems with the method are caused by imperfections of xc potentials it may also be necessary to also consider so-called adiabatic approximations, in which the time dependence enters the xc functional only via the time-dependent (TD) density functional as well as time-or energy-dependent xc functional beyond the adiabatic approximation [481, 491].

Although the focus during this decade has been to introduce functional for specific usage, the new trend is to develop all-purpose functionals.

WEAK INTERACTIONS

Hydrogen bonds (HB) are soft interactions whose bond lengths and angles fluctuate according to local environments and are dependent on the pair of atom groups that forms the extensive donor and acceptor subunits. The major component of hydrogen-bonding interaction is electrostatic. They are crucial for binding affinity and dictating the orientation of an inhibitor binding in the receptor and are thus of great importance to drug design. The bond capacity of HB is essential for bioisostersm. When a moiety of a compound is replaced by a bioisostere, the HB characteristics of the parent has to be matched with the possibility of improvement of drug properties. The strength of hydrogen bond acceptors and donors may vary significantly, and as a result, electron-withdrawing or donating substituents can have opposite effects on the activities of the compounds, via interactions of the inhibitor with the receptor [171].

Many structure-activity relationships (SAR) can be traced to modifications of the hydrogen-bonding interaction of the inhibitor with the receptor. Due to the character of being the property of a group of atoms and having susceptibility to local environments, HB cannot be modeled accurately by a general semiempirical or rule-based method. There are many exceptions, such as steric factors, to be accommodated by a finite set of rules. The directional properties are not isotropic and quite important to both computational studies and practical applications [171].

In three-dimensional structures of biological macromolecular systems such as proteins and nucleic acids, stacking involving aliphatic chains, aromatic rings or cations/anions have been widely observed and known to contribute to thermodynamic stabilization. In many theoretical studies the van der Waals (vdW) energy has been shown to be the primary origin of the stabilization energy for stacking between aromatic rings. In order to evaluate the electron correlation effects more sophisticated ab initio calculations are required such as coupled cluster methods with singles, doubles, perturbation, (CCSD(t) as well as quantum Monte Carlo (QMC) methods. Conventional Hartree-Fock (HF) and traditional density functional theory (DFT) face difficulties estimating the stabilization energy gained by stacking aromatic rings. Good consistency can be obtained with CCSD(t) and some DFT methods such as SAPT. Notwithstanding, the computational cost of using sophisticated approaches for the wdW energy are too large. At the other end, the usage of empirical functions in molecular mechanics (MM) calculations, in order to reduce the computational cost have reportedly yielded inadequate results [333,469].

When halogen atoms act as electrophiles, there are specific molecular interaction which has been recently investigated and known as halogen bonding whose characteristics are parallel with those of hydrogen bonding in terms of strength and directionality [235]. The effective ability of halogen atoms for directing molecular recognition processes became more noticeable in the 1990s, and as a consequence in the last decade, this type of bonding has yielded many applications. Halogen bonding can be important in areas where the control of intermolecular recognition and self-assembly processes plays a central role. There are important implications of halogen bonding, or halogen to oxygen (or nitrogen) which are below or equal to the van der Waals radius sums in biological molecules. The interesting chemical features of halogens make them useful in designing drugs and protein inhibitors. It is also of interest that about half of the molecules applied in high-throughout screening are halogenated. The Protein Data Bank contains over 1000 structures in which the ligands are halogenated yielding d(Cl...O), d(Br…..O) and d(I…O) distances which are less than their respective van der Walls radius sums. There are also many protein structures with halogen bonding angles $< (c - X...O)$ that are larger than 140^0 [235].

Halogen substitution has been indicated to be an important approach for drug design. However, the accurate chemical and structural basis for their contribution to drug-protein affinity and recognition has not been fully elucidated for rational drug design. For small model systems, using high level quantum chemical methods, the key geometrical energetic properties of the halogen bonding interaction yields halogen bonding lengths shorter than the sum of van der Waals radii of the atoms involved. The large size of biological systems prohibits the efficient use of electronic structure methods with a reasonable computational cost. Studies of biological systems, i.e proteins in complex with halogenated ligands, using a two-layer QM/MM Oniom methodology indicates that the halogen-oxygen distances are much less than the van der Waals radius sums. Single-point energy calculations suggest that the interaction becomes comparable in magnitude to classical hydrogen bonding. In addition, the strength of the interactions attenuates in the order H~I > Br >Cl in agreement with characteristics discovered within small model halogen bonded system [235].

For a broad range of biological processes protein-carbohydrate interactions play important roles whereas molecular recognition of target molecules is essential for life processes. Antibodies, enzymes, lectins are among the variety of proteins involved in carbohydrate recognition. X-ray data indicate that through multiple interactions the receptors effectively recognize carbohydrates. Contacts between nonpolar surfaces, networks of hydrogen bonds, polar side chains and main chain amides are essential for protein-carbohydrate recognition. Stacking with aromatic residues can proceed via nonpolar surfaces of carbohydrates [174].

Of particular interest is the recognition by artificial receptors of carbohydrates, i.e carbohydrate-aromatic (CH/π) interactions, which often arise from the sum of repulsive and attractive forces from the inherent properties of each system. In order to understand their roles in the molecular recognition process, a quantitative evaluation of the carbohydrate-aromatic interactions is necessary whereas the origin, dependence, orientation and magnitude plays an essential role. Molecular dynamics, *ab initio* molecular orbital, MP2 and DFT calculations of the carbohydrate-aromatic complexes are of considerable interest. Calculations at the MP2/6-311+G*, MP2/6-31G++**, MP2/6-31G** and CCSD(T) levels indicate the interaction energies depend on the basis sets and electron correlation whereas a CCSD(T) level electron correlation correction and a large basis set close to saturation is necessary for an accurate evaluation of the interaction energy.

A recent *ab initio* calculation of magnitude and nature of carbohydrate-aromatic interactions suggest that the directionality of the carbohydrate-aromatic interaction is weak. The dispersion interaction is the major source of the attraction in the complex. Although the electrostatic contributions to the attraction are relatively small, the size of the interaction energy is not largely different from that of typical hydrogen bonds. Nonetheless, the nature of the carbohydrate-aromatic interaction is very different from those of hydrogen bonds, which have strong directionality due to strong electrostatic interactions. The orientation dependence of the carbohydrate-aromatic interaction is weak due to the small electrostatic contribution to the interaction [174]. Special attention has also been paid to the structure of water molecules on carbohydrate recognition sites of various proteins and many studies support the idea that displacement of these water molecules should have a crucial effect on the binding free energy [167].

A good knowledge of the interactions between active compound and target is essential for the success of rational drug design whereas these interactions are determined by the electron density (ED) which can be determined by X-ray measurements. The problem is however, that for proteins or protein-ligand complexes, high-resolution X-ray diffraction experiments are still extremely demanding. In practice for drug design, in general, only X-ray data of enzyme-inhibitor or enzymes are used providing approximate coordinates which are not sufficiently resolved for ED analysis [80]

The approximate ED in biological environments can also be obtained from crystals of the pure compound assuming that the environment within influences the properties of the inhibitors in a way the enzyme surrounding would. It is not obvious that steric, electrostatic, hydrogen bonding, van der Waals effects, etc govern the stability of crystals as well as enzyme-inhibitor complexes. The confirmation or not of this could aid the molecular recognition process and the differences could also be of interest for using predetermined atomic EDs, in particular if they include the influence of the environment. In principle it would seem that comparison of ED from crystals of enzyme-inhibitor complex and that of an inhibitor should help us elucidate the influence of environments since they yield differences of 0.1 A^{-3} for high-resolution diffraction data sets. For high resolution measurements larger differences are expected whereas it is even more difficult to differentiate between indirect effects of environmental induced changes of the geometrical structure and direct influences of the environment.

The ED from diffraction pattern yield differences due to restricted functions projected in the multipole model. Thus computed EDs yield more reasonable trends than measured ones. Recent work indicates a decrease in differences between theory and experiment with the replacement of Gaussian by Slater-type functions. It is unclear whether effects are artifacts from the differences between experiment and theory or results from the environment. One approach is to compute EDs for different surrounding whereas there would be a strong dependence of computed EDs and Laplacians on the level of sophistication of calculations. However, if we are searching for trends, the dependencies are much smaller.

Periodic HF calculations indicate that the influence of the crystal environment was too small to explain discrepancies although it was strong enough to yield considerable variation in the electrostatic potential (ESP), i.e one of the properties which influence the enzyme-inhibitor process. The enzyme environment via it`s strong catalytic power should influence the ED of the inhibitor. Various investigations concentrate on variations in energies and mechanisms.

Simulation of the various effects were performed with theoretical approaches, incorporating different environments which are represented by electrostatic potentials obtained from molecular mechanics and the inhibitor is described by quantum chemical methods [80]. The potentials incorporate details regarding the molecular nature of the surroundings and the available crystal structure yield the geometrical arrangements of the inhibitors. The conductor-like screening model (COSMO) was used to study the influence of polar solvents and the EDs were determined by gas-phase calculations. The geometries were optimized for various surroundings since steric restrictions which enforce different conformers as well as the enzyme environment leads to ED differences.

Quantum mechanical/molecular mechanical (QM/MM) of various inhibitors in complexes indicates that the ED of the active compound is in general influenced by the environment inside the crystal. This is not true, however, if the geometrical arrangement of the inhibitor in the enzyme differs significantly from that in the crystal. Polar solvent environments provide similar electron distribution whereas EDs computed for gas-phase environments deviate strongly from those in crystal and protein surroundings. Continuum solvation was thus suggested for the determination of the ED of macromolecular systems [80].

For stabilizing structures of proteins, a crucial role is played by noncovalent interactions of which van der Waals (vdW) interactions are a subclass with vdW interactions involving aromatics rings regarded as weakly polar in proteins and as base stacking in nucleic acid chemistry. vDW can be classified as either short-or long-range based on the theory of intermolecular forces whereas perturbation theory can describe the energy as a sum of dispersion energies, induction electrostatic and exchange-repulsion [160]. The van der Waals density functional (vdW-DF) was applied to study hydrogen bonding and stacking interactions between nucleobases. The excellent agreement of the results with high level quantum chemical calculations highlights the use of the vdW-DF for first principles investigations of biologically important molecules.

The results suggest that, in the case of hydrogen-bonded nucleobase pairs, dispersion interactions reduce the cost of propeller twists while having a negligible effects on buckling. In addition, the efficient scaling of DFT methods allowed for the easy optimization of separation distance between nucleobase stacks, indicating enhancements in the interaction energy of up to 3 kcal/mol over previous fixed distance calculations. It is anticipated that these results will be significant for extending the vdW-DF methods to model larger vdW complexes and biological molecules [139].

Exchange-repulsions are short-range predominant but induction, dispersion and electrostatic interactions are strongest. All the contributions can be derived in the multipole approach from electrostatic interactions. Dispersion is a consequence of electron correlation and post-HF methods with large bases sets are necessary to describe vdW since HF theory cannot treat correlation effects.

DFT and MP2 are the quantum chemical methods often used to study vdW in large molecules. MP2 scales with the fifth power of the bases set size and various reduced scaling method have been developed, such as Laplace MP2, local MP2 (LMP2), triatomics-in-molecules MP2 (TRIM MP2), local density fitting MP2 (DF-LMP2), resolution of identity (R1-MP2), R1 version of the local triatomics-in-molecules method (R1-TRIM MP2) pseudospectral numerical technique (PS-MP2), local MP2 theory (PS_MP2) and the efficient method which scales as n3 while recovering 98% of the canonical energy correction (PS-LMP2). One of the weaknesses of DFT include the inappropriate description of London forces whereas the *a posteriori* correction or augmentation of functionals with force-field like dispersion terms, combination, modification and extensions of existing functional are the most frequently applied empirical approaches to overcome the DFT deficiencies which are not always transferable between different systems [158].

The interaction energies of ubiquitous weakly polar interactions in proteins are comparable with those of hydrogen bonds, consequently, they stabilize local secondary and tertiary structures. Some of the most widely-used density functional fails, however, to describe the weakly polar interactions emphasizing the importance of finding and testing functionals which adequately describe and quantify the energetics of such interactions. Recent Investigation of weak polar interactions using meta functional where kinetic energy density is included indicated that the MPW1B95, PWB6K, MPWB1K and PW6B95 performed reasonable well whereas the PWB6K functional was recommended for large systems and the PWPW91 was indicated as a viable alternative to the *ab initio* methods when large complexes are involved.

Calculations of weakly polar interaction energies in polypeptides using DFT and MPT was recently reported. Subsets of various databases were used with BHandHLYP, PWPW91, PS-LMP2 and cc-pVDZ, cc-pVTZ(-f), cc-PVTZ, cc-pvqz(-g), aug-cc-pVDZ, aug-cc-VTGZ(-f) and aug-cc-PvVTZ basis sets. The *a posteriori* counterpoise method was used to correct basis set superposition errors. The BHandHLYP functional indicated good results for various weakly polar interaction and dispersion interactions in agreement with coupled cluster (CCSD(T)) and resolution of identity MP2 (RIMP2) [160,174] methods.

The Lee, Yang and Parr correlation functional combined with the BH functional, which is the result of a linear interpolation between the Slater local exchange and the exact HF yields good results for π-stacking, dispersion and nonbonded interaction energies including charge-transfer complexes. Stacking involving aromatic rings has a significant contribution to the structural stability of biological macromolecules. Recently, a novel computational scheme was reported for accurate and efficient evaluation of π–π and π–σ stacking. In this scheme, the electron density of the aromatic rings is represented by Gaussian-type functions and the parameters involved in the functions are determined by an optimization scheme to reproduce the CCSD(T) results. The computational time is dramatically reduced in comparison with CCSD(T) methods [333].

SELECTED APPLICATIONS OF VARIOUS MODELS TO DRUG DESIGN

During the last decade we have applied many of the methods discussed in this book to Cancer, Aids, Alzheimer, Parkinson and other diseases proposing novel inhibitors [522 -543].

In 2002 we made a theoretical ab initio study of ranitidine [523]. The presence of a heterocyclic ring containing a basic-center linked via a methylene chain to a substituted guanidine or thiourea polar side chain, such as found in the H2-antagonist metiamide, which is an imidazole heterocyclic ring, was often identified as one of the requirements for H2-antagonist activity. In ranitidine, on the other hand, the imidazole ring is substituted for a furan ring, yielding a more active biological H2 antagonist. We used the HF and MP2 methods in order to investigate the open and folded ranitidine conformations and found good agreement with experimental crystallographic data. All our results indicate that, as in metiamide, the folded conformation is also preferred. We have investigated charge distributions, electrostatic, hydrogen bond and solvent effects on stabilizing the conformations and discussed the interactions of ranitidine with the biological receptor.

In 2003 we investigated [524] nucleoside analogs that inhibit human immunodeficiency syndrome (HIV-1) reverse transcriptase such as AZT, d4T, ddI, 3TC and ddC which are chain terminating nucleoside analogs whereas resistance is a major problem. We appealed to atomic charges, regioselective patterns of chemical activity and other indices of biochemical activity that could help us acquire a better understanding of how the drugs work and the mechanism of drug resistance. The HF and DFT methods were used to investigate the above-mentioned nucleoside analogs including diffusion, polarization and correlation effects to obtain fully optimized geometric parameters. The effects of solvents, Mulliken and natural bond orbital charge distributions, vibrational frequencies and hydrogen bond effects were investigated.

In 2004 we reported [525] computer-aided molecular design of novel glucosidase inhibitors for AIDS treatment. At that time statistics suggested that some 20 million people had died and close to 40 million were living with the AIDS disease with 14 thousands infected daily worldwide. Still, only a few pharmaceutics were available for AIDS chemotherapy some of which acts against the virus before entrance into the host cells.

One of these targets is the glucosidase protein which depends on the activity of enzymes such as glucosidase and transferase for the elaboration of the polysaccharides. Several glucosidase inhibitors were investigated whereas the DFT method was used to compute atomic charges and investigate ligand/receptor interactions. Analysis of the interactions of the proposed pharmaceutical, a pseudodisaccharide, with the Thermotoga maritime 4-alpha-glucanotransferase in complex with modified acarbose, the scores from docking as well as the superposition of all the ligands, suggest that our molecular designed pseudo-dissacharide may be a potent glucosidase inhibitor.

In 2004 we also reported [526] a molecular modeling and QSAR study of suppressors of the growth of Trypanasoma cruzi epimastigotes. We used molecular modeling and QSAR tools to study 18 dithiocarbamate suppressors of the growth of Trypanosoma cruzi epimastigotes reported in the literature as superoxide dismutase (SOD) inhibitors. PCA (Principal component analysis) indicated that the descriptors, heat of formation, logarithm of the partition coefficient, superficial area, charge of the nitrogen atom from the ditiocarbamate group as well as charges from the two carbon atoms adjacent to that nitrogen are responsible for the classification between the lower and higher trypanomacid activity. Using docking methods and multiple linear regression methods it was possible to identify the probable bioactive isomers that suppress the growth of T. cruzi epimastiotes. Our best partial least square (PLS) model obtained with the descriptors yields a good correlation between experimental and predicted biological activites and compares with different SODs as possible target for interaction with the dithiocarbamates.

Quantum chemical semi-empirical AM1 and PM3 calculations were performed for the lowest energy conformations of the compounds. The calculated variables were total energy, highest occupied molecular orbital energy (HOMO), lowest unoccupied molecular orbital energy (LUMO), Mulliken's electronegatiity, molecular hardness, molecular softness, atomic charges (from the electrostatic potential), bond orders, heat of formation, polarizability, dipole moment, ionization potential, total surface area, molecular volume, octanol-water partition coefficient (Log P) as well as other topological and three-dimensional molecular descriptors with the purpose of representing different sources of chemical information in terms of size, shape of a molecule, symmetry and atom distribution in the molecule.

In 2004 we also published the work density functional and docking studies of retinoids for cancer treatment [527]. The retinoic acid receptor (RAR) and retinoid X receptor (RXR) are members of the nuclear receptor superfamily. The ligand-binding domain contains the ligand-dependent activation function. The isotypes RAR α β γ are distinct pharmacological targets for retinoids involved in the treatment of various cancers and skin diseases. There is thus considerable interest in synthetic retinoids with isotype selectivity and reduced side effects. We investigated the retinoid acid receptors and three of its panagonists. We carried out DFT as well as the electrostatic potentials calculations. Docking was used to study the interactions between the receptor and the three ligands. A theoretically more potent inhibitor, which can be obtained by modifying one of the retinoic acids investigated, was proposed.

In 2005 we published a work on molecular dynamics, database screening, density functional and docking studies of novel RAR ligands in cancer chemotherapy [528]. We also published in this year our results regarding a rational desing of novel diketoacid-containing ferrocene inhibitors of HIV-1 integrase [529]. In 2005 we reported our research on computer-aided design of a novel ligand for retinoic acid receptor in cancer chemotherapy [530]. Also in this year we published homology modeling and molecular interaction field studies of α-glicosidases as a guide to structure-based design of novel proposed anti-HIV inhibitors [531].

In 2006 we reported [532] the ADMET properties, database screening, molecular dynamics, density functional and docking studies of novel potential anti-cancer compounds. Quantum chemical calculations were performed at the AM1 level, to obtain partial charges, and docking of 350,000 molecules using large databases. Various docking programs were used and compared. In principle all docking applications include four steps, i.e identification and preparation of the receptor site, preparation of the ligands(s), docking the ligand(s) and evaluation of the docked orientations. For the ligands, a flexible algorithm (anchor-first search) was used. Scoring functions used shape, geometry, orientation and force fields. We screened a large database in order to find theoretically more potent RAR ligands (with the largest scoring function). We optimized ~350,000 molecules at the AM1 level in order to obtain geometries and charges for docking calculations. Two promising new ligands with good scores were optimized by DFT. This enables us to have an even better input structure for the next step involving another docking procedure.

Molecular dynamics simulations (MD) were done. From the molecular trajectory of the two systems generated by the molecular dynamics simulations we analyzed the root mean square-deviation of each system with respect to all atoms as well as the trial energy as function of the time. The ADMET (Absorption, distribution, metabolism, excretion and toxicity) properties as well as the parameters of the Rule of Five were investigated. The result of this work is compared with a crystallographic ligand of RAR. Our novel proposed anti-cancer ligand indicates hydrophobic interactions and strong polar interactions with the receptor.

In 2006 we also reported [533] a molecular dynamics, docking, density functional and ADMET studies of HIV-1 reverse transcriptase inhibitors. We noted then that the standard treatment of acquired immune deficiency drugs, that had been licensed for clinical use or subjected to advanced clinical trials, belonged to one of the following three classes (1) nucleoside/nucleotide reverse transcriptase inhibitors (NRTIs), i.e abacavir (ABC), emitricitabine [(-)FTC], zidovudine (AZT), didanosine (ddi), zalcitabine (ddc), savudine (D4T), lamivudine (3TC) and tenofovir disoproxil fumarate; (2) non-nucluseoside reverse transcriptase inhibitors (NNRTIs), i.e emivirine, efavirenz, nevirapine and delavirdine; and (3) protease inhibitors (PIs), i.e lopinavir, nelfinavir, ritonavir, amprenavir, saquinavir and indinavir. Various other events in the HIV replicative cycle can be considered as potential target for chemotherapeutic intervention (1) viral entry through blockade of the viral coreceptors (2) viral adsorption through binding to the viral envelope glycoprotein gp120 (3) viral assembly and disassembly through NCp7 zinc finger-targeted agents (ADA); (4) virus –cell fusion through binding to the viral envelope glycoprotein gp41; (5) proviral DNA integration through integrase inhibitors and (6) viral mRNA transcription through inhibitors of the transcription (transactivation) process. In addition, NRTIs, NNRTIs and PIs have been developed that posses improved metabolic characteristics as well as activity.

Nucleoside analogs constitute a family of biological molecules (ddI, d4T, ddC and 3TC) which play an important role in the transcription process of the human immunodeficiency virus. The normal nucleoside substrates used by reverse transcriptase (RT) to synthetize DNA are mimicked by these nucleoside analogs which lacked a 3'-OH group and consequently act as chain terminators when incorporated in the DNA by RT. Although these nucleoside analogs show good activity as inhibitors of HIV, their long-term usefulness is limited by toxicities. Resistance and mutation are also problems. We did molecular dynamics, density functional with correlation as well as docking of inhibitors of HIV-1 reverse transcriptase RT. We proposed a novel potential HIV-1 RT inhibitor RTI (which theoretically appears to bind in a similar mode as other nucleoside reverse transcriptase inhibitors and in addition introduces new hydrogen bond interactions. Our novel RTI has high docking scores and the molecular dynamics studies as well as the analysis of the ligand-receptor interactions in the active site as well as ADMET properties suggest advantages and specificities for this potential RTI.

In 2006 we also published the book Modern Biotechnology in Medicinal Chemistry and Industry [522].

In 2007 we reported [534] computer-aided molecular design of novel HMG-CoA reductase inhibitors for the treatment of hyhpercholesterolemia [532]. Elevated cholesterol levels are a primary risk factor for the development of coronary artery disease. Dietary changes associated with drug therapy can reduce high serum cholesterol levels and dramatically decrease the risk of stroke and overall mortality. HMG-CoA reductase is an important molecular target of hypolipemic drugs, known as statins, which are effective in the reduction of cholesterol serum levels, attenuating cholesterol synthesis in-liver by competitive inhibition regarding the substrate HMG-CoA. We focused on computer-aided molecular design using density functional theory, flexible docking, molecular dynamics as well as ADMET and synthetic accessibility analyses in order to propose novel potential HMG-CoA reductase inhibitors, designed by bioiososeric modification which are promising for the treatment of hypercholesterolemia.

We also reported [535] in 2007 virtual screening, molecular interaction field, molecular dynamics with explicit water solvation, docking, density functional and ADMET properties of novel AChE inhibitors in Alzheimer's disease (AD). This disease affects approximately 10% of the world's population with 65 years of age, being the most common form of dementia in adults and is characterized by senile plaquets and cholinergic deficits. Many drugs currently used for the treatment of AD are based on the improvement of cholinergic neurotransmission achieved by Acetylcholinestarase (AChE) inhibition, the enzyme responsible for acetylcholine hydrolysis. The complexes of AChE with inhibitors were computer-aided designed by us. Toxicity and Metabolism predictions, flexible docking as well as MIF studies were also made. Using the various models discussed above we proposed novel potential AChE inhibitors for the treatment of Alzheimer's disease.

In 2007 we published the first volume of our Enciclopedia: Current Methods in Medicinal Chemistry and Biological Physics [542].

In 2008 we performed [536] molecular dynamics, flexible docking, virtual screening, ADMET predictions and molecular interaction fields studies to design novel potential MAO-B inhibitors. Monoamine oxidase is a flavoenzyme bound to the mitochondrial outer membranes of the cells, which is responsible for the oxidative deamination of neurotransmitter and dietary amines. It has two distinct isozymic forms, designated MAO-A and MAO-B, each displaying different substrate and inhibitor specificities. They are the well-known targets for antidepressant, Parkinson's disease and neuroprotecive drugs. Optimizations of the compound, flexible docking and virtual screening in large databases were done, scored and ranked. Toxicity predictions were performed and the 'Rule of Five' (RO5) were calculated for these proposals. Usage of the various models allowed us to design new molecules with potential higher selectivity and enzymatic inhibitory activity over MAO-B.

In 2008 we also reported [537] molecular dynamics, density functional, ADMET predictions, virtual screening, molecular interaction field studies for identification and evaluation of novel potential CDK2 inhibitors in cancer therapy. The cyclin-dependent kinases (CDKs) are a class of serine-threonine kinases that are responsible for the progression of cells through the various phases and transitions of the cell cycle. As the name implies, the activity of these kinases as well as their subcellular localization and substrate specificity depend upon the presence of a proteic regulatory subunit called cyclin. We proposed eight novel potential inhibitors of CDK2 which showed interesting structural characteristics that are required for inhibiting the CDK2 activity and show potential as drug candidates for the treatment of cancer. One of the proposals and one of the drug-like compounds selected by virtual screening indicated to be promising candidates for CDK2-based cancer therapy.

In 2008 we also investigated a) the use of virtual screening, flexible docking and molecular interaction fields to design novel HMG-CoA reductase inhibitors for the treatment of hyhpercholesterolemia [538] and b) pharmacokinetic and pharmacodynamic predictions of novel potential HIV-1 integrase inhibitors [539].

In 2008 we published the second volume of our Enciclopedia: Current Methods in Medicinal Chemistry and Biological Physics [543].

In 2009 we published research [540] on computer-aided drug design of novel PLA_2 inhibitor candidates for treatment of snakebites. Phospholipases A_2 (PLA_2) are enzymes commonly found in snake venoms from Viperidase and Elaphidae families which are major components thereof. Many plants are used in traditional medicine as active agents against various effects induced by snakebite. In this work we presented the PLA_2 BthTX-I structure prediction based on homology modeling. In addition, we performed virtual screening in a large database yielding a set of potential bioactive inhibitors. A flexible docking program was used to investigate the interaction fields (MIFs) calculations with the phospholipases model indicating important binding effects. We proposed a theoretically nontoxic, drug-like, and potential novel BthTX-1 inhibitor. These calculations have been used to guide the design of novel phospholipase inhibitors as potential lead compounds that may be optimized for future treatment of snakebit victims as well as other human diseases in which PLA_2 enzymes are involved.

In 2010 we reported computer-aided drug design and ADMET predictions for identification and evaluation of novel potential farnesyltransferase inhibitors in cancer therapy [541]. Ras protein is a cell component that controls growth and multiplication. They are small G proteins that are linked to GDP in rest and linked to GTP when active, whereas the linkage to TTP is temporary. It was previously observed that an abnormal form of the signaling Ras is present in almost 30% of cancers, being more prevalent in both pancreatic and colon cancer. This protein binds in a persistent manner to GTP and cannot promote hyhdrolysis, as occurs normally being thus constantly activated. It is believed than once the Ras proteins are involved in the control of the cell growth and divisions, mutations of these proteins could be related to the development of cancer. Thus, methods capable of neutralizing Ras could be considered useful in the fight against cancer. In this context, protein farneshltransferas (FTase) has been studied as a therapeutic target.

We used various computational methodologies including molecular dynamics, density functional theory, virtual screening, ADMET predictions and molecular interaction field studies to design and analyze four novel potential inhibitors of Farnesyltransferase. Evaluation of two proposals regarding their drug potential as well as lead compounds have indicated them as novel promising FTase inhibitors, with theoretically interesting pharmacotherapeutic profiles, when compared to the very active and most cited FTase inhibitors that have activity data reported, which are launched drugs of compounds in clinical tests. One of our two proposals appear to be a more promising drug candidate and FTase inhibitor, but both derivative molecules indicate potential very good pharmacotherapeutic profiles in comparison with two reference pharmaceuticals. Two other proposals have been selected with virtual screening approaches and by us investigated, which suggest novel and alternatives scaffolds to design future potential FTase inhibitors. Such compounds can be explored as promising molecules to initiate a research protocol in order to discover novel anticancer drug candidates targeting Farnesyltransferase, in the fight against cancer.

ACKNOWLEDGEMENTS

We acknowledge financial assistance from CNPq, Faperj and Fapesp.

REFERENCES

[1]   Devereux M, Popelier PLA and McLay IM. Quantum Isostere Database: A Web-Based Tool using quantum chemical topology to predict bioisosteric replacements for drug design. J. Chem. Inf. Model 2009;49:1497-1513.

[2]   Lima LM, Barreiro EJ. Bioisosterism: a useful strategy for molecular modification and drug design. Curr. Med. Chem. 2005;12:23 -49.

[3]   Thomber CW. The quest for bioisosteric replacements. J. Chem. Inf. Model. 2006;96: 3147 – 3176.

[4]   Bader RFW, Bayles D. Properties of atoms in molecules. Group addiivity. J. Phys. Chem. 2000;104:5579–5589.

[5]   Holliday JD, Jelfs SP, Willett P. Calculation of intersubstituent similarity using R-Group descriptors, J. Chem. Inf. Comput. Sci.. 2003;43:406–411.

[6]   Lewell XQ, Jones AC, Bruce CL, Harper G, Jones MM, McLay IM, Bradshaw. J, Drug rings Database with web interface. A tool for identifying alternative chemical rings in lead discovery programs. J. Med. Chem. 2003;46:3257–3274.

[7]   Haigh JA, Pickup BT, Grant, AJ, Nicholls A. Small molecule shape-fingerprints. J. Chem. Inf. Model. 2005;45:673–684.

[8]   Seber A, Teckentrup A, Briem H, Flexsim R. A virtual affinity fingerprint descriptor to calculate similarities of funcional groups, J. Comput-aided Mol. Des. 2002;16:903-916.

[9]   Watson P, Willett P, Gillet VJ, Verdonk, ML. Calculating the knowledge-based similarity of functional groups using crystallographic data. J. Comput-aided mol. Des. 2001;15:835-857.

[10]   Talete SRL, Todeschini R, Consonni V, Pavan V. Dragon, Molecular modeling software, Milan, Italy..

[11]   Tripos-Associates, SYBYL. Molecular modeling software, version 6.7, St. Louis MO, U.S.A.

[12]   Accelrys TSAR, version 3.3; San Diego, CA, U.S.A. 2005.

[13]   Accelrys Cerius2, version 4.7; San Diego, CA U.S.A. 2005.

[14]   BROOD: OpenEye Scientific Software Inc: Santa Fe, NM, U.S.A. 2006.

[15]   Devereux M, Popelier PLA, McLay LM, Towards an ab intio fragment database for bio-isosterism:dependence of QCT properties on level of theory. Conformation and chemical environment, J. Comput. Chem. 2009;30:1300-1319.

[16]   Devereux M, Popelier PLA,McLay IM. A refined model for prediction of hydrogen bond acidity and basicity parameters from quantum chemical molecular descriptors. Phys. Chem. Chem. Phys. 2009;11:1595-1603.

[17]   Ehresmann B, Martin B, Horn AHC, Clark T, Local molecular properties and their use in predicting reactivity. J. Mol. Model;2003:9:342-347.

[18]   Poater T, Sola M, Duran M, Fradera X. The calculation of electron localization and delocalization indices at the Hartree-Fock, density functional and post-Hartree-Fock levels of theory. Theor. Chem. Acc. 2002, 107, 362-371.[19]   Rafat M, Devereux M, Popelier PLA. Rendering of quantum topological atoms and bonds. J. Mol. Graphics Modell. 2005;24:111-120.

[20]   Chaudry UA, Popelier PLA. Estimation of pK$_a$ using quantum topological molecular similarity (QTMS) descriptors: Appplication to carboxylic acids, anilines and phenols. J. Org.Chem. 2004;69:233-241.

[21]   Popelier PLA, Chaudry UA, Smith PJ. Quantum topological molecular similarity. Part 5. Further developments with an application to the toxicity of polychlorinated dibenzo-p-dioxins. J. Chem. Soc. 2002;2: 231-1237.

[22]   Popelier PLA, Smith PJ. QSAR models based on quantum topological molecular similarity. Eur. J. Med. Chem. 2006;41:862-873.

[23]   Platts JA. Theoretical prediction of hydrogen bond basicity. Phys. Chem. Chem. Phys. 2000;2:3115-3120.

[24]   Platts JA, Butina D, Abraham MH, Hersey A. Estimation of molecular linear free energy relation descriptors using a group contribution approach. J. Chem. Inf. Comput. Sci. 2000;39: 835-845.

[25]   Kalgutkar AS, Gardner I, Obach RS, Shaffer CL, Callegari E, Henne KR, Mutih AE, Dalvie DK, Lee JS, Nakai Y, O'Donnell JP, Boer J, Garriman, SP. A comprehensive listing of bioactivaion pathways or of organic functional groups. Curr. Drug. Metab. 2005:6:161-225.

[26]   WDI, World Drug Index, Derwent Information; 1996.

[27]   Kosugi T, Nakanishi I and Kitaura K. Binding free energy calculations of adenosine deaminase inhibitor and the effect of methyl substitution in inhibitors. J. Chem. Inf. Model. 2009;49: 615– 622.

[28]   Knight JL and Brooks III CL. λ-dynamics free energy simulation methods J. Comput. Chem.. 2009;30:1692–1700.

[29]   Kostjukov VV, Khomytova NM and Evstigneev MP. Partition of thermodynamic energies of Drug-DNA complexation. Biopolymers 2009;91:773– 789.

[30]   Mulakala C and Kaznessis YN. Path-integral method for predicting relative binding affinities of protein-ligand complexes. J. Am. Chem. Soc. 2009;131: 4521–4528.

[31]   Oostenbrink C. Efficient free energy calculations on small molecule host-guest systems – A combined linear interaction energy/one-step perturbation approach. J. Comput. Chem. 2009;30: 212 -221.

[32]   Nervall M, Hanspers P, Carlsson J, Boukharta L and Aqvist J. Predicting binding modes from free energy calculations. J. Med. Chem. 2008;51:2657–2667.

[33]   Cossins BP, Foucher S, Edge CM and Essex JW. Assessment of nonequilibrium free energy methods. J. Phys. Chem. B 2009;113:5508–5519.

[34]   Banavali NK, Im W, Roux B. Electrostastic free energy calculations using the generalized solvent boundary potential method. J. Chem. Phys. 117:7381-7388.

[35]   Chipot C, Rozanska X, Dixit SB. Can free energy calculations be fast and accurate at the same time? Binding of low-affinity, nonpeptide inhibitors to the SH2 domain of the Src protein. J. Comput. Aided Mol. Des. 2005;19:765-770.

[36]   Jarzynski C. Nonequilibrium equality for free energy differences. Phys. Rev. Lett. 1997; 78:2690-2693.

[37]   Shirts MR, Hooker EB and Pande VS. Equilibrium free energies from nonequilibrium measurements using maximum-likelihood methods. Phys. Rev. Lett. 91:140601-140604

[38]   Zeevaart JG, Wang L, Thakur VV, Leung CS, Rives JT, Bailey CM, Domacal RA, Anderson KS and Jorgensen WL. Optimization of azoles as anti-human immunodeficiency virus agents guided by free-energy calculations. J. Am. Chem. Soc. 2008;13:9492-9499.

[39]   Gilson MK and Zhou HX. Calculation of protein-ligand binding affinities. Annu. Rev. Biophys. Biomol. Struct. 2007;36:21-42.

[40]   Laurie ATR and Jackson RM. Methods for the prediction of protein-ligand binding sites for structure-based drug design and virtual ligand screening. Current protein and peptide science 2006;7:395-406.

[41]   Wang W; Wang J, Kollman PA. What determines the van der Waals coefficient β in the LIE (linear energy) method to estimate binding ree energies using molecular dynamics simulations. Proteins 1999;34:395-402.

[42]   Shirts MR and Pande VS. Comparison of efficiency and bias of free energies computed by exponential averaging, the Bennett acceptance ratio and thermodynamic integration. The Journal of Chemical Physics 2005;122:144107-144108.

[43]   Zhou R, Friesner RA, Ghosh A, Rizzo RC, Jorgensen WL, Levy RM. New linear interaction mehod for binding affinity calculations using a continuum solvent model. J. Phys. Chem. B 2001;105:10388-10397.

[44]   Grater F, Schwarzl SM, Dejaegere A, Fischer S, Smith JC. 2005; Protein/ligand binding free energies calculated with quantum mechanics/molecular mechanics. J. Phys. Chem. B. 2005;109:10474-10483.

[45]   Wu D and Kofke DA. Phase-space overlap measures.I. Fail-safe bias detection in free energies calculated by molecular simulation. The Journal of Chemical Physics 2005;54103-54110.

[46]   Woods CJ and Essex JW. Enhanced configurational sampling in binding free-energy calculations. J. Phys. Chem. B 2003;107:13711-13718.

[47]   Woods CJ, Essex JW and King MA. The development of replica-exchange-based free-energy methods. J. Phys. Chem. B 2003;107:13703-13710.

[48]   Foloppe N and Hubbard R. Towards predictive ligand design with free-energy based computational methods. Current medicinal chemistry. 2006;13:3583-3608.

[49]   Wu D and Kofke A. Rosenbluth-sampled nonequilibrium work method for calculation of free energies in molecular simulation. The Journal of Chemical Physics 2005;122:204104-204113.

[50]   Pohorille A, Chipot C. Eds. Free energy calculatiohns-Theory and applications in chemistry and biology; Springer: Heidelberg, 2007.

[51]   Zwanzig RW. High-temperature equation of state by a perturbation method. I. Nonpolar gases. J. Chem. Phys. 1954;22:1420-1426.

[52]   Beutler TC, Mark AE, van Schaik RC, Gerber PPR, van Gunsteren WF. Avoiding singularities and numerical instabilities in free energy calculations based on molecular simulations. Chem. Phys. Lett. 1994;222:529-539.

[53]   Áqvist J, Medina C, Samuelsson JE. A new method for predicting binding affinity in compter-aided drug design. Protein Eng. 1994;7:385-391.

[54]   Oostenbrink BC, Pitzera JW, Van Lipzig MMH, Meerman, JHN, van Gunsteren WF. Simulations of the estrogen receptor ligand-binding domain: Affinity of natural ligands and Xenoestrogens. J. Med. Chem. 2000;43;4594-4605.

[55]   Oostenbrink C, van Gunsteren WF. Free energies of binding of polychlorinated biphenyls to the estrogen receptor from a single simulation. Proteins 2004;54:237-246.

[56]   Woods CJ, Manby FR and Mulholland AJ. An efficient method for the calculation of quantum mechanics/molecular mechanics free energies. The J. of Chem. Phys. 2008; 128:14109-14117.

[57]   Kumar S, Payne PW, Vasquez M. J. Method for free-energy calculations using iterative techniques. J. Comput. Chem. 1996;17:1269-1275.

[58]   Michel J, Verdonk ML and Essex JW. Protein-ligand complexes: Computation of the relative free energy of different scaffolds and binding modes. J. Chem. Theory and Computation. 2007;3:1645-1655.

[59]   Hansmann UHE. Parallel tempering algorithm for conformational studies of biological molecules. Chem. Phys. Lett. 1997;281:140-150.

[60]   Faloppe N, Hubbard R. Towards predictive Ligand design with free-energy based computational methods? Curr. Med. Chem. 2006;13:3583–3608.

[61]   Ashbaugh HS, Asthagiri D. Single ion hydration free energies: A consistent comparison between experiment and classical molecular simulation. J. Chem. Phys. 2008;129:204501– 204506.

[62]   Guo Z, Brooks CL III, Kong X. Efficient and flexible algorithm for free energy calculations using the λ-dynamics approach. J. Phys. Chem. B 1998;102:2032-2036.

[63]   Biletti-Putzer R, Yang W, Karplus M. Generalized ensembles serve to improve the convergence of free energy simulations. Chem. Phys. Lett. 2003;377:693-641.

[64]   Damodaran KV, Banba S, Brooks CL III. Application of multiple topology λ-dynamics to a host-guest system β-Cyclodextrin with substituted benzenes. J. Phys. Chem. B. 2001;105:9316-9322.

[65]   Banba S, Brooks CL III. Free energy screening of small ligands bindng to an artificial protein cavity. J. Chem. Phys. 2000;113:3423-3433.

[66]   Brooks BR, Bruccoleri RE, Olafson BD, Sates DJ, Swaminuthan S, Karplus M. CHARMM:a program for macromolecular energy, minimization and dynamics calculations J. Comp. Chem. 1983;4:187-217.

[67]   Pitera J, Kollman PA. Designing an optimum guest for a host using mutimolecule free energy calculations: Predicting the best. J. Am Chem. Soc. 1998;120:7557-7567.

[68]   Guo Z, Brooks CL III. Rapid screening of binding affinities:Application of the λ-dynamics method to a trypsin-inhibitor system. J. Am. Chem. Soc. 1998;120:1920-1921.

[69]   Zoete V, Michielin O, Karplus M. Protein-ligand binding free energy estimation using molecular mechanics and continmuum electrostatics. Application to HIV-1 protease inhibitors. J. Comput.-Aided Mol. Des. 2003;17:861-880.

[70]   Wu D, Kofke DA, Phase-apsce overlap measures. II. Design and implementation of staging methods for free-energy calculations. J. Chem. Phys. 2005;123:84109–84110.

[71] Mobley DL, Graves AP, Chodera JD, McReynolds AC, Stoichet BK and Dill KA. Predicting absolute ligand binding free energies to a simple model site. J. Mol. Biol. 2007;371:1118-1134.

[72] Pearlman DA, Koffman PA. The lag between the Hamiltonian and the system configuration in fre energy perturbation calculations. J. Chem. Phys. 1989;91:7831-7839.

[73] Lee MS, Salsbury FR, Brooks CL. Constant-pH molecular dynamics using continuous titration coordinates. Proteins 2004;56:738-752.

[74] Abrams JB, Rosso L, Tuckerman ME. Efficient and precise solvation free energies via alchemical adiabatic molecular dynamics. J. Chem. Phys. 2006;125;74115–74127.

[75] Bitetti-Putzer, Dinner AR, Yang W, Karplus M. Conformational sampling via a self-regulating effective energy surface. J. Chem. Phys. 2006;124:174901-174915.

[76] Pitera JW, Kollman PA. Exhaustive mutagenesis in silico:multicoordinate free energy calculations on proteins and peptides. Proteins. 2000; 41;385–397.

[77] Cross JB, Thompson DC, Rai BK, Baber JC, Fan KY, Hu Y, Humblet C. Comparison of several molecular docking programs: pose prediction and virtual screeing accuracy. J. Chem. Inf. Model 2009;49:1455–1474.

[78] Fukinishi H, Teramoto R, Takada TG and Shimada J. Bootstrap-based consensus scoring method for protein-ligand docking. J. Chem. Inf. Model. 2008;48: 988–996.

[79] Stroganov OV, Novikov FN, Stroylov VS, Kulkov V and Chilov GG. Lead Finder: An approach to improve accuracy of protein-ligand docking, binding energy estimation and virtual screening. J. Chem. Inf. Model 2008;48:2371–2385.

[80] Mladenovic M, Arnone M, Fink RF and Engels B. Environmental effects on charge densities of biologically active molecules: Do molecule crystal environments indeed approximate protein surrounding. J. Phys. Chem. B 2009;113:5072–5082.

[81 Harpsoe K, Liljefors T, Balle T. Prediction of the binding mode of biarylpropsylsufonamide allosteric AMPA receptor modulators based on docking, GRID molecular interaction fields and 3D-QSAR analysis. Journal of Molecular Graphics and Modelling 2008;26:874-883.

[82] Butler KT, Luque FJ and Barril X. Toward accurate relative energy predictions of the bioactive conformation of drugs. J. Comput. Chem. 2009;30:601–610.

[83] Marcou G, Rognan D. Optimizing fragment and scaffold docking by use of molecular interaction fingerprints. J. Chem. Inf. Model. 2007;47:195-207.

[84] Areej M, Hammad A and Taha MO. Pharmacophore modeling, quantitative structure-activity relationship analysis and shape-complemented *in silico* screening allow access to novel influenza neuraminidase inhibitors. J. Chem. Inf. Model. 2009;49:978-996.

[85] Loving K, Salam NK and Woody Sherman. Energetic analysis of fragment docking and application to structure-based pharmacophore hyphothesis generation. J. Comput. Aided Mol. Des. 2009;23:541-554.

[86] Chaudhaery SS, Roy KK and Saxena AK. Consensus superiority of the pharmacophore-based alignment over maximum common substructure (MCS): 3D-QSAR studies on carbamates as acetylcholinesterase inhibitors. J. Chem. Inf. Model. 2009;49:1590-1601.

[87] Du qs, Huang RB, Wel YT, Pang ZW, Du LQ and Chou KC. Fragment-based quantitative structure-activity relationship (FB-QSAR) for fragment-based drug design. J. Comput Chem. 2009;30:295–304

[88] Hert J, Keiser MJ, Irwin JJ, Oprea TI and Shoichet BK. Quantifying the relationships among drug classes. J. Chem. Inf. Model. 2008;48:755–765.

89] Rastelli G, Degliesposti G, Del Rio A and Sgobba M, Binding estimation after refinement, a new automated procedure for the refinement and rescoring of docked ligands in virtual screening. Chem. Biol. Drug Des. 2009;73:283–286.

[90] Roberts BC and Mancera RL. Ligand-protein docking with water molecules. J. Chem. Inf. Model. 2008;48:397–408.

[91] Illingworth CJR, Morris GM, Parkers KEB, Snell CR and Reynolds CA. Assessing the role of polarization in docking. J. Phys. Chem. A 2008;112:12157–12163.

[92] Vajda S and Kozakov D. Convergence and combination of methods in protein-protein docking. Current opinion in structural biology 2009;19:164–70.

[93] Moffat K, Gillet VJ, Whittle M, Bravi G, Leach ARA. Comparison of field-based similarity searching methods:CatShape, FBSS and ROCS. J. Chem. Inf. Model. 2008; 48:719-729.

[94] Huang Z, Wong CF and Wheeler RA. Flexible protein-flexible ligand docking with disrupted velocity simulated annealing. Proteins 2008;71:440–454.

[95] Seifert MH. Robust optimization of scoring functions for a target class. J. Comput Aided Mol. Des. 2009;23:633-644.

[96] Thompson DC, Denny A, Nilakantan R, Humblet C, McCarthy DJ and Feyfant E. CONFIRM:connecting fragments found in receptor molecules. J. Comput Aided Mol. Des. 2008; 22:761–772.

[97]   Vewnhorst J, Nunez S, Terpstra JW and Kruse CG. Assessment of scaffold hopping efficiency by use of molecular interaction fingerprints. J. Med. Chem. 2008;51:3222–3229.

[98]   Potemkin VA, Pogrebnoy AA and Grishina MA. Technique for energy decomposition in the study of "receptor-ligand" complexes. J. Chem. Inf. Model. 2009;49:1389–1406.

[99]   Perdih A, Hodoscek M and Solmajer T. MurD ligase from E. coli: Tetrahedral intermediate formation study by hybrid quantum mechanical/molecular mechanical replica path method. Proteins 2009;74:744–759.

[100]   Angelopoulos N, Hadjiprocopis A and Walkinshaw MD. Bayesian model averaging for lligand discovery. J. Chem. Inf. Model. 2009;49:1547-1557.

[101]   Lounkine E and Bajorath J. Topological fragment index for the analysis of molecular substructures and their topological envirolnment in active compounds. J. Chem. Inf. Model. 2009;49:162–168.

[102]   Rarey M, Kramer B, Lengauer T, Klebe G. A fast flexible docking method using a incremental construction algorithm. J. Mol. Biol. 1996;261:470-489.

[103]   Welch W, Ruppert J, Jain AN. Hammerhead: Fast, fully automated docking of flexible ligands to protein binding sites. Chem. Biol. 1996;3:449-462.

[104]   Jones G, Wiletti P, Glen RC, Leach AR, Taylor R. Development and validation of a genetic algorithm for flexible docking. J. Mol. Biol. 1997;267:727-748.

[105]   Morris GM, Goodsell DS, Halliday R, Huey R, Hart WE, Belew RK, Olson AJ. Automated docking using a Lamarckian genetic algorithm and an empirical binding free energy function. J. Comput. Chem. 1998;19:1639-1662.

[106]   Baxter CA, Murray, CW, Clark DE, Westhead DR, Eldridge, MD. Flexible docking using Tabu search and an empirical estimate of binding affinity. Proteins. 1998;33:367-382.

[107]   Liu M, Wang S. MCDOCK: A Monte Carlo simulation approach to the molecular docking problem. J. Comput..-aided Mol. Des. 1999;13:435-451.

[108]   Perola E, Xu K, Kollmeyer TM, Kaufmann SH, Prendergast FG, Pang YP. Successful virtual screening of a chemical database for farnesltranferase inhibor leads. J. Med. Chem. 2000;43:401-408.

[109]   Ewing TJ, Makino S, Skillman AG, Kuntz ID. DOCK 4.0: search strategies for automated molecular docking of flexible molecule databases. J. Comput-Aided Mol. Des. 2001;15:411-428.

[110]   Zavodsky MI, Sanschagrin PC, Korde RS, Kuhn LA. Distilling the essential features of a protein suface for improving protein, ligand docking, scoring and virtual screening. J. Comput. Aided Mol. Des. 2002;16:883-902.

[111]   Jain AN: Surflex:Fully automatic flexible molecular docking using a molecular similarity-based search engine. J. Med. Chem. 2003;46:499-511.

[112]   Friesner RA, Banks JL, Murphy RB, Halgren TA, Klicic JJ, Mainz DT, Repasky MP, Knoll EH, Shelly M, Perry JK, Shaw DE, Francis P, Shenkin PS. Glide: a new approach for rapid, accurate docking and scoring.1. Method and assessment of docking accuracy. J. Med. Chem. 2004;47:1739-1749.

[113]   Kellenberger E, Rodrigo J, Muller P, Rognan D. Comparative evaluation of eight docking tools for docking and virtual screening accuracy. Proteins 2004;57:225-242.

[114]   Beeley NRA, Sage C. GPCRs:an update on structural approaches to drug discovery. Targets 2003;2:19-25.

[115]   Felts AK, Gallicchio E, Wallqvist A, Levy RM. Distinguishing native conformations of proteins from decoys with an effective fre energy estimator based on the OPLS all-atom force field nd the Surface Generalized Born solvent model. *Proteins* 1002; 48:404-422.

[116]   Kroemer RT, Vulpetti A, McDonald JJ, Rohrer DC, Trosset JY, Giordanetto F, Cotesta S, McMartin C, Kihlen M, Stouten PFW. Assessment of docking poses:Interactions-based accuracy classification (IBAC) versus crystal structure deviations. J. Chem. Inf. Comput. Sci. 2004; 44:871-881.

[117]   Kontoyianni M, Sokil GS, McClelan LM. Evaluation of library ranking efficacy in virtual screening. J. Comput. Chem. 2005;26:11-22.

[118]   Warren GL, Andrews CW, Capelli AM, Clarke B, LaLonde J, Lambert MH, Lindvall M, Nevins N, Sermus SF, Senger S, Todesco G, Wall ID, Woolven JM, Peishoff, Head MS. A critical assessment of docking program and scoring functions. J. Med. Chem. 2006;49:5912-5931.

[119]   Charifson PS, Corkery JJ, Murcko MA, Walters WP. Consensus scoring: A method for obtaining improved hit rates from docking databases of three-dimensional structures into proteins. J. Med. Chem. 1999;42:5100-5109.

[120]   Biassantz C, Folkers G, Rognan D. Protein-based virtual screening of chemical datbases: 1. Evaluation of different docking/scoring combinations. J. Med. Chem. 2000;43:4759-4767.

[121]   Stahl M, Rarey M. Detailed analysis of scoring functions for virtual screening. J. Med. Chem. 2001;44:1035-1042.

[122]   Clark RD, Strizhev A, Leonard J. Blake JF, Mathew JB. Consensus scoring for ligand/protein interactions. J. Mol. Graph. Model. 2002;44:1035-1042.

[123] Wang R, Lu Y, Wang S. Comparative evaluation of 11 scoring functions for molecular docking. J. Med. Chem. 2003;46:2287-2303.

[124] Jacobsson M, Liden P, Stjernachantz E, Bostrom H, Norinder U. Improvement structure-based virtual screening by multivariate analysis of scoring data. J. Med. Chem. 2003; 46:5781-5789.

[125] Verdonk ML, Berdini V, HartshornMJ, Mooij WTM, Murray CW, Taylor TD, Watson P. Virtual screening using protein-ligand docking:Avoiding artificial enrichment. J. Chem. Inf. Comput. Sci. 2004;44:793-806.

[126] Yang JM, Chen YF, Shen TW, Kristal BS, Hsu DF. Consensus scoring criteria for improving enrichment in virtual screening. J. Chem. Inf. Model. 2005;45:1134-1146.

[127] Breiman L. Bagging predictors. Machine Learning 1996;24:123-140.

[128] Bryngelson JD, Onuchic JN, Socci ND, Wolynes PG. Funnels, pathways and the energy landscape of protein folding:a synhesis. Proteins 1995;21:167-195.

[129] Koretke KK, Luthey-Schulten ZA, Wolynes PG. Self-consistently optimized energy functions for protein structure prediction by molecular dynamics. Proc. Natl. Acad. Sci. USA 1998; 95:2932-2937.

[130] Fukunishi H, Watanabe O, Takada S. On the Hamiltonian replica exchange method for efficient sampling of biomolecular systems:Application to protein structure in structure prediction. J. Chem. Phys. 2002;116:9058-9067.

[131] Chikenji G, Fujitsuka Y, Takada S. Shaping up the protein folding funnel by local interaction:Lesson from a structure prediction study. Proc. Natl. Acad. Sci. USA 2006;103:3141-3146.

[132] Fujitsuka Yk, Chikenji G, Takada S. SimFold energy function fior de novo protein structure predictin:Consensus with Rosetta. Proteins 2006;62:381-396.

[133] Jin W, Kambara O, Sasakawa H, Tamura A, Takada S. De novo design of foldable proteins with smoth folding funnel:automated negative design and experimental verifications. Structure 2003;11:581-590.

[134] Liu Z, Dominy BN, Shaknovich EI. Structural Miing:Self consistent design on flexible protein-peptide docking and transferable binding affinity potential. J. Am. Chem. Soc. 2004; 126:8515-8528.

[135} Camacho CJ, Vajda S. Protein docking along smooth association pathways. Proc. Natl. Acad. Sci. USA 1001;98:10636-10641.

[136] Teramot R, Fudunishi H. Supervised consensus scoring for docking and virtual screening. J. Chem. Inf. Model 2007;47:526-534.

[137] Bohm HF. Prediction of binding constants of protein ligands: A fast method for the prioritization of hits obtained from de novo design or 3D database search programs. J. Comput-Aided Mol. Des. 1998;12:309-323.

[138] FlexX. Version 1.12.21. BioSolvelTgMBh:Sankt Augustin, Germany.

[139] Pei J, Wang Q, Zhou J and Lai L. Estimating protein-ligand binding free energy:atomic salvation parameters for partition coefficient and salvation free energy calculation. Proteins: Structure, function and bioinformatics 2004; 57:651-664.

[140] Higo J, Nakasako M. Hydration structure of human lysozyme investigated by molecular dynamics simulation and cryogenic X-ray crystal structure analyses:on the correlation between crystal water sites, solvent density and solvent dipole. J. Comput. Chem. 2002;23:1323-1336.

[141] Poornima CS, Dean PM. Hydration in drug design. 1. Multiple hydrogen-bonding features of water molecules in mediating protein-ligand interactions. J. Comput-Aided Mol. Des. 1995;9:500-512.

[142] Nakasako M. Large-scale networks of hydrating water molecules around bovine beta-trypsin revealed by cryogenic X-ray crystal structure analysis. J. Mol. Biol. 1999; 289:547-564.

[143] Hendlich M, Bergner A, Gunter J, Klebe G. Relibase: Design and development of a database for comprehensive analysis of protein-ligand interactions. J. Mol. Biol. 2003;326:607-620.

[144] Lu Y, Wang R, Yang CY, Wang S. Analysis of ligand-bound water molecules in high-resolution-cryhstal structures of protein-ligand complexes. J. Chem. Inf. Model. 2007;47:668-675.

[145] Poormina CS, Dean PM. Hydration in drug design 2. Influence of local site surface shape on water binding. J. Comput-Aided Mol. Des. 1995;9:513-520.

[146] Chung E, Henriques D, Renzoni D, Zvelebil M, Bradshaw JM, Waksam G, Robinson CV, Ladbury JE. Mass spectrometic and thermodynamic studies reveal the role of water molecules in complexes formed between SH2 domains and tyrosyl phosphopeptides. Struct. Fold. Des. 1998;6:1141-1151.

[147] Yakomizo T, Higo J, Nakasako M. Patterns and networks of hydrogen-bonds in the hydration structure of human lysozyme. Chem. Phys. Lett. 2005;410:31-35.[148] Sreenivasan U, Axelsen PH. Buried water in homologous serine proteases. Biochemistry 1992;31:12785-12791.

[149] Loris R, Sas PP, Wyms L. Conserved waters in legume lectin crystal structures. The importance of bound water for the sequence-structure relationship within the legume lectin family. J. Biol. Chem. 1994;269:26722-26733.

[150] Shaltiel S, Cox S, Taylor SS. Conserved water molecule contribute to the extensive network of interactions at the active site of protein kinase. Proc. Natl. Acad. Sci. USA 1998; 95:484-491.

[151] Davis AM, Teague SJ, Kleywegt GJ. Application and limitations of X-ray crystallographic data in structure-based ligand and drug design. Angew. Chem. Int. Ed. 2003;42:2718-2736.

[152] Sanschagrin PC, Kuhn LA. Cluster analysis of consensus water sites in thrombin and trypsin shows conservation between serine proteases and contributions to ligand specificity. Protein Sco. 1998;7:2054-2064.

[153] Loris R, Langhorst U, De Vos, Decanniere K, Bouckaert J, Maes D, Transue TR, Steyaert J. Conserved water molecules in a large family of microbial ribonucleases. Proteins 1999; 36:117-134.

[154] Ogata K, Wodak SJ. Conserved water molecules in MHC class-1 molecules and their putative structural and functional roles. Protein Eng. 2002;15:697-705.

[155] Prasad BVLS, Suguna K. Role of water molecules in the structure and function of aspartic proteinases. Acata Crystallogr. Sect. D. Biol. Crystallogr. 2002;58:250-259.

[156] Catalyst 4.11;Accelrys; San Diego, CA, 2005.

[157] Phase, 3.0207:Schrodinger LLC, New York, 2008.

[158] Csontos J, Palermo NY, Murphy RF and Lovas S. Calculation of weakly polar interaction energies in polypeptides using density fuctional and local Moller-Plesset perturbation theory. J. Comput. Chem. 2008;20:1344–1352

[159] Faerman CH, Karplus PA. Consensus preferred hydration sites in six FKBP12-drug complexes. Proteins 1995;23:1-11.

[160] Levoye A, Jockers R. Alternative drug discovery approaches for orphan GPCRs. Drug Discovery Today 2008; 1:52-58.

[161] Poormina CS, Dean PM. Hydration in drug design 3. Conserved water molecules at the ligand-binding sites of homologous proteins . J Comput-aided Mol. Des. 1995;9:521-531.

[162] Babor M, Sobolev V, Edelman M. Conserved positions for ribose recognition. Importance of water bridging interactions among ATP, ADP and FAP-protein complexes. J. Mol. BIol. 2002;323:523-532.

[163] Bottoms CA, Smith PE, Tanner JJ. A structurally conserved water molecule in Rossman dinucleotide-binding domains. Protein. Sci. 2002;11:2125-2137.

[164] Powers RA, Schoichet BK. Structure-based approach for binding site identification on AmpC beta-lactamase. J. Med. Chem. 2002;45:3222-3234.

[165] Huang K, Lu W, Anderson S, Laskowski M, James MNG. Water molecules participate in proteinase-inhibitor interactions:crystal structure of Leu18, Ala18 and Gly18 vaiants of turkey ovomujcoid inhibitor third domain complexed with Streptomyces griseus proteinase B. Protein Sci. 1995;4:1985-1997.

[166] Gauto DF, Di Lella S, Guardia CMA, Estrin DA and Marti MA. Carbohydrate-binding proteins: Dissecting ligand structures through solvent environment occupancy. J. Phys. Chem. B 2009;113:8717-8724.

[167] Bostrom J, Hogner A, Schmitt S. Do structurally similar liands bind in a similar fashion. J. Med. Chem. 2006;49:6716-6725.

[168] Palomer A, Perez JJ, Navea S, Llorens O, Pascual J, Garcia L, Mauleon D. Modeling cyclooxygenase inhibition. Implication of active site hydration on the selectivity of ketoprofen analogues. J. Mod. Chem. 2000;43:2280-2284.

[169] Rejto PA, Verkhivker GM. Mean field analysis of FKBP12 complexes with FK06 and rapamycin implications for a role of crystallographic water molecules in molecular recognition and specificity. Proteins 1997;28:313-324.

[170] Bondesson L, Miikkelsen KV, Luo Y, Garberg P, Agren H. Density functional theory calculations of hydrogen bonding energies of drug molecules. J. of Mol. Struct. 2006;776:61-68.

[171] Ni H, Sotriffer CA, McCammon JA. Ordered water and ligand mobility in the HIV-integrase-5CETEP complex: a molecular dynamics study. J. Med. Chem. 2001;44:3043-3047.

[172] Lemieux RU. How water provides the impetus for molecular recognition in aqueous solution. Acc. Chem. Res. 1996;29;373-380.

[173] Finley JB, Atigadda VR, Duarte F, Zhao JJ, Brouilette M J, Air GM, Luo M. Novel aromatic inhibitors of influenza virus neuraminidase make selective interactions with conserved residues and water molecules in the active site. J. Mol. Biol. 1999;293:1107-1119.

[174] Tsuzuki S, Uchimaru T and Mikami M. Magnitude and nature of carbohydrate-aromatic interactions: ab initio calculations of fucose-benzene complex. J. Physics. Chem. B. 2009;113: 5617–5621

[175] Pastor M, Cruciani G, Watson KA. A strategy for the incorporation of water molecules present in a ligand binding site into a three-dimensional quantitative structure-activity relationship analysis. J. Med. Chem. 1997;40:4089-4012.

[176] Wang T, Wade RC. Comparative binding energy (COMBINE) Analysis of influenza neuraminidase-inhibitor complexes. J. Med. Chem. J. med. Chem. 2001;44:961-497.

[177] McGovern SL and Shoichet BK. Docking and scoring in virtual screening for drug discovery:methods and applications. Nat. Rev. Drug. Discov. 2004;3:935-949.

[178] Pujadas G, Palau J. Molecular mimicry of substrate oxygen atoms by water molecules in the β-anylase active site. Protein Sci. 2001;10:1645-1657.

[179] Cramer CJ and Truhlar DG. A universal approach to solvation modeling. Accounts of Chem. Research 2008; 41:760-768.

[180] Antes I, Merkwirth C, Lengauer TJ. POEM:Parameter Optimization using ensemble methods:Application to target specific scoring functions. J. Chem. Inf. Model. 2005;45:1291-1302.

[181] Lloyd DG, Garcia-Sosa AT, Alberta IL, Todorov NP, Mancera RL. The effect of tightly bound water molecules on the structural interpretation of lignd-derived pharmacophore models.J. Comput-aided Mol. Des. 2004;18:89-100.

[182] Dunitz JD. The entropic cost of bound water in crystals and biomolecules. Science 2004; 264:670-671.

[183] Dunitz JD. Win some, loose some:enthalphic-entropic compensation in weak intermolecular interactions. Chem. Biol. 1995;2:709-712.

[184] Ladlury JE, Just add water! The effect of water on the specificity of protein-ligand binding sites and its potential application to drug design. Chem. Biol. 1996;3:973-980.

[185] Schnecke V, Kuhn LA. Virtual screening with solvation and liqand-induced complementarity. Perspect. Drug. Discov. Des. 2000;20:171-190.

[186] Li Z, Lazaridis T. Thermodynamic contributions of the ordered waer molecule in HIV-1 protease. J. Am. Chem. Soc. 2003;125:6636-6637.

[187] Cozzini P, Fornabaio M, Marabotti A, Abraham DJ, Kellogg GE, Mozzarelli A. Free energy of ligand binding to protein:evaluation of the contribution of water molecules by computational methods. Curr. Med. Chem. 2004;11:3093-3118.

[188] Kriz Z, Otyepka M, Bartova I, Koda J. Analysis of CDK2 active site hydration: a method to design new inhibitors. Proteins 2004;55:258-274.[

[189] Lu Y, Yand CY, Wang S. Binding free energy contributions of interfacial waters in HIV-1 protease/inhibitor complexes. J. Am. Chem. Soc. 2006;128:11830-11839.

[190] Helms V, Wade RC. Hydration energy landscape of the active site cavity of cytochrome P450. Proteins 1998;32:381-396.

[191] Fornabano M, Spyrakis F, Mozzarelli A, Cozzini P, Abraham DJ, Kellogg GE. Simple, intuititve calculations of free energy of binding for proton-ligand complexes. 3. The free energy contribution of structural water molecules in HIV-1 protease complexes. J. Med. Chem. 2004; 47:4507-4516.

[192] Helms V, Wade RC. Computational alchemy to calculate absolute protein-ligand binding free energy. J. Am. Chem. Soc. 1998;120:2710-2713.

[193] Hamelberg D, McCammon JA. Standard free enegy of releasing a localized water molecule from the binding pockets of proteins:double-decoupling method. J. Am. Chem. Soc. 2004;126:7683-7689.

[194] Li Z, Lazaridis T. Effects of water displacement on binding thermodynamics: concanavalin A. J . Phys. Chem. B 2005;109:662-670.

[195] Burillari C, Taylor J, Viner R, Essex JW. Classification of water molecules in protein binding sites. J. Am. Chem. Soc. 2007;129:2577-2587.

[196] Ehrlich L, Reczko M, Bohr H, Wade RC. Prediction of protein hydration sites from sequence by modular neural networks. Protein Eng.1998;11:11-19.

[197] Henchman RH, McCammon JA, Extracting hydration sites around proteins from explicit water simulations. J. Comput. Chem. 2002;23:861-869.

[198] Schymkovitz JWH, Rousseau F, Martins IC, Ferkinghoff-Borg J, Stgricher F, Serramo L. Prediction of waer and metal binding sites and their affinities by using the Fold-X force field. Proc. Natl. Acad. Sci. USA 2005;102:10147-10152.

[199] Raymer ML, Sanschagrin PC, Punch WF, Venkataraman S, Goodman ED, Kuhn LA, Predicting conserved water-mediated and polar ligand interactions in proteins using a K-neares-neihbors genetic algorithm. J Mol. Biol. 1997;265:445-464.

[200] Korveylesi T, Dennis S, Silberstein M, Bown L, Vajda S. Algorithms for computational solvent mapping of proteins. Proteins 2003;51:340-351.

[201] Carugo O, Bordo D. How many water molecules can be detected by protein crystallography. Acta Crystallogr. Sect. D: Biol. Crystallography 1999;55:479-483.

[202] Carugo O, Argos P. Acessibility to internal cavities and ligand binding sies monitored by protein crystallographic thermal factors. Proteins 1998;31:201-213.

[203] Armadasi A, Spyrakis F, Cozzini p, Abraham DJ, Kelllogg GE, Mozzarelli A. Mapping the energetics of water-protein and water-ligand interactions with the 'natural' HNT force field: predictive tools for characterizing the roles of water in biomolecules. J. Mol. Biol. 2006; 358:289-309.

[204] Garcia-Sosa AT, Mancora RL, Dean PM. WaterScore:a novel method for distinghuishing between bound and displaceble water molecules in the crystal sructure of the binding site of protein-ligand complexes. J. Mol. Model. 2003;9:172-182.

[205] Carugo O. Correlation between occupancy and B factor of water molecules in protein crysal structures. Protein Eng. 1999;12:1021-1024.

[206] Eilmes A and Kubisiak P. Relative complexation energies for Li$^+$ ion in solution:molecular level solvation versus polarizable continuum model study. J. Phs. Chem A. 2010. DOI 10.1021/jp9077359a

[207] Kelly CP, Cramer CJ and Truhlar DG. Aqueous solvation free energies of ions and ion-water clusters based on an accurate value for the absolute aqueous solvation free energy of the proton. 2006;110:16066-16081.

[208] Chen JM, Xu SL, Wawrzaj ZM Basaab GS, Jordan DB. Structure-based design of potent inhibitors of scytalone dehydrase displacement of a water molecule from the active site. Biochemistry 1998;37:17735-1774.

[209] Holdgate GA, Tunnincliffe A, Ward WHJ, Weston SA, Rosenbrock G, Barth PT, Taylor IWF, Pauptit RA, Timms D. The entropic penalty of ordered water accounts for weaker binding of the antibiotic novobiocin to a resistant mutant of DNA gyrase: a thermodynamic and crystallographic study. Biochemistry 1997;36:9963-9673.

[210] Teramoto R, Fukunishi H. Supervised consensus scoring for docking and virtual screening. J. Chem. Inf. Model. 2007:47:526-534.

[211] Mikol V, Papageorgious C, Borer X. The role of water molecules in the structure-based design of (5-hydroxnorvaline) 2-cyclosporine-synthesis, biological activity and crystallographic analysis with cyclophilin-A. J. Med. Chem. 1995;36:3361-3367.

[212] Picket SD, Sherborne BS, Wilkinson T, Bennett J, Borkasakoti N, Boradhurst M, Hurst D, Kilford I, McKinnell M, Jones PS, Discovery of novel low molecular weight inhibitors of IMPDH via virtual needle screening. Bioorg. Med. Chem. Lett. 2003;13:1691-1694.

[213] Mancera RL. De novo ligand design with explicit water molecules:an application to bacterial enuraminadase. J. Comput-Aided Mol.Des. 2002;16-479-499.

[214] Garcia-Sosa AT, Mancera RL. The effect of tightly-bound water molecules on scaffold diversity in the computer-aided de novo ligand design of CKD-2 inhibitors. J. Mol. Model. 2006;12:422-431.

[215] Cherbavaz DB, Lee ME, Sroud RM, Koschi DE. Active site water molecules revealed in the 2.1 angstrom resolution structure of a site-directed mutant of isocitrate dehydrogenase. J. Mol. Biol. 2000;295:377-385.

[216] Garcia-Sosa AT, Firth-Clark S, Mancera RL. Including tightly-bound water molecules in de novo drug design. Exemplification through the in silico generation of poly(ADP-ribose)polylmerase ligands. J. Chem. Inf. Model. 2005;45:624-633.

[217] Rarey J, Kramer B, Lengauer T. The particle concept:placing discrete water molecules during proton-ligand docking predictions. Proteins 1999;34;17-28.

[218] Taha MO, Dahabiyeh LA, Bustanji Y, Zalhoum H, Saleh S. Combining ligand-based pharmacophore modeling, QSAR analysis and in-silico screening for the discovery of new potent hormone sensitive lipase inhibitors. J. Med. Chem. 2008; 51:6478-6494.

[219] Rao MS, Olson AJ. Modelling of inhibitor complexes:A computational flexible docking approach. Proteins 1999;34:173-183.

[220] Minke WE, Diller DJ, Hol WG, Verlinde CL. The role of waters in docking strategies with incremental flexibility for carbohydrate derivatives:heat-labile enterotoxin, a multivalent test case. J. Med. Chem. 1999;42:1778-1788.

[221] Osterberg F, Morris GM, Sanner MF, Olson AJ, Goodsell DS. Automated docking to multiple target structures:incorporation of protein mobility and structural water heterogeneity in AutoDock. Proteins 2002;46:34-40.

[222] Floriano WB, Vaidehi N, Zamanakos G, Goddard WA, III. Hier VLS. Hierarchical docking protocol for virtual ligand screening of large-molecule databases. J. Med. Chem. 2004;47, 56-71.

[223] Bellocchi D, Macchianulo A, Constantino G, Pellicciar R. Docking studies on PARP-1 inhibitors:insights into the role of a binding pocket water molecule. Bioorg. Med. Chem. 2005; 13:1151-1157.

[224] Yang JM, Chen CC. GEMDOCK: A generic evolutionary method for molecular docking. Proteins 2002;55:288-304.

[225] de Graaf C, Pospisil P, Wouter P, Folkers G, Venneule NPE. Binding mode prediction of cytochrome P450 and thymidine kinase protein-ligand complexes by consideration of water and rescoring in automated docking. J. Med. Chem. 2005;48:2308-2318.

[226] Verdonk ML, Chessari G, Cole JC, Hartshorn MJ, Murray CW, Nisink JWM, Taylor RD, Taylor R. Modeling water molecules in protein-ligand docking using GOLD. J. Med. Chem. 2005;48:6504-6515

[227] de Graff C, Oostenbrink C, Keizers PHJ, van der Wijst T, Jongejan A, Vermeulen NPE. Catalytic site prediction and virtual screening of cytochrome P450 2D6 substrates by consideration of water and rescoring in automated docking. J. Med. Chem. 2006;49:2417-2430.

[228] Harsborn MJ, Verdonk ML, Chessari G, Brewerton SC, Mooij WTM, Mortenson PN, Murray CW. Diverse, high-quality test set for the validation of protein-lignd docking performance. J. Med. Chem. 2007;50:726-741.

[229] de Graff C, Oostenbrink NPE. Catalytic side prediction and virtual screening of cytochrome P450 2D6 substrates by consideration of water and rescoring in automated docking. J Med. Chem. 2006,49:2417-2430.

[230] Mancer RL, Kallblad PK, Todorov NP. Ligand-protein docking using a quantum stochastic tunneling optimization method. J. Comput. Chem. 2004;25:858-864.

[231] Sun XM, Wei XG, Wu XP, Ren Y, Wong NB and Li WK. Cooperative effect of solvent in the neutral hydration of ketenimine:an ab initio study using the hybrid cluster/continuum model. J. Phys. Chem. A 2010;114:595-602.

[232] Klebe G. Virtual ligand screening:strategies, perspectives and limitations. Drug Discovery Today 2006;11:580-594.

[233] Leong MK, Chen YM, Chen HBk and Chen PH, Development of a new predictive model for interactions with human Cytochrome P450 2A6 using pharmacophore ensemble/supprot vector machine (PhE/SVM) approach. Pharmaceutical Research 2009;26:987-1000.

[234] Lu Y, Wang Y, Yang H, Yan X, Luo X, Jiang H and Zhu W. Halogen bonding–a novel interaction for rational drug design. J. Med. Chem. 2009;52: 2854–2862

[235] Benighaus T, DiStasio RA, Lochan RC, Chai JD, Head-Gordon M. Semiempirical Double-Hybrid Density functional with improved description of long-range correlation. J. Phys. Chem A. 2008;112:2702-2712.

[236] Markt P, Schuster D, Kirchmair J, Laggner C, Langer T. Pharmacophore modeling and parallel screening for PPAR ligands. J. Comput. Aided Mol Des. 2007;21:575-590.

[237] Todorov NP, Mancera RL, Monthoux PH. A new quantum stochastic tunneling method for ligand protein docking. Chem. Phys. Lett. 20003;369:257-263.

[238] LigPrep, version 2.1. Schrodinger LLC:New York, 2007.

[239] Moitessier N, Englebienne P, Lee D, Lawandi J, Corbeil CR. Towards the development of universal, fast and highly accurae docking/scoring methods: a long way to go. Br. J. Pharmacol. 2008;153:S7-S26.

[240] Totrov M, Abagyan R. Flexible protein-ligand docking by global energy optimization in internal coordinates. Proteins:Struct. Funct. Genet. 1997;29:215-220.

[241] Tietze S, Apostolakis J. GlamDock:development and validation of a new docking tool on several thousand protein-ligand complexes. J. Chem. Inf. Model. 2007;47:1657-1672.

[242] Sutherland J, O`Brien L, Weaver D. Pruned receptor surface models and pharmacophores for three-dimensional database searching. J. Med. Chem. 2004;47:3777-3787.

[243] Ortuso F, Langer T, Alcaro S. GBPM:GRID-based pharmacophore model:concept and application studies to protein-protein recognition. Bioinformatics 2006;22:1449-1455.

[244] S teuber H, Zentgraf M, Gerlach C, Sotrifter CA, Heine A, Klebe G. Expect the unexpected or caveat for drug designers:multiple structure determinations using aldose reductase crystals treated under varying conditions. J. Mol. Biol. 2006;363:174-187.

[245] Thomsen R, Christensen MH. MolDock:A new technique for high-accuracy molecular docking. J. Med. Chem. 2006;49:3315-3321.

[246] Oshiro CM, Kuntz ID, Dixon JS Flexible lignd docking using a genetic algorithm. J. Comput. Aided Mol. Des. 1997;9:113-130.

[247] Rarey M, Kramer B, Lengauer T. Multiple automatic base selection:Protein-ligand docking based on incremental construction without manual intervention. J. Comput Aided Mol. Des. 1997;11:369-384.

[248] Kramer B, Rarey M, Lengauer T. Evaluation of the FLEXX Incremental construction algorithm for protein-ligand docking. Proteins:Struct. Funct. Genet. 1999;37:228-241.

[249] Taha MO, Aandil AM, Zaki DD, AlDamen MA. Ligand based assessment of factor Xa binding site flexibility via elaborate pharmocophore exploration and genetic algorithm-based QSAR modeling. Eur. J. Med. Chem. 2005;40:701-727.

[250] Zsoldos Z, Reid D, Simon A, Sadjad SB, Johnson AP. EHiTS: A new fast, exhaustive flexible ligand docking system. J. Mol. Graphics. Model. 2007;7:421-435.

[251] McMartin C, Bohacek RS. QXP:Powerful, rapid computer algorithms for structure-based drug design. J. Comput. Aided. Mol. Des. 1997;11:333-344.

[252] Venkatachalam, CM, Jiang X, Oldfield T, Waldman M, LigandFit: a novel method for the shape-directed rapid docking of ligands to protein active sites. J. Mol. Graphics Modell. 2003; 21:289-307.

[253] Friesner RA, Murphy RB, Repasky MP, Frye LL, Greenwood JR, Halgren TA, Sanschagrin PC, Mainz DT Glide: A new approach for rapid, accurate docking and scoring. 1. Method and assessment of docking accuracy. J. Med. Chem. 2004;47:1739-1749.

[254] Friesner RA, Banks JL, Murphy RB, Halgren TA, Klicic JJ, Mainz DT, Repasky MP, Knoll EH, Shelly M, Perry JK, Shaw DE, Francis P, Shenkin PS. Extra precision glide:docking and scoring incorporating a model of hydrophobic enclosure for protein-ligand complexes. J. Med. Chem. 2006;49:6177-6196.

[255] Cole JC, Murray cw, Nissink JWM, Taylor RD, Taylor R. Comparing protein-ligand docking programs is difficult. Proteins:Struct. Funct. Bioinformat. 2005;60:325-332.

[256] Khedkar SA, Malde AK, Coutinho EC, Srivastava S. Pharmacophore modeling in drug Discovery and development:an overview. Med. Chem. 2007; 3:187-197.

[257] Nissink JWM, MurrayC, Hartshorn M, Verdonk ML, Cole JC, Tahylor RA. New test set for validating predictions of protein-ligand interaction. Proteins:Struct. Funct. Genet 2002;49:457-471.

[258] Hartshorn MJ, Verdonk ML, Chessari G, Brewerton SC, Mooij WTM, Mortenson PN, Murray CW. Diverse, high quality test set for the validationof protein-ligand docking performance. J Med. Chem. 2007;50:726-l741.

[259] Jain AN, Nicholls A. Recommendaions for evaluation of computational methods. J. Comput. Aided. Mol. Des. 2008;22:133-139.

[260] Kellenberger E, Rodrigo J, Muller P, Rognan D. Comparative evaluation of eight docking tools for docking and virtual screening accuracy. Proteins:Sturct. Funct. Bioinformat. 2004; 57:225-242.

[261]Kontoyianni M, McClellan LM, Sokol GS. Evaluation of docking performance: Comparative data on docking algorithm. J. Med. Chem. 2004;47:558-565.

[262] Yoon S, Smellie A, Hartsough DD, Filikov A. Surrogate docking:structure-based virtual screening at high throughput speed. J. Comput-Aided Mol. Des. 2005;19:483-497.

[263] Graves AP, Brenk R, Shoichet BK. Decoys for Docking. J Med. Chem. 2006;48:3714-3728.

[264] Huan N, Shoichet BK, Irwin JJ. Benchmarking sets for molecular docking. J. Med. Chem. 2006;49:6789-6801.

[265] Neria E, Fischer S, Karplus M. Simulation of activation free energies in molecular systems. J. Chem. Phys. 1996;195:1902-1921.

[266] Mehler EL. Self-consistent, free energy based approximatiton to calculate pH dependent electrostatic effects in proteins. J. Phys. Chem. 1996; 100:16006-16018.

[267] Gallicchio E, Zhang LHY, Levy RM. The SGB/NP hydration free energy model based on the surface generalized born solvent reaction field and novel nonpolar hydration free energy estimators. J. Comput. Chem. 2002;23:517-529.

[268] Stouten PFW, Frommel C, Nakamura H, Sander C. An effective solvation term based on atomic occupancies for use in protein simujlations. Mol. Simul. 1993;10:97-120.

[269] Payne AWR, Glen RC. Molecular recognition using a binary genetic search algorithm. J. Mol. Graph. 1993;11:74-91.

[270] Block P, Sotriffer CA, Dramburg I, Klebe G. AffinDB: a freely accessible database of affinities for protein-ligand complexes from the PDB. Nucleic Acids Res. 2006; 34:D522-D526.

[271] Wang R, Fang X, Lu Yang CY, Wang S. The PDBbind Database: Methodologies and updates. J. Med. Chem. 2005;48:4111-4119.

[272] Nicholls A, Grant JA. Molecular shape and electrostatics in the encoding of relevant chemical information. J. Comput. Aided Mol. Des. 2005;48:1489-1495.

[273] Zhang JW, Aizawa M, Amari S, Iwasawa Y, Nakano T, Nakata K. Development of KiBank, a database supporting structure-bsed drug design. Comput. Biol. Chem. 2004;28:401-407.

[274] Bender A, Mussa HY, Glen RC, Reiling S. Similarity searching of chemical databases using atom environment descriptors (MOL-PRINT 2D):evaluation of performance. J. Chem. Inf. Comput. Sci. 2004;44:1708-1718.

[275] Jain AN. Bias, reporting and sharing:computational evaluation of docking methods. J. Comput-aided Mol. Des. 2008,22:201-212.

[276] Lipinski CA, Lombardo F, Dominy BW, Freeney PJ. Experimental and computational approaches to estimate solubility and permeability in drug discovery and development settings. Adv. Drug. Delivery Rev. 1997;23:3-25.

[277] Zhu K, Pincus DL, Zhao S, Friesner RA. Long loop prediction using the protein local optimization program. Proteins:Struct. Funct. Bioinformat 2006;65:438-452.

[278] Chilov GG, Stroganov OV, Svedas VK. Molecular modeling studies of substrate binding by penicillin acylase. Biochemistry (Moscow) 2008;73:56-54.

[279] Overington JP, Al-Lazikani B, Hopkins AL. How many drug targets are there. Nat. Rev. Drug Discovery 2006;5:993-996.

[280] Abagyan RA, Totrov MM, Kuznetsov DA. ICM:A new method for structure modeling and design: Applications to docking and structure prediction from the distorted native conformation. J. Comput. Chem. 1994;15:488-506.

[281] Ekins S, Mestres J, Testa B. In silico pharmacology for drug discovery:applications to target and beyond.Br. J. Pharmacol. 2007;152:21-37.

[282] Hou TJW, Chen L, Xu X. Automated docking of peptides and proteins by using a genetic algorithm combined with a tabu search. Protein Eng. 1999;12:639-647.

[283] Wang R, Wang S. How does consensus scoring work for virtual library screening: An idealized computer experiment. J. Chem. Inf. Model. 2001;41:1422-1426.

[284] Rawal RK, Kumar A, Siddiqi MI, Katti SB. Molecular docking studies on 4-thiazolidones as HIV-1RT inhibitors. J. Mol. Model. 2007;13:155-161.

[285] ROCS:version 2.3.1.;Openeye Scientific Software Inc. Santa Fe, NM, 2007.

[286] Evrard GX, Langer GG, Perrakis A, Lamzin VS. Assessment of automatic lilgand building in RP/wARP. Acta Crystallogr. 2007;D63:108-117.

[287] Pye CC and Ziegler T. An implementation of the conductor-like screening model of solvation within the Amsterdam density functional package.Theor. Chem. Acc. 1999; 101:396-408.

[288] Dadrass OG, Sobhani AM, Shafiee A, Mahmoudian M. Flexible ligand docking studies of matrix metalloproteinase inhibitors using Lamarckian genetic algorithm. Dari 2004;12:1-10.

[289] Ballester PJ, Richards WG. Ultrafast shape recognition to search compound databases for similar molecular shapes. J. Comput. Chem. 2007; 28;1711-1723.

290] Laskowski RA, Rullmann JA, MacArthur MW, Kaptein R, Thornton JM. AQUA and PROCHECK-NMR:programs for checking the quality of protein structures solved by NMR. J. Biomol. Nmr 1996;8:477-486.

[291] Gold, version 3.1.;CCDC:Cambridge, UK, 2006.

[292] Sippl MJ. Recognition of errors in three-dimensional structures of proteins. Proteins 1993; 17:355-362.

[293] Laskowski RA, McArthur MW, Moss DS, Thornton JM. PROCHECK-aprogram to check the sterochemical quality of protein structures. J. Appl. Crystallogr. 1993;26:283-291.

[294] EON, version 2.3.1:Openehye Scientific Software Inc: Santa Fe, NM, 2007.

[295] Omega, version 2.2.1; Openeye Scientific Software Inc:Santa Fe, NM, 2007.

[296] Muchmore SW, Debe DA, Metz JT, Brown SP, Martin YC, Jajduk PJ. Application of belief theory to similarity data fusion for use in analog searching and lead hopping. J. Chem. Inf. Model. 2998;48:941-948.

[297] Pipeline Pilot, version 5.01.1.100;Scitegic:San Diego, CA, 2006.

[298] Lee MC, Yang R, Duan Y. Comparison between generalized-Born and Poisson-Boltzmann methods, in Physics based scoring functions for protein structure prediction. J. Moll. Model. 2005;12:101-110.

[299] Koehler RT, Villar HO.. Statstical relationships among docking scores for different protein binding sites. J. Comput. Aided Mol. Des. 2000;14:23-37.

[300] Iwase K, Hirono S. Estimation of active conformations of drugs by a new molecular superposing procedure. J.Comput. Aided Mol. Des. 1999;13:499-512.

[301] Hu S, Andreani R, Robbins A, Muegge I. Evaluation of docking/scoring approaches: a comparative study basd on MMP3 inhibitors. J. Comput. Aided Mol. Des. 2000,14:435-448.

[302] Kubinyl H. Combinatorial and computational approaches in structure-based drug design. Curr. Opin. Drug. Discovery Dev. 1998;1:16-27.

[303] Olsen L, Petterson I, Hemmingsen L. Docking and scoring of metallo-beta-lactamase inhibitors. J. Comput. Aided Mol. Des. 2004;18:287-302.

[304] Glide Xp, 2.0207; Schrodinger LLC, New York, 2008.

[305] Klebe G. Foundation review: Virtual ligand screening:strategies, perspectives and limitations. Drug Discovery today. 2006;11:580-594.

[306] Potemkin VA, Arslambekov RM, Bartashevich EV, Grishina MA, Belik AV, Perspicace S, Guccione S. Multiconformational method for analyzing the biological activity of molecular structures. J. Struct. Chem. 2002;43:1045-1049.

[307] Kubinyi H, Hamprecht FA, Mietzner T. Three-dimensional quantitative similarity-activity relationships (3D QSiAR) from real similarity matrices. J. Med. Chem. 1998;41:2553-2564.

[308] Potemkin VA, Grishina MA. A new paradigm for pattern recognition of drugs. J. Comput. Aided Mol. Des. 2008;22:489-505.

[309] Potemkin VA, Bartashevich EV, Belik AV. New approaches to prediction of thermodynamic parameters of substances using molecular data. Russ. J. Phys. Chem. 1996; 70:411-416.

[310] Cheng JF, Zapf J, Takedomi K, Fukushima C, Ogiju T, Zhang SH, YHang G, Sakurai N, Barbosa M, Jack R, Xu K. Combination of virtual screening and high throughput gene profiling for identification of novel liver X receptor modulators. J. Med. Chem. 2008;51:2057-2061.

[311] Potemkin VA, Grishina MA, Bartashevich EV. Modeling of drug molecule orientation within a receptor cavity in the BiS algorithm framework. J. Struct. Chem. 2007;48:155-160.

[312] Tsirelson V, Stash A, Zhurova E, Zhurov V, Pinkerton AA, Zavodnik V, Shutalev A, Gurskaya G, Rykounov A, Potemkin V. Electron-density Properties of the functionally-substituted hydro-pyrimidines. Acta Crystallogr. Sect A. Found. Crystallogr. 2005; A61, C427.

[313] Cosgrove da, Bayada DM, Johnson AP. A novel mehod of aligning molecules by local surface shape similarity. J. Comput. Aided Mol. Des. 2000;14:573-591.

[314] Huang N, Kalyanaraman C, Irwin JJ and Jacobson MP. Physics-based scoring of protein-ligand complexes:enrigthment of know inhibitors in large-scale virtual screening. J. Chem. Inf. Model. 2006;46:243-253.

[315] Grant JA, Gallardo MA, Pickup BT. A fast method of molecular shape comparison: A simple application of a Gaussian description of molecular shape. J. Comput. Chem. 1996; 17:1653-1666.

[316] Ritchie DW, Kemp GJL. Protein docking using spherical polar Fourier correlations. Proteins; Struct. Funct. Bionf. Genet 2000; 39:178-194.

[317] Putta S, Beroz P. Shapes of things:computer modeling of molecular shape in drug discovery. Curr. Top. Med. Chem. 2007; 27:1514-1524.

[318] Sutherland JJ, Nandigam RK, Erickson JA, Vieth M. Lessons in molecular recognition.2. Assessing and improving cross-docking accuracy. J. Chem. Inf. Model. 2007;47:2293-2302.

[319] Mortier WJ, Van Genechten K, Gasteiger J. Electronegativity equalization-application and parametrization. J. Am. Chem. Soc. 1985;107:829-835.

[320] Grishina MA, Bartashevich EV, Potemkin VA, Belik AV. Genetic algorithm for predicting structures and properties of molecular aggregates in organic substances. J. Struct. Chem. 2002; 43:1040-1043.

[321] Bartashevic EV, Potemkin VA, Grishina MA, Belik AV. A method for multiconformation modeling of the three-dimentsional shape of a molecule. J. Struct. Chem. 2002;43:1033-1039.

[322] Perola E. Minimizing false positives in kinase virtual screens. J. Chem. Theory Comput. 2006;64:422-435.

[323] Machicado C, Lopez-Llano J, Cuesta-Lopez, Bueno M and Sancho J. Design of ligand binding to an engineered protein cavity using virtual screening and thermal up-shift evaluation. J. Comp.-Aided Mol. Des. 2005;19:421-443.

[324] Brenk R, Vetter SW, Boyce SE, Goodin DB and Shoichet BK. Probing molecular docking to a charged model binding sitge. J.Mol. Biol. 2006;357:1449-1470.

[325] Musah RA, Jensen GM, Burke SW, Rosenfeld RJ and Goodin DB. Artificial protein cavities as specific ligand-binding templates:characterization of an engineered heterocyclic catin-binding site that preserves the evolved specificity of the parent protein. J. Mol. Biol. 2002; 315:845-857.

[326] Gohlke H and Klebe G. Statistical potentials and scoring functions applied to protein-ligand binding. Curr. Opin. Struct. Biol. 2001;11:231-235.

[327] Nabuurs SB, Wagener M, de Vlieg J A flexible approach to induced fit docking. J. Med. Chem. 2007.49:5885-5594.

[328] Jorgensen WL. Efficient drug led discovery and optimization. Acc. Chem. Research. 2009; 42:724-733.

[329] Wei BQ, Weaver LH, Ferrari AM, Matthews BW and Schoichet BK. Testing a flexible-receptor docking algorithm in a model binding site.J. Mol. Biol. 2004; 337:1161-1182.

[330] Chang CE and Gilson MK. Free energy entropy and induced fit in host-guest recognition :calculations with the second-generation mining minima algorithm. J. Am. Chem. Soc. 2004; 126:13156-13164.

[331] Chen J, Lai L. Pocket v.2: Further developments on receptor-based pharmacophore modeling. J. Chem. Inf. Model. 2006;47:2684-2691.

[332] Jorgensen WL. The many roles of computation in drug discovery. Science 2004;303:1813-1818.

[333] Hagiwara Y and Tateno M. A novel computational scheme for acurate and efficient evaluation of π stacking. J. Phys Condens. Matt. 2009;21:245103-245108.

[334] Congreve M, Chessari G, Tisi D, Woodhead AJ. Recent developments in fragment-based drug discovery. J. Med. Chem. 2008; 51:3361-3680.

[335] Das Debananda, Koh Yasuhiro, Tojo Y, Ghosh AK and Musuya H. Prediction of potency of protease inhibitors using free energy simulations with polarizable quantum mechanics-based ligand and a hybrid water model. J. Chem. Inf. Mode 2009;49:2851-2862.

[336] Rao CB, Subramanian J and Sharma SD. Managing protein flexibility in docking and its applications. Drug Discovery Today 2009;14:394-400.

[337] Subramanian J, Sharma S and B-Rao C. A novel computational analysis of ligand-induced conformational changes in the ATP binding sites of cyclin dependent kinases. J. Med. Chem. 2006;49:5434-5441.

[338] Subramanian J, Sharma S, Chandrika BR. Modeling and selection of flexible proteins for structure-based drug design:backbone and side chain movements in p38 MAPK. ChemMed Chem. 2008;3:336-344.

[339] Sherman W, Day T, Jacobson MP, Friesner RA and Farid R. Novel procedure for modeling ligand/receptor induced fit effects. J. Med. Chem. 2006; 49:534-553.

[340] Cavasotto CN and Abagyan R. Protein flexibility in ligand docking and virtual screening to protein kinases. J Mol. Bio. 2004;337:209-225.

[341] Muegge I, Oloff S. Advances in virtual screening. Drug Discovery Today. Technol 2006; 3:405-411.

[342] Sousa SF, Fernandes PA, Ramos MJ. Protein-ligand docking:current status and future challenges. Proteins 2006;7:259-269.

[343] Ferrara P, Gohlke H, Price DJ, Klebe G, Brooks CL III. Assessing scoring functions for protein-ligand interactions.J. Med. Chem. 2004;47:3032-3407.

[344] Jacobson MP, Kaminski GA, Friesner RA and Rapp CS. Force field validation using protein side chain rediction . J. Phys. Chem. B 2002;106:11673-11680.

[345] Tan L, Lounkine E, Bajorath J. Similarity search using fingerprints of molecular fragments involved in protein-ligand interactions. J. Chem. Inf. Model. 2008; 48:2308-2312.

[346] Englebienne P, Flaux H, Kuntz DA, Corbeil CR, Gerber-Lemaire S, Rose DR, Moitessier N. Evaluation of docking programs for predicting binding of Golgi a-nmannosidase II inhibitors :a comparison with crystallography. Proteins:Struct. Funct. Bionf. 2007;69:160-176.

[347] Bissantz C, Folkers G, Rognan D. Protein-based virtual screening of chemical databases. 1. Evaluation of different docking/scoring combinations. J. Med. Chem. 2000;43:4759-4767.

[348] Szilagyi A, Skolnick J. Efficient prediction of nucleic acid binding function from low-resolution protein structures. J. Mol. Biol. 2006; 358:922-933.

[349] Schulz-Gasch T, Stahl M. Binding site characteristics in structure-based virtual screening:evaluation of current docking tools. J. Mol. Model. 2005;9:47-57.

[350] Stoichet BK. Virtual screening of chemical libraries. Nature 2004; 432:862-865.

[351] Lyne PD, Lamb ML, Saeh JC. Accurate prediction of the relative potencies of members of a series of kinase inhibitors using molecular docking and MM-GBSA scoring. J. Med. Chem. 2006;49:4805-4808.

[352] Wolber G, Langer T. LigandScout:3-D pharmacophores derived from protein-bound ligands and their use as virtual screening filters. J. Chem. Inf. Model. 2005;45:160-169.

[353] McGaughey GB, Sheridan RP, Bayly CI, Culberson JC, Kreatsoulas C, Lidnsley S, Mairov V, Truchon JF, Cornell WD. Comparison of topological, shape and docking methods in virtual screening. J. Chem. Inf. Model. 2007;47:1504-1519.

[354] Zhou Z, Felts AK, Friesner RA, Levy RM. Comparative performance of several flexible docking programs and scoring functions: Enrichment studies for a diverse set of pharmaceutically relevant targets. J. Chm. Inf. Model. 2007;47:1599-1608.

[355] Deng W, Verlinde CLMJ. Evaluation of different virtual screening programs for docking in a charged binding pocket. J. Che. Inf. Model. 2008;48:2010-2020.

[356] Kellenberger E, Foata N, Rognan D. Ranking target in structure-based virtual screening of three-dimensional protein libraries:Methods and problems. J. Chem. Inf. Model. 2008;48:1014-1025.

[357] Sheridan RP, McGaughey GB, Cornell WD. Multiple protein structures and multiple ligands:effects on the apparent goodness of virtual screening results. J. Comput. Aided Mol. Des. 2008;22:257-265.

[358] Bursulaya BD, Torrov M, Abagyan R, Brooks CL III. Comparative study of several algorithms for flexible ligand docking. J. Comptu. Aided Mol. Des. 2004;17:755-763.

[359] Sheridan RP, Kearsley SK. Why do we need so man chemical similarity search methods. Drug Discovery Today 2002;7:903-911.

[360] Perola E, Walters WP, Charifson PS. A detailed comparison of current docking and scoring methiods on systems os pharmaceuticl relevance. Proteins:Struct. Funct. Bioinf. 2004; 56:235-249.

[361] Lee HS, Choi J, Kufareva I, Abagyan R, Filikov A, Yang Y and Yoon S. Optimization of high throughput virtual screening by combining shape-matching and docking methods. J. Chem. Inf. Model. 2008;48:489-497.

[362] Onodera K, Satou K, Hirota H. valuations of molecular docking programs for virtual screening. J. Chem. Inf. Model. 2007;47:1609-1618.

[363] Wolber G, Seidel T, Bendix F, Langer T. Molecule-pharmacophore modeling and three-dimensional database searching for drug design using catalyst. Curr. Med. Chem. 2008;13:23-29.

[364] Kristam R, Gillet VJ, Lewis RA, Thorner D. Comparison of conformational analysis techniques to generate pharmacophore hypotheses using catalyst. J. Chem. Inf. Model. 2005;45:461-476.

[365] Nicholls A. What do we know and when do we know it. J. Comput- Aided Mol. Des. 2008; 22:239-255.

[366] Liebeschuetz JW. Evaluating docking programs:keeping the playing field level. J. Comput.Aided Mol. Des. 2008;22:229-238.

[367] Dror O, Shulman-Peleg R, Nussinov R, Wolfson HJ. Predicting molecular interactitons in silico.I. A guide to pharmacophore identification and its applications to drug design. Curr. Med. Chem. 2004;11:71-90.

[368] Kirchmair J, Markt P, Distinto S, Wolber G, Langer T. Evaluation of the performance of 3D virtual screening protocols; RMSD compasions, enrichment assessments, and decoy selection. What can we learn from earlier mistakes. J. Comput-Aided Mol. Des. 2008;22:213-228.

[369] Good AC, Oprea Ti. Optimization of CAMD techniques 3. Virtual screening enrichment studies:a help or hindrance in tool selection. J. Comput-Aided Mol. Des. 2008;22:169-178.

[370] Hecker EA, Duraiswami C, Andrea TA and Diller DJ. Use of catalyst pharmacophore models for screening of large combinatorial libraries. J. Chem. Inf. Comput. Sci. 2002;42:1204-1211.

[371] Irwin JJ. Community benchmarks for virtual screening. J. Comput Aided Mol. Des. 2008; 22:193-199.

[372] Hawkins PCD, Warren GL, Skillman AG,. How to do an evaluation:pitfalls and traps. J. Comput. AIDED Mol. Des. 2008;22:191-192.

[373] Alcaro S, Gasparrini F, Incani O, Mecucci S, Misiti D, Pierini M, Villani CA. `quase-flexible` automatic docking processing for studying stereoselective recognition mechanisms. Part I. Protocol validation. J. Comput. Chem. 2000;21:515-530.

[374] Guner O, Clement O, Kurogi Y. Pharmacophore modeling and three dimensional database searching for drug design using catalyst:recent advances. Curr. Med. Chem. 2004;11:2991-3005.

[375] corina. Version 1.82: Molecular Networks GmbH:Erlangen Germany, 1997.

[376] Maestro, version 7.5.116; Schrodinger. LLC: Portland QR, USA 2006.

[377] Shoichet BK, Bodian DL, Kuntz ID. Molecular docking using shape descriptors. J. Comput. Chem. 1992;13:380-397.

[378] Ewing TJA, Kuntz ID Critical evaluation of search algorithms for automated molecular docking and database screening J. Comput. Chem 1997;18:1175-1189.

[379] Moustakas DT, Llang PT, Pegg S, Pettersen E, Kuntz ID, Brooijmans N, Rizzo RC. Development and validation of a modular extensible docking program:DOCK 5. J. Comput. Aided Mol.. Des. 2006;20:601-619.

[380] Desjarlais RL, Sheridan RP, Seibel GL, Dixon JS, Kuntz ID, Venkatarahavan. Using shape complementarity as an initial screen in designing ligands for a receptor binding site of known three-dimensional structure. J. Med. Chem. 1988;31:722-729.

[381] Norinder U, Bergstrom CAS, Prediction of ADMET properties. ChemMedChem 2006; 1:920-937

[382] Kirchmair J, Wolber C, Laggner C, Langer T. Comparative analysis of protein-bound ligand conformations with respect to catalysts`s conformational space subsampling algorithms. J. Chem. Inf. Model. 2005;23:129-138.

[383] Boehm HJ. Ludi:rule-based atomatic design of new substituents for enzyme inhibitor leads. J. Comput-aided Mol. Des. 1992;6:593-606.

[384] Barreiro G, Kim JT, Guimaraes CRW, Bailey CM, Domaoal RA, Wang L, Anderson KS, Jorgensen WL. From docking false-positive to active anti-HIV agent. J. Med. Chem. 2007; 50:5324-5329.

[385] Dixon SL, Smondyrev AM, Knoll EH, Rao SN, Shaw DE, Friesner   RA. PHASE:a new engine for pharmcophore perception, 3D QDSAR model development, and 3D database creening:1. Methodology and preliminary results. J. Comput-Aided Mol. Des. 2006;20:647-71.

[386] Halgren TA, Murphy RB, Friesner RA, Beard HS, Frye LL, Pollard WT, Banks JL. Glide: A new approach for rapid accurate docking and scoring. 2. Enrichment factors in database screening. J. Med. Chem. 2004;l47:1750-1759.

[387] Elridge MD, Murray CW, Auton TR, Paolini GV, Mee RP. Empirical scoring functions. 1. The development of a fast empirical scoring function to estimate the binding affinity of ligands in receptor complexes. J. Comput. Aided Mol. Des. 1997;11:425-445.

[388] Kurogi Y, Guner OF. Pharmacophore modeling and three dimensional database searching for drug design using catalyst. Curr. Med. Chem. 8;2007; 3:187-197.

[389] Kirchmair S, Ristic K, Eder P, Markt G, Wolber C, Laggner T. Larger, fast and efficient *in silico 3D screening:*toward maximum computational efficiency of pharmacophore-biased and shape based approaches. J. Chem Inf. Model 2007;47:2182-2196.

[390] Proudfoot JR. The evolution of synthetic oral drug properties. Bioorg. MEed. Chem. Lett 2005; 1:920-937.

[391] Joseph-McCarthy D, Tomas BEIV, Belmarsh M, Moustakas D, Alvarez JC. Pharmacophore-based molecular docking to account for ligand flexibility. PROTEINS: Struct. Funct. Bioinf. 2003;51:172-188.

[392] Joseph-McCarthy D, McFadyen IJ, ZOou J, Walker G, Alvarez JC. Pharmacophore-based molecular docking; A practical guide. Drug Discovery Ser. 2005;1:327-347.

[393] Rush TS, Manas ES, Tawa GJ, Alvarez JC. Solvation-based scoring for high-throughpt docking. Drug Discovery Ser. 2005;1;249-277.

[394] Joseph-McCarthy D, Alvarez JC. Automated generation of MCSS-derived pharmacophoric DOCK site pints for searching multiconformation databases. Proteins;Stuct. Funct. Genet. 2003; 51:189-202.

[395] Thompson DC, Hublet C, Joseph-McCarthy D. Investigation of MM-PBSA rescoring of docking poses. J. Chem. Inf. Model. 2008;48;1081-1091.

[396] Jain An Surflelc-Dock 2.1: Robust performance from ligand energetic modeling, ring flexibility and knowledge-based seach. J. Comput.-Aided Mol. Des. 2007;21:281-306.

[397] Pham TA, Jain AN. Parameter Estimation for scoring protein-lignd interactions using negative training data. J. Med. Chem 2006;49:5856-5868.

[398] Verkhivker Gm, Bouzida D, Gehlhaar DK, Rejto PA, Arthurs S, Colson AB, Feer ST, Llarson V, Luty BA, Marone , Rose PW. Deciphering common failures in molecular docking of ligand-proetin complexes. J. Compujt-Aidd Mol. Des. 2000;14:731-751.

[399] Triballeau N, Acher F, Brabet I, Pin JP, Bertrand HO. Virtual screening workflow development guided by the 'Receiver Operatin characteristic' curve approach. Application to high-throughput docking on metabotropic glutamine receptor subtye 4. J. Med. Chem. 2005; 48:2534-2547.

[400] Jain AN. Ligand-based structural hypothesis for virtual screening. J. Med. Chem. 2004; 47:947-961.

[401] Truchon JF, Bayly CI. Evaluating virtual screening methods:good and bad metrics for the early recognition problem. J. Chem. Inf. Model. 2007;488-508.

[402] Salazar PF and Seminario JM. Identifying receptor-ligand interactions through an ab initio approach. J. Phys. Chem. B 2008;112;1290-1292.

[403] Brown SP and Muchmore SW. Large-scale application of high-throughput molecular mechanics with Poisson-Boltzmann Surface area for routine physics-based scoring of protein-ligand complexes. J. Med. Chem 2009;52:3159-3165.

[404] Kim R and Skolnich J. Assessment of programs for ligand binding affinity prediction. J. comput. Chem 2008;29:1316-1311.

[405] Yusuf D, Davis AM, Kleywegt GJ and Schmitt S. An alternative method for the evaluation of docking performance:RSR vs RMSD. J. Chem. Inf. Model. 2008;48:1411-1422.

[406] Elkins S, Mesres J and Testa B. Insilico pharmacology for drug discovery:Mehods for virtual ligand screening and profiling . Br. J. Pharmacol 2007;152:9-20.

[407] Leach AR, Shoichet BK and Peishoff CE. Prediction of protein-ligand interactions. Docking and scoring:Successes and gaps. J. Med. Chem. 2006;49:5851-5855.

[408] Cummings MD, Deslarlais RL, Givvs AC, Mohan V and Jaeger EP. Comparison of automated docking programs as virtual screening tools. J. Med. Chem. 2005; 48:962-976.

[409] Kowvat EM and Langer T. Impact of scoring functions on enrichment in docking-based virtual screening: An application study on rennin inhibitors. J. Chem. Inf. Comput. Sci. 2004; 44:1123-1129.

[410] Zhang Q and Muegge I. Scaffold hopping through virtual screening using 2d and 3d descriptors: Ranking, voting and consensus scoring. J. Med. Chem. 49:1536-1548.

[411]Rosenfield RJ, Goodsell DS, Musah RA, Morris GM. Goodin DB, Olson AJ. Automated docking of ligands to an artificial active site:augmenting crystallographic analysis with computer modeling. J. Comput. Aided Mol. Des. 2003;17:525-536.

[412] Kuhn B, Gerber P, Schulz-Gasch T, Stahl M. Validation and use of the MM-PBSA approach for drug discovery. J. Med. Chem. 2005; 48:4040-4948.

[413] Lyne PD, Lamb ml, Saeh JC Accurate prediction of the relative potencies of members of a series of kinase inhibitors using molecular docking and MM-GBSA scoring. J. Med. Chem. 2006; 49:4805-4808.

[414] Weis A, Katebzadeh K, Soderhjeim P, Nilsson I, Ryed U. Ligand affinities predicted with the MM/PBSA method: dlependence on the simujlation method and the force field. J. Med. Chem. 2006;49:6596-6606.

[415] Case DA, Cheatham TE, III, Darden T, Gohlke H, Luo R, Merz KM, Onufirev A, Simmerling C, Wang B, Woods RJ. The Amber biomolecular simulation programs. J. Comput. Chem. 2005;26:1668-1688.

[416] Brown SP, Muchmore SW. Rapid estimation of relative protein-ligand binding affinities using a high-throughput version of MM-PBSA. J. Chem. Inf. Model, 2007;47:1493-1503.

[417] Huey R, Morris GM, Olson AJ, Goodsell DS. A semi empirical fre energy force field wih chanrge-based desolvation. J. Comput. Chem.2007:28:1145-1152.

[418] Ferrari AM, Degliesposti G, Sgobba M,Rastelli G. Validation of an automated procedure for the prediction of relative free energies of binding on a set of aidose reductase inhibitors. Bioorg Med. Chem. 2007; 15:7865-7877.

[419] Huang N, Shoichet BK, Irwin JJ. Benchmarking sets for molecular docking. J. Med. Chem. 2006;49:6789-6801.

[420] Cavasotto CN, Kovacs JA, Abagyan RA. Representing receptor flexibility in ligand docking through relevant normal modes. J. Am. Chem. Soc. 2005;127:9632-9640.

[421] Neves MA, Dinis TC, Colombo , Sa e Melo ML. Fast three dimensional pharmacophore virtal sceening of new potent non-steroid aromatase inhibitors. J. Med. Chem. 2009;52:143-150.

[422] Ferrari AM, Wei BQ, Costantino L, Shoichet BK. Soft docking and multiple receptor conformations in virtual screening. J. Med. Chem. 2004;47:5076-5084.

[423] Feig M, Karanicolas J, Brooks CI III. MMTSB tool set:enhanced sampling and multiscale modeling methods for applicaions in structural biology. J. Mol. Graph. Mod. 2004;22:377-395.

[424] Frisch MI, Trucks GW, Schlegel HB, Scuseria GE, Robb MA, Cheeseman JR, Montgomery JA, Jr. Vreven T, Kudin KN, Burant jc, Millam JM, Iyengar SS, Tornasi J, Barone V, Mennucci B, Cossi M, Scalmani G, Rega N,Petersson GA, Nakatsuji H, Hada M, Ehara M, ooa K, Fukuda R, Hasegawa J, Ishida M, Nakajima T, Honda Y, Kiao O, Nakai H, Klene M, Li X, Know JE, Hrachian HP, Cross JB,Bakken V, Adarno C, Jaramillo j, Gomperts R, Stratmann RE, Yajev O, usin AJ, Cammi R, Pomelli C, Ochterski JW, Ahyala PY, Morokuma K, Voth GA, Salvador P, Dannenberg JJ, Zakrzewski VG Dapprich S, Daniels AD, Srain MC, Farkas O, Malick DK, Rabuck AD, Raghavachari K, Foresman JB, Ortiz JV, Cui Q,

Baboul AG, Clifford S, Cioslowski J, Stefanov BB, Liu G, Liashenko A, Piskorz P, Komaromi I, Martin Rl, Fox DJ, Keith T, AL-Laham MA, Peng CY, Nanaaklara A, Challacombe M, Gill PMW, Johnson B, Chen W, Won MW, Gonzale C, Pople JA, Gaussian 03 Revision C.02. Wallingford, CT;Gaussian, 2004.

[425] Chocholousova J, Feig M. Balancing an accurate representation of the molecular surface in generalized born formalisms with integrator stability in molecular dynamics simulations. J. Comp. Chem. 2006;28:719-729.

[426] Kovacs JA, Cavasotto CN, Abagyan R. Conformational sampling of protein flexibilith in generalized coordinates: application to ligand docking. J. Comput. Theor. Nanosci: 2005;2:354-361.

[427] Wiley EA, Deslongchamps G. PostDock: A novel visualitation tool for the analysis of molecular docking. Comput Visual Sci. 2009;12:1-7.

[428] Brooijmans, N, Kuntz ID. Molecular recognition and docking algorithms. Ann. Rev. BIOPHYS. Biomol. Struct. 2003;335-373.

[429] Halperin I, Ma B, Wolfson H, Nussinov R, Principles of docking: an overview of search algorithms and a guide to scoring functitons. Proteins 2002;47:409-443.

[430] Jain AN, Virtual screening in lead discovery and optimization. Curr. Opin. Drug. Discovery Dev. 2004;7:396-403.

[431] Orry AJW, Abagyan RA and Cavasotto CN. Structure-based development of target-specific compound libraries. Drug Discov. Today 2006; 11:261-266.

[432] Chiang YK, Kuo CC, Wu YS, Chen CT, Coumar MS, Wu JS, Hsieh HP, Chang CY, Jseng HY, Wu MH, Leou JS, Song js, Chang JY, Lyu PC, Chao YS and Wu SY. Generation of ligand-based pharmacophore model and virtual screening for identification of novel tubulin inhibitors with potent anticancer activity. J. Med. Chem. 2009;52:4221-4223.

[433] Teague SJ. Implications of protein flexibility for drug discovery. Nat. Rev. Drug Discovery 2003;2:527-541.

[434] Gregori-Puigjane E, Mestres J. SHED:Shannon entropy descriptors from topological feature distributions. J. Chem. Inf. Model. 2006;46:1615-1622.

[435] Mizutani MY, Takamatsu Y, Ichinose T, Nakamura K, Itai A. Effecive handling of induced-fit motion in flexible docking. Proteins 2006; 63:878-891.

[436] Zhao H. Scaffold selection and scaffold hopping in lead generation: a medicinal chemistry perspective. Drug Discovery Today 2007;12:149-155.

[437] Irwin JJ, Schoichet BKI. ZINC: A free database of commercially available compounds for virtual screening. J. Chem. Inf. Model. 2005;45-177-182.

[438] Hawkins PC, Skillman AG, Nicholls A. Comparison of shape-matching and docking as virtual screening tools. J. Med. Chem. 2007;50:74-82.

[439] Guner OF. History and evolution of the pharmacophore concept in computer-aided drug design. Cure. Topics Med. Chem. 2002;2:1321-1332.

[440] Hert J, Willett p, Wilon DJ, Acklin P, Azzaoui K, Jacoby E, Schuffenbauer A. New methods for ligand-based virtual screening: use of daa fussion and machine leaning to enhance he effectiveness of similarity searching. J. Chem. Inf. Model. 2006;46:462-470.

[441] Barker EJ, Buttar D, Cosgrove da, Gardiner EJ, Kits P, Willett P, Gillet VJ. Scaffold hopping using clique detection applied to reduced graphs. J. Chem. Inf. Model. 2006; 46:503-511.

[442] Graves AP, Shivakumar DM, Boyce SE, Jacobson MP, Case DA and Shoichet BK. Rescoring docking hit lists for model cavity sites: predictions and experimental testing. J. Mol. Biol.; 2008;377:914-934.

[443] Kang L, Li H, Jiang H and Wang X. An improved adaptive genetic algorithm for protein-ligand docking. J. Comput. Aided Mol. Des 2009;23:1-12.

[444] [Pastor M, Cruciani G, McLay Iain, Pickett S and Clementi S. Grid-Independent descriptors (GRIND); A novel class of alignent-independent three-dimensional molecular descriptors. J. Med. Chem. 2000;43:3233-3243.

[445] Weisel M, Proschak E, Schneider G. PocketPicker:analysis of ligand binding-sites with shape descriptors. Chem. Cent. J. 2007;1:1-17.

[446] GRID V.17:Molecular Discovery Ltd. West Way House. Elms Parade. Oxford. 1999.

[447] ALMOND v.2.0: Multivariate Infometric Analysis S.R.1. Viale del Castagni. 16.Perugia 2000.

[448] Durán Ángel, Martínez G C and Pastor M. Development and validation of Amanda, a new algorithm for selecting highly relevant regions in molecular interaction fields, J. Chem. Inf. Model. 2008;48:1813 -1823.

[449] Sciabola s, Stanton RV, Mills JE, Floco MM, Baroni M, Cruciani G, Perrucio F and Mason JS. High-throughput virtual screening of proteins using GRID molecular interaction fields. Bioinformatics 2009;25:3185-3200.

[450] Baroni M, Cruciani G, Sciabola S, Perruccio F and Mason JS. A common referene framework for analyzing/comparing proteins and ligand . Fingerprints for ligands and proteins (FLAP);Theory and application. J. Chem. Inf. Model. 2007;47:279-294.

[451] Ghersi D and Sanchez R. EasyMIFs and SiteHOUND: a tookit for the identification of ligand-binding sites in protein structures. Structural bioinformatics. 2009;23:3185-3186.

[452] Mullins E, Liu YA, Ghaderi A and Fast SD. Sigma Profile Database for predicting solid solubility in pure and mixed solvent mixtures for organic pharmacological compounds with cosmo-based thermodynamic methods. Ind. Eng. Chem. Res 2008;47:1707-1725.

[453] Sun XM, Wei XG, Wu CXP, Ren Y, Wong NB and Li WK. Cooperative effect of solvent in the neutral hydration of ketenimine:An ab initio study using the hybrid cluster/continuum model. J. Phys. Chem. A 2010;114:595-602.

[454] Shivakumar D, Deng Y and Roux B. Computations of absolute solvation free energies of small molecules using explicit and implicit solvent model. J. of Chem. Theory and Computation. 2009;5:919-930.

[455] Reddy MR, Singh UC, Erion MD. LJ.Ab initio quantum mechanics-bsed free energy perturbation method for calculating relative salvation free energies. Comput. Chem. 2007; 28:491-494.

[456] Reddy MR and Erion MD. Relative binding affinities of fructose-1.6-bisphosphatase inhibitors calculated using a quantum mechanics-based free energy perturbation method. J. Am. Chem. Soc. 2007;129:9296-9297.

[457] Deng Y and Roux B. Computation of binding free energy with molecular dynamics and grand canonical Monte Carlo simulations. The Journal of Chemical Physics. 2008;128:115103-115111.

[458] Lerner MG, Meagher KL and Carlson HA. Automatied clustering of probe molecules from solvent mapping of protein surfaces: new algorithms applied to hot-spot mapping and structure-based drug design. J. Comput. Aided Mol. Des. 2008;22:727–736.

[459] Hodak M, Chisnell R, Lu W and Bernholc J. Functional implications of multistage copper binding to the prion protein. PNAS 2009;106:11756-11581.

[460] Shen J, Quiocho FA. Calculation of binding energy differences for receptor-ligand systems using the Poisson-Boltzmann method. J. Comp. Chem. 1995;16:445-453.

[461] Kollman PA, Massova I, Reyes C, Kuhn B, Huso OS, Chong L, Lee M, Lee T, Duan Y, Wang W, Donini AO, Cieplack, Srinivasan P, Case J, Cheatham TE. Calculating structures and free energies of complex molecules:combining molecular mechanics and continuum models. Acc. Chem. Res. 2000; 33:889-897.

[462] Tounge BA, Reynolds CH. Calculation of the binding affinity of β-secretase inhibitors using the linear interaction energy method. J. Med. Chem. 2003;46:2074-2082.

[463] Cavalli A, Carloni P and Recanatini M. Tartet-related applications of first principles Quantum Chemical Methods in Drug Design. Chemical Reviews. 2006;106:3497-3519.

[464] Jorgensen WL, Maxwell DS, Tirado-Rives J. Development and testing of the OPLS All-Atom Force Field on Conformational Energetics and Properties of organic liquids. J. Am. Chem. Soc. 1996;118:11225-11236.

[465] Cornell WD, Cieplak P, Bayly CI, Gould IR, Merz KM, Ferguson DM, Spellmeyer DC, Fox TG, Caldwell JW, Kollman PA. A second generation force field for the simulation of proteins, nucleic acids and organic molecules. J. Am. Chem. Soc. 1996;117:5179-5197.

[466]   MacKerell AD Jr, Bashford D, Bellott M, Dunbrack RL Jr, Evanseck JD, Field MJ, Fisher S, Gao J, Guo H, Ha S, Joseph-McCarthy D, Kuchnir L, Kuczera K, Lau FTK, Mattos C, Michnick, S, Ngo T, Nguyen DT, Prodhorn B, Reiher WE III, Roux B, Schlenkrich M, Smith JC, Stote R, Straub J, Watanabe M, Wiorkiewicz-Kuczera J, Yin D, Karplus M. All-atom empirical potential for molecular modeling and dynamics studies of proteins. J. Phs. Chem. B. 1998;102:3586-3616.

[467] Warshel A. Computer simulations of enzyme catalysis: Methods, progress and insights. Annu. Rev. Biophys. Biomol. Struct. 2003;32:425-443.

[468] Car R, Parinello M. Unified approach for molecular dynamics and density-functional theory. Phys. Rev. Lett. 1985;55:2471-2474.

[469] Waller MP, Robertazzi A, Plats JA, Hibbs DE, Williams PA. Hybrid densitgy functional theory for π-stacking interactions:Application to benzenes, pyridines and DNA bases. J. Comput. Chem. 2006;27:491-504.[470] Hohenberg P, Kohn W. Inhomogeneous electron gas. Physical Review B 1964;136:864-871.; Kohn W, Sham L. Self-consistent equations including exchange and correlation effects. J. Phys. Rev. A 1965;149:1133-1138.

[471] Dans PD and Coitiño, Density functional theory characterization and descriptive analysis of cisplatin and related compounds. J. Chem. Inf. Model. 2009;49:1407-149.

[472] Guadarrama P, Soto-Castro D and Otero JR. Performance of DFT hybrid functional in the theoretical treatment of H-bonds:Analysis term-by-term. International Journal of Quantum Chemistry 2007;108:229-237.

[473] Koch W, Holthausen MC. A Chemist's Guide to density functional theory: Wiley-VCH; Weinheim, Germany 2000.

[474] Parr RG, Yang W. Density functional theory of the electronic structure of molecules. Annu. Rev. Phys. Chem. 1995;46:701-728.

[475] Parr RG, Yang W. Density-functional theory of atoms and molecules. Oxford University Press: Oxford, UD, 1989.

[476] Scuseria GE, Staroverov VN. In Theory and applications of computational chemistry: The first forty years; Dykstra CE, Frenking G, Kim KS, Scuseria GE, Eds. Elsevier :Amsterdam; 2005.

[477] de Proft F, Sablon N, Tozer DJ, Geerlings P. Calculation of negative electron affinity and aqueous anion hardness using Kohn-Sham HOMO and LUMO energies. Faraday Discuss. 2007;135:151-159.

[478] Becke AD. Density-functional thermochemistry. III. The role of exact exchange. J. Chem. Phys. 1993;98:5648-5652.

[479] Schwabe T, Grimme S. Phys. Chem. Chem. Phys. Double-hybrid density functional with long-range dispersion correctitons:higher accuracy and extended applicability. 2007;9:3397-3406.

[480] Van Caillie C, Amos RD. Geometric derivatives of excitation energies using SCF and DFT. Chem. Phys. Lett. 1999;308:249-255.

[481] Scalmani G, Frisch MJ, Mennucci B, Tomasi J, Cammi R, Barone V. Geometries and properties of excited states in the gas phase and in solution: Theory and application of a time-dependent density functional theory polarizable continuum model. J. Chem. Phys. 2006;124, 94107-94122.

[482] Grimme S, Steinmetz M, Korth M. How to compute isomerization energies of organic molecules with quantum chemical methods. J. Org. Chem. 2007;72:2118-2126.

[483] Schreiner PR. Angew. Chem. Int. Ed. Relative energy computations with approximate density functional theory- A caveat. Chem. Int. Ed. 2007;46:4217-4219.

[484] Polo V, Grafenstein J, Krala E, Cremer D. Long-range and short-range Coulomb correlation effects as simulated by Hartree–Fock, local density approximation, and generalized gradient approximation exchange functional. Theor. Chem. Acc. 2003:109:22-35.

[485] Handy NC, Cohen AJ. Left-right correlation energy. Mol. Phys. 2001;99:403-412.

[486] Xu X, Zhong Q, Muller RP, Goddard WA, III. An extended hybrid density functional (X3LYP) with improved descriptions of nonbond interactions and thermodynamic properties of molecular systemsJ. Chem. Phys. 2005;122:14105-14129.

[487] Perdew JP, Burke K, Ernzerhof M. Phys. Generalized Gradient Approximation Made Simple. Phys. Rev. Lett. 1996;77:3865-3868.

[488] Quintal MM, Karton A, Iron MA, Boese AD, Martin JML. Benchmark Study of DFT Functionals for Late-Transition-Metal Reactions. J. Phys. Chem. A 2006;110:709-716.

[489] Boese AD, Martin JML. Development of density functionals for thermochemical kinetics. J. Chem. Phys. 2004;121:3405-3416.

[490] Schirmer J, Dreuw A. Critique of the foundations of time-dependent density-functional theory. Phys. Rev A. 2007;75:22513-22529.

[491] Dreuw A, Head-Gordon M. Single-Reference ab Initio Methods for the Calculation of Excited States of large Molecules Chem. Rev. 2005;105:4009-4037.

[492] Sancho-Garcia JC. Assessing a new nonempirical density functional. J.Chem. Phys. 2006; 124:124112-12422

[493] Marques MAL, Gross EKU. The electron gas in TDDFT and SCDT. Annu. Rev. Phys. Chem. 2004;55:427-455.

[494] Vydrov OA, Scuseria GE. Assessment of a long-range corrected hybrid functional. J. Chem. Phys. 2006;125:234109-234118

[495] Furche F, Perdew JP. The performance of semilocal and hybrid density functionals in 3d transiion-metal chemistry. J. Chem. Phys. 2006;124:44103 44130.

[496] Zhao Y and Truhlar DG. Density functionals with broad applicability in chemistry. Acc. Chem. Res 2008;41:157-167.

[497] Tirado-Rives J, Jorgensen WL Performance of B3LYP density functional methods for a large set of organic molecules. J. Chem. Theor. Commun. 2008;4:297-306.

[498] Hao MH. Theoretical calculation of hydrogen-bonding strength for drug molecules. J. of Chem. Theory and Computation. 2006;2:363-872.

[499] Bouteiller Y, Poully JC, Desfrancois C and Gregoire G. Evaluation of MP2, DFT and DFT-D methods for the prediction of infrared spectra of peptides. J. Phys. Chem. A 2009;113:6301-6307.

[500] Minenkov Y, Occhipinti G and Jensen VR. Metal-phosphine bond strengths of the transition metals: A challenge for DFT. J. Phys. Chem. A;2009;113:11833-11844

[501] Wang YG. Examination of DFT and TDDFT Methods II. J. Phys. Chem. A 2009; 113:10873-10879.

[502] Scuseria GE, Staroverov VN. Progress in the development of exchange-correlation functionals. In Theory and application of computational chemistry: The first 40 years. Dykstra CE, Frenking G, Kim KS, Scuseria GE, EDs, Elsevier:Amsterdam, 2005.

[503] Y, Truhlar DG. The MO6 suite of densiy functionals for main group thermochemistry, thermochemical kinetics, noncovalent interactions, excited states and transition elements. Theor Chem. Acc. 2008 published online D0i.10..1007/s00214-007-0310-x.

[504] Zhao Y, Schultz NE, Truhlar DG. Design of density functionals by combining the method of constraint satisfaction with parametrization for thermochmistry, thermochemical kinetics and noncovalent interactions. J. Chem. Theory Comput. 2006;2:364-382.

[505] Mori-Sanchez P, Cohen AJ, Yan W. Many-electron self-interaction error in approximate density functionals. J. Chm. Phys. 2006;124:91102-91104.

[506] Perdew JP, Ruzsinsky A, Tão J, Staroverov VN, Scuseria GE, Csonka GI. Prescriptor for the design and selection of density functional approximaions. J. Chem. Phys. 2005;123:62201-62209.

[507] Xu X, Goddard WA. The X3LYP extended functional to acurate decriptions of nonbond ineractions, spin states and thermochemical poperties. Proc. Ntl. Acad. Sci. USA; 2004; 101:2673-2677.

[508] Grimme S. Semiempirical GGA-type densityy functional constructed with a long-range dispersion corection. J. Comput. Chem. 2006;27:1787-1799.

[509] Sato TA, Tsuneda T, Hirao K. A density-funtional study on π-aromatic interactions. J. Chem. Phys 2005;123:104307-1043010.

[510] Jurecka P, Ceerny J. Hotza P, Salahub DR. DFT augmented with an empirical dispersion term. J. Comput. Chem. 2007;28:555-569.

[511] Check CE, Gilbert TM. Progressive systematic underestimation of reaction energies in the B3LYP model as the number of C-C bonds increases. J. Org. Chem. 2005;60:9828-9834.

[512] Zhao Y, Truhlar DG. A density functional that accounts for medium-range correlation energies in organic chemistry. Org. Lett. 2006;8:5653-5756.

[513] Woodrich MD, Corminbouef C, Schreiner PR, Fokin AA and Schleyer PVR. How accurate are DFT treatments of organic energies? Org. Lett. 2007;9:1851-1854.

[514] Schultz N, Zhao Y, Truhlar DG. Dnsity functional for inorganometallic and organometallic chemistry. J. Phys. Chem. A 2005;109:11127-11143.

[515] Harvey JN. On the accuracy of DFT in transition metal chemistry. Annu. Rep. Prog. Chem. Sct 2006;104:4811-4 815.

[516] Zhao Y and Truhlar DG. Design of density functionals that are broadly accurate for hermochemistry, thermochemical kinetics and nonbound ineractions. J. Phys. Chem. A 2005; 109:5656 – 5667.

[517] Zhao Y, Truhlar DG. How well can new-generation density functionals methods describe stacking interactions in biological systems. Phys. Chem. Chem. Phys. 2005;8:2701-2705.

[518] Zhao Y, Tishchenko O, Truhlar DG. How well can density functional methods describe hydrogen bonds to π acceptors? J. Phys. Chem. B 2005;109:19046-19051.

[519] Hamprecht FA, Cohen AJ, Tozer DJ, Handy NC. Development and assessment of new exchange-correlation functional. J. Chem. Phys. 1998;199:6264-6271.

[520] Kobayashi R, Amos RD. The application of CAM-B3lyp to the charge-transfer band problem of the zincbacteriochlorin-bacteriochlorin complex. Chem. Phys. Lett. 2006;420:106-109.

[521] Thonhauser T, Cooper VR, Li S, Puzder A, Hyldguard P, Langreth DC. Van der Waals density functional: Self-consistent potential and the nature of the van der Waals bond. Phys. Rev. B 2007:74:125112-125123.

[522] Modern biotechnology in medicinal chemistry and industrry; 2006; Editor: Carlton A. Taft, Research Signpost, Kerala, India.

[523] Martins JBL, Perez MA, Silva CHTP, Taft CA, Arissawa M, Longo E, Mello PC, Stamato FMLG and Tostes JGR. Theoretical ab initio study of ranitidine. International Journal of Quantum Chemistry. 2002;90:575-586.

[524] Arissawa M, Taft CA, Felcman J. Investigation of nucleoside analogs with anti-HIV activity. International Journal of quantum chemistry 2003;93:422-432.

[525] C. H. T. P. Silva and C. A. Taft. Computer-aided molecular design of novel glucosidase inhibitors for AIDS treatment. Journal of biomolecular structure and dynamics. 2004;22:59-63.

[526] Silva CHTP, Sanches SM and Taft CA. A molecular modeling and QSAR study of suppressors of the growth of Trypanasoma cruzi espimastigotes. J. Mol. Graph and Modelling 2004;23:89-97.

[527] Silva CHTP, Almeida P, Taft CA. Density functional and docking studies of retinoids for câncer treatment. J. Mol. Model 2004;10:38-43.

[528] Silva CHTP and Taft CA. Molecular dynamics, database screening, density functional and docking studies of novel RAR ligands in cancer chemotherapy 2005;117:73-77.

[529] da Silva CHTP, Del Ponte G, Neto AF, Taft CA. Rational desing of novel diketoacid-containing ferrocene inhibitors of HIV-1 integrase. Bioorganic Chemistry. 2005;33:274-284.

[530] Silva CHTP, Leopoldino AM, Silva EHT, Espinoza VAA and Taft CA. Computer-aided design of a novel ligand for retinoic acid receptor in cancer chemotherapy. Int. J. of Quantum. Chem. 2005; 102:1131-1135.

[531] Silva CHTP, Carvalho I and Taft CA. Homology modelling and molecular interaction Field studies of α-glucosidases as a guide to structure-based design of novel proposed anti-HIV inhibitors. J. of Computer-Aided Molecular Design. 2005; 1983-92.

[532] Silva CHTP and Taft CA. ADMET properties, database screening, Molecular dynamics, density functional and docking studies of novel potential anti-cancer compunds. J. of Biomolecular structure & dynamics.2006;24:263-268.

[533] Silva CHTP and Carvalho I. Molecular dynamics, docking, density functional and ADMET studies of HIV-1 reverse transcriptase inhibitors. J. of Theoretical and Computationa Chemistry 2006;5:579-586.

[534] da Silva VB, Andrioli WJ, Carvalho I, Taft CA and Silva CHTP. Computer-aided molecular design of novel HMG-CoA reductase inhibitors for the treatment of hyhpercholesterolemia. 2007;6:811-821.

[535] Silva CHTP, Carvalho I and Taft CA. Virtual screening, molecular interaction field, molecular dynamics docking, density functional and ADMET properties of novel AchE inhibitors in Alzheimer's disease. J. OF Biomolecular Structure & Dynamics. 2007;24:515-523.

[536] Braun GH, Jorge DMM, Ramos HP, Alves RM, Guilliati S, Samppaio SV, Taft and Silva CHTP.Molecular dynamics, flexible docking, virtual screening. ADMET predictions and molecular interaction field studies to design novel potential MAO-B inhibitors. J. of Biomolecular structure & dynamics 2008;25:347-355.

[537] da Silva VB, Kawano DF, Gomes AS, Carvalho I, Taft CA, Silva CHTP. Molecular dynamics, density functional, ADMET predictions, virtual screening and molecular interaction Field studies for identification oand evaluation of novel potential CDK2 inhibitors in câncer therapy. J. Phys. Chem. A 2008;112:8902-8910.

[538] Silva CHTP, DA Silva VB and Taft CA. Use of virtual screening, fleible docking and molecular interaction fields to design novel HMG-CoA reductase inhibitors for the treatment of hypercholesterolemia. J. Phys. Chem. A 2008;112:2007-2011.

[539]Silva CHTP, da Silva VB and Taft CA. Pharmacokinetic and pharmacodynamic predictions of novel potential HIV-1 integrase inhibitors.Drug metabolism letters 2008;2:256-260.

[540] Hage-Mellin LIS, Silva CHTP, Semighini EP, Taft CA and Sampaio SV. Computer-aided drug design of novel PLA_2 inhibitor candidates for treatment of snakebite. J. of Biomolecular Structure & dynamics 2009;27:27-36.

[541] Silva CHTP, da Silva VB, Resende J, Rodrigues PF, Bononi FC, Benevenuto CG and Taft CA, J. of Molecular Graphics and Modeling. 2010; 28:513-523.

[542] Current Methods in Medicinal Chemistry and Biological Physics;2007, Vol. 1, Editors Carlton A. Taft and Carlos H. T. P. Silva, Research Signpost, Kerala, India.

[543] Current Methods in Medicinal Chemistry and Biological Physics. 2008, Vol. 2. Editors Carlton A. Taft and Carlos H. T. P. Silva, Research Signpost, Kerala, India..

CHAPTER 2

The Role of Glycogen Synthase Kinase 3β in Alzheimer's Disease, with Implications in Drug Design

Adriana Mieco Namba and Carlos Henrique Tomich de Paula da Silva

School of Pharmaceutical Sciences of Ribeirão Preto, University of São Paulo, Av. do Café, s/n, Monte Alegre, 14040-903, Ribeirão Preto, São Paulo, Brazil

Abstract: The main neuropathological hallmark of Alzheimer's disease (AD) is the accumulation of aberrant hyperphosphorylated microtubule-associated protein tau, forming the intracellular neurofibrillary tangles and the extracellular deposits of β-amilóide peptide (βA). Glycogen Synthase Kinase-3β (GSK-3β), a serine/threonine kinase, has emerged as one of the most attractive therapeutic targets for the treatment of AD. This enzyme has been linked to all the primary abnormalities associated with Alzheimer's disease, including hyperphosphorylation of the microtubule-associated protein tau, which contributes to the formation of neurofibrillary tangles, and its interactions with others Alzheimer's disease-associated proteins. Thus, the significant role of GSK-3β in essential events in the pathogenesis of AD makes this kinase an attractive therapeutic target for neurological disorders. This chapter explores the nature and the structure of this promising enzyme, focusing on the structure-based design of new GSK-3β inhibitors.

INTRODUCTION

Alzheimer's disease (AD) [1-3] is a chronic, neurodegenerative disorder which is characterized by progressive memory loss and impairments in language and behaviour that ultimately leads to death. At autopsy, the AD brain is characterized by a number of important pathological changes, including selective neuronal and synaptic losses [4], intracellular neurofibrillary tangles (NFTs) and extracellular senile plaques [5]. The senile plaques are mainly composed of the 40–42 amino acid-long amyloid β-peptide (Aβ) in fibrillar form, called Aβ-40 and Aβ-42, respectively, which are produced by proteolytic cleavage of the amyloid β-protein precursor (APP) [6-9], through sequential cleavages by two proteases, β- and γ-secretase.

The neurofibrillary tangles are polymers of paired helical filaments generated by the aggregation of protein tau in the abnormal hyperphosphorylated state [10-15]. Tau is a microtubule-associated protein that stabilizes microtubules within neurites and axons [16]. Microtubules are the essential components of the cytoskeleton; they are responsible for the formation and maintenance of the neuronal morphology and their specific connections. The microtubule associated proteins contribute to regulate the dynamism and stability of the microtubules, and therefore they are essential to maintain the correct function of the microtubules. The hyperphosphorylated tau of the paired helical filaments is highly insoluble and is incapable of binding to microtubules and promoting microtubules assembly. Consequently, tau abnormal phosphorylation causes the loss of tau function, microtubule instability, and neurodegeneration in AD brain [17,18].

Early-onset Alzheimer's, an usual form of dementia that strikes people younger than age 65, is linked to three genes: APP gene on chromosome 21 and Presenilins 1 (PS1) and 2 (PS2), located on chromosome 14 and 1, respectively. Missense mutations in PS1, PS2 or APP changes the proteases activities, increasing the production of the Aβ-42 [19-28]. Aβ-42 is the species initially deposited in plaques in the brain, contributing to cell death and neuronal loss. [29-31].

The etiology of AD has not yet been established for most of the cases known as the 'sporadic' forms of AD [32]. The most widely accepted hypothesis regarding the pathogenesis of AD is the so-called 'amyloid cascade' hypothesis [2,6,25,33], which proposes that abnormal processing of APP and the subsequently increased production, aggregation and deposition of Aβ-peptides are the primary events in AD. Fibrillar aggregates of the β-amyloid peptide would then act as neurotoxic agents, causing tau hyperphosphorylation, NFT formation, synaptic degeneration and neuronal cell death [2,33]. Studies have shown that large numbers of amyloid plaques are found in some cognitively normal elders, suggesting that Aβ deposition may not always result in dementia [32]. Thus, tau hyperphosphorylation becomes a crucial point in the 'amyloid cascade' hypothesis.

One of the more prominent sites in tau protein is Thr231, which is phosphorylated by the enzyme glycogen synthase kinase 3 beta, GSK-3β, an active serine/threonine kinase [34,35]. Phosphorylation of Thr231 which is increased after prephosphorylation of Ser235, plays a significant role in regulating tau's ability to bind and stabilize microtubules, because it changes tau conformation [36,37].

GSK-3β IN ALZHEIMER'S DISEASE

GSK-3β has emerged as an attractive therapeutic target for the treatment of several neurological diseases, including Alzheimer's disease [38-40]. This enzyme is a proline-directed serine/threonine kinase that was originally identified as a result of its role in glycogen metabolism regulation, CNS being the tissue with the highest GSK-3β levels [41]. It is one of the two isoforms of GSK-3 that are highly expressed in the brain, consisting of 420 amino acids (~ 47-kDa) [41].

GSK-3β is believed to influence Alzheimer's disease pathology at multiple levels. This enzyme can phosphorylate tau on residues that contribute to paired helical filament formation [42-46]. It is associated with PS1 toxicity and with cleavage of APP, which leads to amyloid plaque formation [47-51]. In addition, GSK-3β has been shown to bind presenilin-1; mutant PS-1 expression increases GSK-3β activity and, consequently, tau phosphorylation in cells [50,51].

Both *in vitro* and *in vivo* studies have demonstrated that inhibition of GSK-3β, by either pharmacological or genetic means, can reverse hyperphosphorylation of tau and prevent behavioral impairments in mice [50,52-57].

STRUCTURAL ASPECTS OF GSK-3β

The crystal structure of GSK-3β has been solved by several groups [58-60] and the analysis of its structure has provided insight into both its regulation of the kinase activity and its preference for pre-phosphorylated substrates. Fig. **1** illustrates the dimeric structure of apo, nonphosphorylated GSK-3β, solved at 2.7 Å resolution (PDB code: 1I09), by molecular replacement [60].

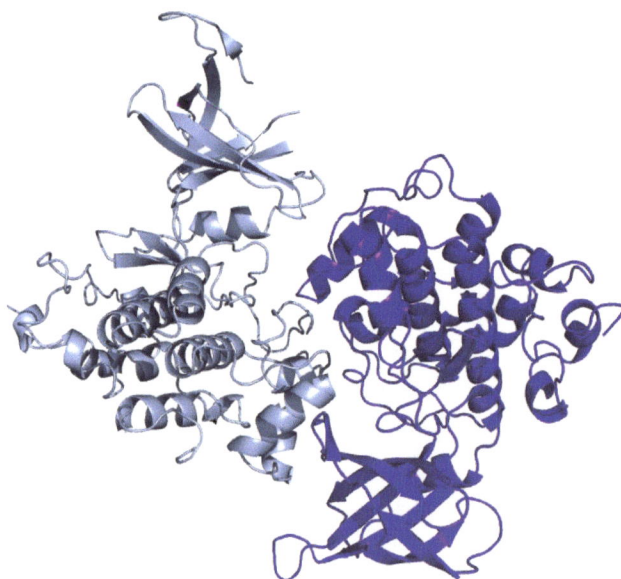

Figure 1: Dimeric structure of apo GSK-3β, solved by X-ray diffraction at 2.7 Å resolution [18].

The main dimeric sites are residues Asp260 to Val263 at the N-terminus of an α-helix (262–273) from one monomer, which interacts with Tyr216 to Arg220 at the end of the activation segment of the other. Direct polar interactions are limited to an ion pair between Asp260 and Arg220, and main chain to main chain hydrogen bonds between the peptide carbonyls of Asp260 and Val263 with the peptide nitrogens of Arg220 and Tyr216, respectively. The hydrophobic face of the side chain of Tyr216 interacts with a hydrophobic patch formed by Ile228, Phe229, Gly262, Val263, and Leu266 from the other monomer. There are overall shape complementarities at the interface but few other direct contacts. Several solvent-bridged interactions are evident. In general, dimer formation buries ~2358 Å^2 of accessible surface [59].

The overall shape is shared by all kinases [61,62], consisting of an N-terminal β-strand domain (residues 25-138) and a C-terminal α-helical domain (residues 139-343) [60]. The N-terminal domain is formed by a seven-stranded β sheet curved over on itself to form a closed orthogonal β barrel. The 5th and 6th strands of the barrel are connected by a short α-helix (residues 96-102) that consists of two turns. This helix is conserved in all kinases, whereas two of its residues play key roles in the catalytic activity of the enzyme. Arg96 is involved in the alignment of the two domains. Glu97 is positioned in the active site and forms a salt bridge with Lys85, a key residue in catalysis. The N-terminal domain connects to the remainder of the protein via an α-helix (residues 138-149) extending from the end of the 7th strand [60].

The activation loop (residues 200–226) runs along the surface of the substrate binding groove. The C-terminal 39 residues (residues 344–382) are outside the core kinase fold and forms a small domain that packs against the α-helical domain. The ATP (adenosine triphosphate) binding site (substrate-binding pocket) is at the interface of the α-helical and β-strand domain and is bordered by the glycine-rich loop and the hinge. It contains three basic residues, i.e. Arg96, Arg180 and Lys205, that bind the phosphate anion on the primed Ser/Thr residue in the substrate motif [59,60].

CATALYTIC ACTIVITY AND REGULATION OF GSK-3β

The catalytic activity of protein kinases depends upon the correct orientation of the catalytic groups contributing to the transfer of the γ-phosphate group from ATP to a Ser, Thr, or Tyr side chain of the protein substrate. Another factor is the accessibility and correct positioning of the groups forming the substrate peptide binding site, which provides affinity and specificity for the substrate [59,63].

GSK3-β has two phosphorylation sites, that influence the catalytic activity of the protein. Ser9 is the phosphorylation site for AKT, and the phosphorylation of this residue inactivates GSK3-β. Phosphorylation of Tyr216, located on the activation loop, increases the catalytic activity.

The substrate specificity of GSK3β is unusual. Recognition of substrates by the GSK-3β usually requires prior phosphorylation of the substrate. Analysis of phosphorylated sites by GSK-3β [59] (see Table **2**) suggests a preference for sequences of the type: Ser/Thr–X–X–X–Ser/Thr, where the C-terminal serine or threonine is already phosphorylated [64-66], so that prior phosphorylation of the n+4th residue facilitates phosphorylation of the nth residue.

GSK-3β function can be regulated at many levels [38,67]. GSK-3β can be negatively regulated by phosphorylation at the N-terminal domain (Ser9 residue), which acts as a pseudo-substrate that blocks the access of substrates to the catalytic site [68] or can be activated through phosphorylation of Tyr216 in the T-loop domain, which facilitates the access of substrates to the catalytic site [69]. In addition, the activity of this protein can be controlled through its intracellular distribution [70], and by its interaction with many other proteins [71] or potential inhibitors [69].

GSK-3β INHIBITORS

Regarding the high therapeutical potential of targeting GSK-3β in many different pathologies, the search for its inhibitors is a very active field in both academic centers and pharmaceutical companies. For approximately the last fifty years the drug lithium has been the mainstay for the treatment of bipolar disorder, with a beneficial effect often observed in approximately 60–80% of patients and with no tolerance or sensitivity been developed during many years of treatment [72-74]. GSK-3β was first linked to bipolar disorder in 1996 by the discovery that lithium is a direct inhibitor of GSK-3β [75]. They found that lithium inhibited GSK-3β with an IC50 of approximately 2 mM, slightly larger than the therapeutic concentration range of lithium in serum, which is approximately 0.5–1.5 mM [75]. Subsequently, GSK-3β was shown to be inhibited by lithium both in intact cells [76] and in mammalian brain *in vivo* [44].

Among the multiple effects in the brain due to lithium, there is the inhibition of GSK-3β induced tau phosphorylation. Lithium reversibly reduced tau phosphorylation at therapeutic concentrations, and even at high concentrations did not alter the neuronal morphology [77]. In addition, lithium prevents the neuronal death induced by the fibrillary β-amyloid. Neuroprotection appears to be mainly due to GSK-3β inhibition [78]. Another ionic compound, zinc, has been shown to non-competitively inhibit GSK-3β and induce an increase in glucose transport activity in mouse adipocytes [79]. However, because of the non-selective nature of lithium and zinc, the metabolic actions of these ions cannot be ascribed solely to inhibition of GSK-3β. For this reason, several classes of highly selective GSK-3β inhibitors have been developed.

At present, several GSK-3β inhibitors have been described, with IC50 values in the nanomolar range (Table **1** and Fig. **2**) [48] whereas most of the observed effects are *in vitro* and cellular studies.

Pyrazines, pyrimidines, bisindolemaleimides, hymenialdisine, paullones, indirubins, and anilinomaleimides have been developed as ATP competitive GSK-3β inhibitors, while thiadiazolidinones were reported to be the first ATP noncompetitive GSK-3β inhibitors. Soon after crystallization of GSK-3β [59,60,82], the enzyme was cocrystallized with some inhibitors, which provided an understanding of their mechanism of interaction within the ATP-binding pocket.

The 2.4 Å crystal structure of GSK-3β with the non-hydrolyzable ATP analog adenyl imidodiphosphate (AMP-PNP), pdb code: 1PYX, provides a logical starting point for understanding how ATP-mimetic inhibitors interact with GSK-3β [82] (Fig. **3**). AMP-PNP binds in the cleft formed between the N- and C-terminal lobes of GSK-3β, with the adenine group making hydrogen bonds with the hinge residues Asp133 and Val135. In addition to the polar interactions, the adenine group also makes hydrophobic interactions with GSK-3β residues Ile62, Val70, Ala83, Val110, Leu132, Tyr134 and Leu188 (Fig. **2**).

The ribose group of AMP-PNP interacts with GSK-3β through a single hydrogen bond between O3' and the carbonyl oxygen of Glu185. No direct hydrogen bonds are observed between O2' and GSK-3 β residues.

This is in contrast to what was observed for several other protein kinase complexes with nucleotides, in which a hydrogen bond is formed with a conserved residue near the hinge.

In GSK-3β, this residue is Thr138 and although it seems possible for a threonine to make this type of hydrogen bond, it is not the case in this structure.

Instead, the Oγ of Thr138 is directed away from the ribose group, making a hydrogen bond with the backbone nitrogen of Arg141.

Lys85 hydrogen bonds to the α- and β-phosphates of AMP-PNP and also forms a salt-bridge with a kinase-conserved glutamate (Glu97) from the C-helix.

"Mg1" coordinates four oxygen atoms; one from each of the α- and γ-phosphates and one from each of the kinase conserved residues Asn186 and Asp200. "Mg2" shows octahedral coordination of six oxygen atoms; one from each of the β- and γ-phosphates, both carboxylate oxygen atoms from Asp200 and two water molecules.

In addition, the kinase conserved residue Lys183 (catalytic loop) extends up towards the γ-phosphate making hydrogen bonds with a γ-phosphate oxygen and a carboxylate oxygen of another kinase conserved residue Asp181 (catalytic loop).

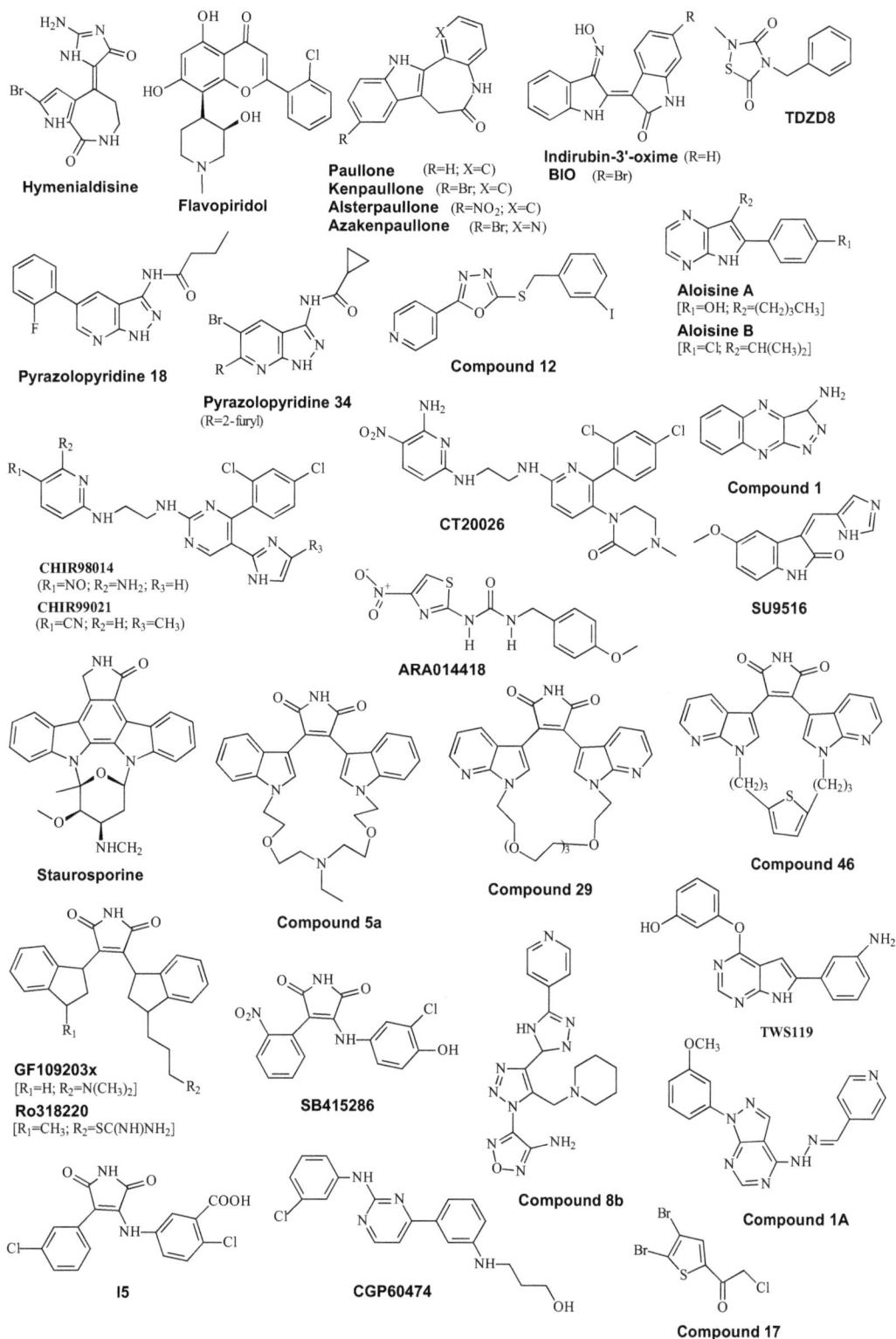

Figure 2: Structures of some of the most studied pharmacological inhibitors of GSK-3β.

No direct interactions are observed between the AMP-PNP phosphate groups and the nucleotide-binding loop of GSK-3β. Instead the loop interacts with the phosphate groups through bridging water molecules and shields the phosphate groups from the bulk solvent.

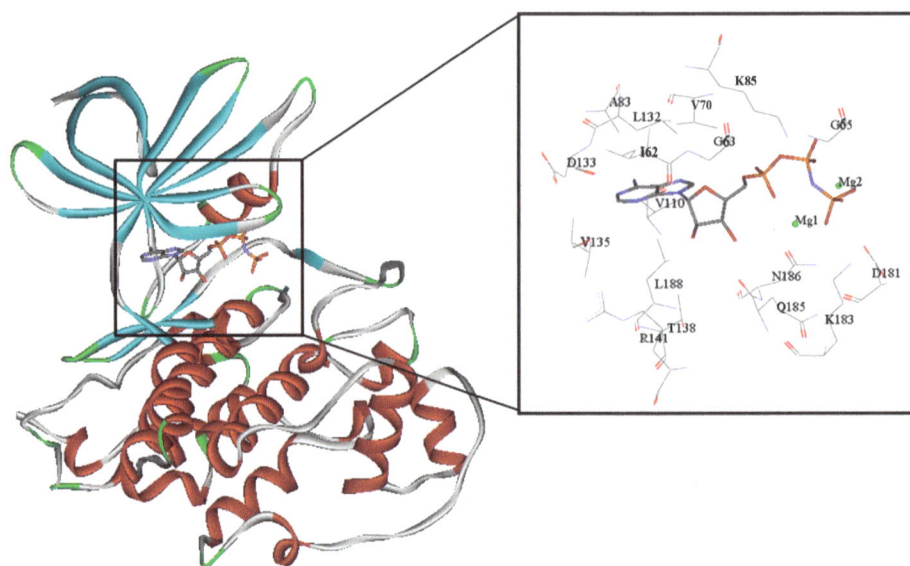

Figure 3: The 2.4 Å crystal structure of GSK-3β monomer complexed with AMP-PNP.

Table 1: Pharmacological inhibitors of GSK-3β

INHIBITOR	CLASS	IC50 (μM)	REF
Hymenialdisine	Pyrroloazepine	0.010	[88]
Flavopiridol	Flavone	0.450	[89]
Kenpaullone	Benzazepinone	0.023	[90,91]
Alsterpaullone	Benzazepinone	0.004	[90,91]
Azakenpaullone	Benzazepinone	0.018	[92]
Indirubin-3'-oxime	Bis-Indole	0.022	[89]
6-Bromoindirubin-3' oxime	Bis-Indole	0.005	[84,85]
6-Bromoindirubin-3'-acetoxime	Bis-Indole	0.010	[84,85]
Aloisine A	Pyrrolopyrazine	0.650	[93]
Aloisine B	Pyrrolopyrazine	0.750	[93]
TDZD8	Thiadiazolidinone	2.000	[80]
Compound 12	Pyridyloxadiazole	0.390	[94]
CHIR98014	Aminopyrimidine	0.00058	[95]
CHIR99021 (CT99021)	Aminopyrimidine	0.007	[95]
CT20026	Aminopyridine	0.004	[96]
Compound 1	Pyrazoloquinoxaline	1.000	[97]
SU9516	Oxindole (indolinone)	0.330	[98]
ARA014418	Thiazole	0.104	[83]
Staurosporine	Bisindolylmaleimide	0.089	[99]
Compound 5[a]	Bisindolylmaleimide	0.018	[99]
Compound 29	Azaindolylmaleimide	0.034	[100]
Compound 46	Azaindolylmaleimide	0.036	[101]
GF109203x (bisindolylmaleimide I)	Bisindolylmaleimide	0.190	[102]
Ro318220 (bisindolylmaleimide IX)	Bisindolylmaleimide	0.003-0.038	[102,103]
SB216763	Arylindolemaleimide	0.075	[104]
SB415286	Anilinomaleimide	0.13	[104,105]
I5	Anilinoarylmaleimide	0.160	[82]
CGP60474	Phenylaminopyrimidine	0.010	[106]
Compound 8b	Thiazole	0.280	[107]
TWS119	Pyrrolopyrimidine	0.030	[108]
Compound 1[a]	Pyrazolopyrimidine	0.016	[109]
Compound 17	Chloromethyl thienyl ketone	1.00	[81]

Analysis of the GSK-3β structure indicates that the major difference between the phosphorylated and unphosphorylated form is the rotamer conformation of the Tyr216. Phosphorylation causes an ~ 120° rotation of the tyrosine side chain and repositioning of the side chains of Arg220 and Arg223, to hydrogen bond to the phosphate group of Tyr216.

Despite the wide chemical diversity, most pharmacological inhibitors of GSK-3 β share common properties [48]: (i) they have a low molecular weight (< 600), (ii) they are rather flat, hydrophobic heterocycles, (iii) most, but not all [80,81], act by competing with ATP in the ATP-binding site of the kinase (lithium acts directly by competing with magnesium, but also indirectly by increasing the inhibitory phosphorylation of Ser9 of GSK-3β [75]), (iv) they essentially bind through hydrophobic interactions and 2–3 hydrogen bonds with the kinase, and (v) the backbone carbonyl and amino side-chains of Val135 act as an H-bond acceptor and H-bond donor, respectively, to the inhibitors, whereas the backbone carbonyl of Asp133 often acts as an H-bond acceptor [82–87].

It's likely that substituted aminopyrimidine molecules developed by Chiron Corporation were the first synthetic molecules specifically reported as GSK-3β inhibitors.

But what is more frequent until now for discovering new GSK-3β inhibitors, are the screening programs with the specific objective of finding GSK-3β inhibitory activity in other compounds previously reported with other biological properties.

This is the case of the inhibitors hymenialdisines, paullones, indirubins, and maleimide derivatives.

STRUCTURE-BASED VIRTUAL SCREENING AND NOVEL GSK-3B INHIBITORS

Structure-based approaches have been used to provide insights into the structural and binding environment based on the key interactions shown by selective and nonselective ATP-competitive GSK-3β inhibitors. Several other computational approaches have also been employed for the design and development of the GSK-3β inhibitors such as Quantitative Structure Activity Relationship (QSAR) studies, pharmacophore map generation, molecular field approaches and other methods [110-115].

A number of drug discovery programs have yielded small-molecule ATP-competitive inhibitors that are presently in various stages of development [48]. For the purpose of finding biologically active and novel compounds and providing new ideas for drug-design, virtual screening has been successfully employed in recent years [113-115]. Structure based pharmacophore mapping [116,117] has been extensively applied in the initial phase of drug discovery programs [113-115]. A pharmacophore model postulates that there is an essential three dimensional (3D) arrangement of functional groups that a molecule must have to be recognized by the binding pocket. It collects common features distributed in 3D space that is intended to represent groups in a molecule that participate in important interactions between drugs and their active sites. Hence, a pharmacophore model provides crucial information about how well the common features of a subject molecule overlap the hypothesis model.

Kim and co-workers [115] applied ligand-based sequential virtual screening [118], which was started with the Catalyst/HipHop [119] pharmacophore based virtual screening and was followed by additional screening model. HipHop finds common feature pharmacophore models among a set of highly active compounds thus carrying out a qualitative model without the use of activity data, which represents the essential 3D arrangement of functional groups common to a set of molecules for interacting with a given biological target.

The training GSK-3β inhibitors used by Kim and co-workers for pharmacophore generation [115] are displayed in Fig. **4**. The best pharmacophore query was comprised of three hydrogen bond acceptors, one hydrogen bond donor, and one hydrophobic feature. The alignment of compound 4P with the best pharmacophore model and docking into the active site of crystal structure of GSK-3β (PDB code: 1I09) using FlexX docking software [120], showed that the hydrogen bond acceptor and donor features on the maleimide ring are generated from hydrogen bond with Asp133 and Val135, respectively. In addition, the hydrogen bond acceptor on the pyrazine ring was consistent with the fact that such features interacts with the backbone of Asp200 burying into the hydrophobic pocket. The hydrogen bond acceptor on the substitution butyl-alcohol came from the interaction with the NH of Gln185.

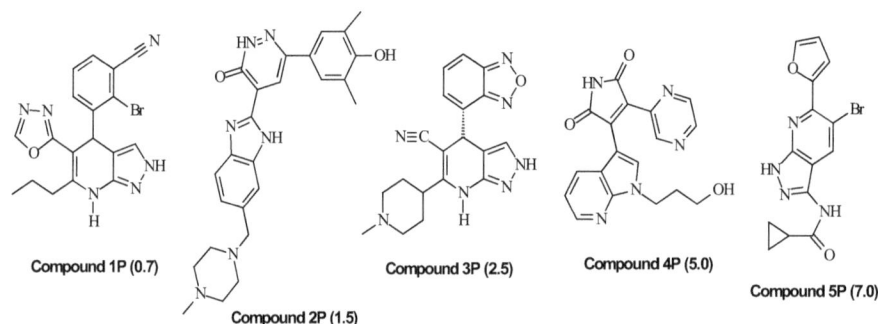

Figure 4: The structures and activities (IC$_{50}$, nM) of the training GSK-3β inhibitors used for pharmacophore generation.

In the next step, the authors applied virtual screening with the models and an external library: ChemDiv. Pre-processing of the total library was carried out to reduce the time-consuming conformation generation step of pharmacophore-based virtual screening. The final 56 hit compounds were carefully selected considering docking pose, structural diversity, and synthetic accessibility. Based on the percentage inhibition values, a total of seven compounds were selected and the activities evaluated by IC50 value (Fig. **5**). The best hit compound 7 fulfilled the best pharmacophore, by matching perfectly three hydrogen bond acceptors and one donor. The docking pose and conformation of the compound showed good alignment with the results from the ligand-based approach. It also showed the conserved interactions with important residues, such as Asp133, Val135, and Arg141, as in the other crystal complexes. In this study, a successful virtual screening application was presented revealing novel, micromolar GSK-3β inhibitors.

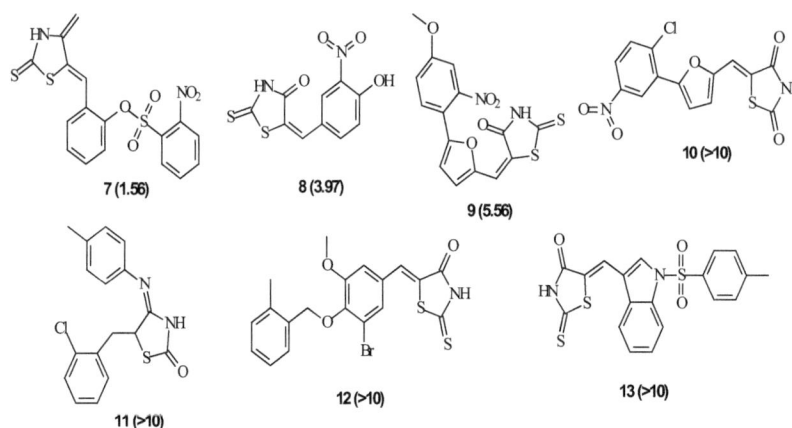

Figure 5: The structures and activities (IC$_{50}$, µM) of the hit compounds from ligand-based sequential virtual screening with external library.

According to the Binding Database (BindingDB) [44-47], a public, web-accessible repository that currently holds ~ 20000 experimentally determined binding affinities of protein–ligand complexes, there are ~560 GSK-3β complexes with inhibitors, which have biologic activity reported.

The PDB has currently 11 structures of GSK-3β complexed with different inhibitors, with information about the bioactive conformations that can provide pharmacophore hypotheses.

However, the selectivity of most GSK-3β inhibitors is not well known, making this enzyme an attractive target for design and development of potential inhibitors that can act more selectively in the inhibition of the formation of both neurofibrillary tangles and amyloid plaques, the two main pathological features of Alzheimer's disease.

REFERENCES

[1]   Alzheimer A. Über eigenartige Krankheits fälle des späteren Alters, Z. Gesamte Neurol. Psychiat. 1911; 4: 356–385.

[2]   Yankner BA. Mechanisms of neuronal degeneration in Alzheimer's disease, Neuron. 1996; 16, 921–932.

[3]   Kang J, Lemaire HG, Unterbeck A, Salbaum JM, Masters CL, Gzeschik KH, Multhaup G, Beyreuther K, Müller-Hill B. The precursor of Alzheimer's disease amyloid A4 protein resembles a cell-surface receptor, Nature, 1987; 325, 733-736.

[4]   Morrison JH, Hof PR, Life and death of neurons in the aging brain. Science, 1997; 278: 412–419

[5]   Hardy J, A hundred years of Alzheimer's disease research. Neuron 2006; 52: 3–13.

[6]   Selkoe DJ. The cell biology of beta -amyloid precursor protein and presenilin in Alzheimer's disease. Trends Cell Biol 1998; 8: 447-453.

7]   Lee SJ, Liyanage U, Bickel PE, Xia W, Lansbury PJ, Kosik KS. A detergent-insoluble membrane compartment contains A beta in vivo, Nat. Med. 1998; 4: 730-734.

[8]   Selkoe, DJ, Schenk D. Alzheimer's disease: molecular understanding predicts amyloid-based therapeutics, Annu. Rev. Pharmacol. Toxicol. 2003; 43: 545-584

[9]   Masters CL, Simm G, Weinman NA, Multhaup G, McDonald BL, Beyreuther K, Amyloid Plaque. Core Protein in Alzheimer Disease and Down Syndrome, Proc. Natl. Acad. Sci. USA, 1985; 82: 4245-4249.

[10]   Grundke-Iqbal I, Iqbal K, Tung YC, Quinlan M, Wisniewski HM, Binder LI. Abnormal phosphorylation of the microtubule-associated protein tau (tau) in Alzheimer cytoskeletal pathology. Proc. Natl. Acad Sci USA, 1986; 83: 4913–4917.

[11]   Grundke-Iqbal I, Iqbal K, Quinlan M, Tung YC, Zaidi MS, Wisniewski HM. Microtubule-associated protein tau. A component of Alzheimer paired helical filaments. J. Biol. Chem. 1986; 261: 6084–6089.

[12]   Iqbal K, Grundke-Iqbal I, Smith AI, George L, Tung YC, Zaidi T. Identification and localization of a τ peptide to paired helical filaments of Alzheimer disease. Proc. Natl. Acad. Sci. USA, 1989; 86: 5646–5650.

[13]   Lee VM, Balin BJ, Otvos LJ, Trojanowski JQ. A major subunit of paired helical filaments and derivatized forms of normal Tau. Science 1991; 251: 675–678.

[14]   Selkoe DJ, Alzheimer's Disease: A Central Role for Amyloid, J. Neuropathol. Exp. Neurol. 1994; 53: 438–447.

[15]   Nagy Z, Esiri MM, Jobst KA, Morris JH, King EMF, McDonald B, Litchfield S, Smith A, Barnetson L, Smith AD. Relative Roles of Plaques and Tangles in the Dementia of Alzheimer's Disease: Correlations Using Three Sets of Neuropathological Criteria, Dementia 1995; 6, 21-31.

[16]   Lovestone S, Reynolds CH. The phosphorylation of tau: a critical stage in neurodevelopment and neurodegenerative processes. Neuroscience, 1997: 78, 309–324.

[17]   Goedert M, Crowther RA, Garner CC. Molecular characterization of microtubule-associated proteins tau and MAP2. Trends Neurosci. 1991; 14(5):193-199.

[18]   Lee VMY, Goedert M, Trojanowski JQ, Neurodegenerative taupathies, Annu. Rev. Neurosci. 2000; 24: 1121-1159.

[19]   Rossor NM, Newman S, Frackowiak SR, Lantos P, Kennedy AM. Alzheimer's disease families with amyloid precursor protein mutations, Ann. N. Y. Acad. Sci. 1993; 695: 198-202.

[20]   Campion D, Flaman MJ, Brice A, Hannequin D, Dubois B. Martin C. et al., Mutations of the presenilin I gene in families with early-onset Alzheimer's disease, Hum. Mol. Genet. 1995; 4: 2373-2377.

[21]   Cruts M, Hendriks L, van Broeckhoven C. The presenilin genes: a new family involved in Alzheimer's disease pathology. Hum. Mol. Genet. 1996; 5: 1449-1455.

[22]   Levy-Lahad E, Wasco W, Poorkaj P, Romano DM, Oshima J, Pettingell WH, Yu CE, Jondro PD, Schmidt SD, Wang K. et al., Candidate gene for the Chromosome 1 familial Alzheimer's disease locus, Science, 1995; 269: 973-977.

[23]   Rogaev EI, Sherrington R, Rogaeva EA, Levesque G, Ikeda M, Liang Y, Chi H, Lin C, Holman K, Tsuda T, et al., Familial Alzheimer's disease in kindred with missens mutations in a gene on chromosome 1 related to the Alzheimer's disease type 3 gene. Nature, 1995; 376: 775-778.

[24]   Ezquerra M, Carnero C, Blesa R, Oliva R. A Novel Presenilin 1 Mutation (Leu166Arg) Associated With Early-Onset Alzheimer Disease, Arch. Neurol., 2000; 57: 485-488.

[25]   Selkoe DJ. Translating cell biology into therapeutic advances in Alzheimer's disease. Nature, 1999; 399: A23-A31.

[26]   Takashima A, Honda T, Yasutake K, Michel G, Murayama O, Murayama M, Ishiguro K, Yamaguchi H, Activation of tau protein kinase I/glycogen synthase kinase-3beta by amyloid beta peptide (25-35) enhances phosphorylation of tau in hippocampal neurons. Neurosci. Res. 1998; 31: 317-323.

[27]   Balaraman Y, Limaye AR, Levey AI, Srinivasan S, Glycogen synthase kinase 3beta and Alzheimer's disease: pathophysiological and therapeutic significance. Cell. Mol. Life Sci., 2006; 63:1226-1235.

[28]   Borchelt DR, Ratovitski T, van Lare J, Lee MK, Gonzales V, Jenkins NA, Copeland NG, Price DL, Sisodia SS. Accelerated amyloid deposition in the brains of transgenic mice coexpressing mutant presenilin 1 and amyloid precursor proteins. Neuron 1997; 19: 939–945.

[29]   Loo TD, Copani A, Pike JC, Whittemore RE, Walencewicz AJ, Cotman CW. Apoptosis is induced by B-amyloid in cultured central nervous system neurons. Proc. Natl. Acad. Sci. USA, 1993; 90: 7951-7955.

[30] Yaar M, Zhai S, Pilch FP, Doyle MS, Eisenhauer BP, Fine ER, et al., Binding of beta-amyloid to the p75 neurotrophin receptor induces apoptosis - A possible mechanism for Alzheimer's disease. J. Clin. Invest. 1997; 100: 2333-2340.

[31] Estus S, Tucker MH, van Rooyen C, Wright S, Brigham FE, Wogulis M. et al., Aggregated amyloid-beta protein induces cortical neuronal apoptosis and concomitant "apoptotic" pattern of gene induction, J. Neurosci., 1997; 17: 7736-7745.

[32] Álvarez G, Muñoz Montaño JR, Satrustegui J, Ávila J, Bogónez E, Díaz-Nido J, Regulation of tau phosphorylation and protection against beta-amyloid-induced neurodegeneration by lithium. Possible implications for Alzheimer's disease. Bipolar Disord. 2002; 4(3): 153-165

[33] Hardy JA, Higgins GA, Alzheimer's disease: The amyloid cascade hypothesis, Science 1992; 256: 184-185.

[34] Embin, N, Rylatt DB, Cohen P. Glycogen synthase glycogen synthase kinase 3_beta: structural basis for phosphatekinase-3 from rabbit skeletal muscle. Seperation from cyclic- primed substrate specificity and autoinhibition. Eur. J. Biochem. 1980; 107: 519–527.

[35] Goedert M, Jakes R, Crowther RA, Cohen P, Vanmechelen E, Vandermeeren M, Cras P. Epitope mapping of monoclonal antibodies to the paired helical filaments of Alzheimer's disease: identification of phosphorylation sites in tau protein. Biochem. J., 1994; 301: 871-877.

[36] Jicha GA, Lane E, Vincent I, Otvos L Jr., Hoffmann R, Davies PA. A conformation- and phosphorylation-dependent antibody recognizing the paired helical filaments of Alzheimer's disease. J. Neurochem. 1997; 69(5): 2087-2095.

[37] Daly NL, Hoffmann R, Otvos LJr, Craik DJ. Role of phosphorylation in the conformation of tau peptides implicated in Alzheimer's disease, Biochemistry, 2000; 39(30): 9039-9046.

[38] Avila J, Hernández F. GSK-3 inhibitors for Alzheimer's disease. Expert Rev. Neurother. 2007; 7(11): 1527-1533.

[39] Martinez A. Preclinical efficacy on GSK-3 inhibitors: towards a future generation of powerful drugs, Med. Res. Rev. 2008; 28(5): 773-796.

[40] Hopper C, Killick R, Lovestone S. The GSK3 hypothesis of Alzheimer's disease. J. Neurochem. 2008; 104(6): 1433-1439.

[41] Woodgett J.R. Molecular cloning and expression of glycogen synthase kinase-3/factor A. Embo J., 1990; 9(8): 2431-2438.

[42] Lovestone S, Reynolds CH, Latimer D, Davis DR, Anderton BH, Gallo JM, Hanger D, Mulot S, Marquardt B, Stabel S. Alzheimer's disease-like phosphorylation of the microtubule-associated protein tau by glycogen synthase kinase-3 in transfected mammalian cells. Curr. Biol., 1994; 4: 1077–1086.

[43] Hong M, Chen DC, Klein PS, Lee VM, Lithium reduces tau phosphorylation by inhibition of glycogen synthase kinase-3. J. Biol. Chem. 1997; 272: 25326-25332.

[44] Muñoz-Montaño JR, Moreno FJ, Avila J, Diaz-Nido, J, Lithium inhibits Alzheimer's disease-like tau protein phosphorylation in neurons. FEBS Lett. 1997; 411: 183-188.

[45] Spittaels K, Van den Haute C, Van Dorpe J, Geerts H, Mercken M, Bruynseels K, Lasrado R, Vandezande K, Laenen I, Boon T, Van Lint J, Vandenheede J, Moechars D, Loos R, Van Leuven F, J. Biol. Chem. 2000; 275: 41340–41349.

[46] Lucas JJ, Hernandez F, Gomez-Ramos P, Moran MA, Hen R, Avila J. Decreased nuclear beta-catenin, tau hyperphosphorylation and neurodegeneration in GSK-3beta conditional transgenic mice. EMBO J. 2001; 20: 27–39.

[47] Engel T, Hernandez F, Avila J, Lucas JJ. Full reversal of Alzheimer's disease-like phenotype in a mouse model with conditional overexpression of glycogen synthase kinase-3. J. Neurosci., 2006; 26: 5083-5090.

[48] Meijer L., Flajolet M, Greengard P. Pharmacological inhibitors of glycogen synthase kinase 3, Trends Pharmacol. Sci. 2004; 25: 471-480.

[49] Phiel CJ, Wilson CA, Lee VM, Klein PS. GSK-3alpha regulates production of Alzheimer's disease amyloid-beta peptides, Nature. 2003; 423: 435-439.

[50] Takashima A, Murayama M, Murayama O, Kohno T, Honda T, Yasutake K, Nihonmatsu N, Mercken M, Yamaguchi H, Sugihara S, Wolozin B, Presenilin 1 associates with glycogen synthase kinase-3beta and its substrate tau. Proc. Natl. Acad. Sci. USA 1998; 95: 9637-9641.

[51] Zhang Z, Hartmann H, Do VM, Abramowski D, Sturchler-Pierrat C, Staufenbiel M, Sommer B, van de Wetering M, Clevers H, Saftig P, De Strooper B, He X, Yankner BA. Destabilization of beta-catenin by mutations in presenilin-1 potentiates neuronal apoptosis. Nature 1998; 395: 698 –702.

[52] Perez M, Hernandez F, Lim F, Diaz-Nido J, Avila J, Chronic lithium treatment decreases mutant tau protein aggregation in a transgenic mouse model. J. Alzheimers Dis. 2003; 5: 301-308.

[53] Engel T, Goni-Oliver P, Lucas JJ, Avila J, Hernandez F, Chronic lithium administration to FTDP-17 tau and GSK-3beta overexpressing mice prevents tau hyperphosphorylation and neurofibrillary tangle formation, but pre-formed neurofibrillary tangles do not revert. J. Neurochem. 2006; 99: 1445-1455.

[54] Le Corre S, Klafki HW, Plesnila N, Hubinger G, Obermeier A, Sahagun H, Monse B, Seneci P, Lewis J, Eriksen J, Zehr C, Yue M, McGowan E, Dickson DW, Hutton M, Roder HM. An inhibitor of tau hyperphosphorylation prevents severe motor impairments in tau transgenic mice, Proc. Natl. Acad. Sci. USA, 2006: 103, 9673-9678.

[55]   Nakashima H, Ishihara T, Suguimoto P, Yokota O, Oshima E, Kugo A, Terada S, Hamamura T, Trojanowski JQ, Lee VM, Kuroda S. Chronic lithium treatment decreases tau lesions by promoting ubiquitination in a mouse model of tauopathies, Acta Neuropathol 2005; 110: 547-556.

[56]   Noble W, Planel E, Zehr C, Olm V, Meyerson J, Suleman F, Gaynor K, Wang L, LaFrancois J, Feinstein B, Burns M, Krishnamurthy P, Wen Y, Bhat, R, Lewis J, Dickson D, Duff K, Inhibition of glycogen synthase kinase-3 by lithium correlates with reduced tauopathy and degeneration in vivo, Proc. Natl. Acad. Sci. USA 2005; 102: 6990-6995.

[57]   Gong CX, Iqbal K. Hyperphosphorylation of microtubule-associated protein tau: a promising therapeutic target for Alzheimer disease. Curr. Med. Chem. 2008; 15(23): 2321-2328.

[58]   Bax B, Carter PS, Lewis C, Guy AR, Bridges A, Tanner R, Pettman G, Mannix C, Culbert AA, Brown MJ, Smith DG, Reith AD. The structure of phosphorylated GSK-3beta complexed with a peptide, FRATtide, that inhibits beta-catenin phosphorylation. Structure, 2001; 9:1143-1152.

[59]   Dajani R, Fraser E, Roe SM, Young N, Good V, Dale TC, Pearl LH. Crystal structure of glycogen synthase kinase 3 beta: structural basis for phosphate-primed substrate specificity and autoinhibition. Cell, 2001; 105(6): 721-732.

[60]   ter Haar E, Coll JT, Austen DA, Hsiao HM, Swenson L, Jain J. Structure of GSK3beta reveals a primed phosphorylation mechanism. Nat. Struct. Biol., 2001; 8: 593-596.

[61]   Hanks SK, Quinn AM, Hunter T. The protein kinase family: conserved features and deduced phylogeny of the catalytic domains. Science 1988; 241: 42–52.

[62]   Hanks SK, Quinn AM. Protein kinase catalytic domain sequence database: identification of conserved features of primary structure and classification of family members. Methods Enzymol. 1991; 200: 38–62.

[63]   Johnson LN, Noble MEM, Owen DJ. Active and inactive protein kinases: structural basis for regulation. Cell 1996; 85: 149-158.

[64]   Fiol CJ, Haseman JH, Wang YH, Roach PJ, Roeske RW, Kowalczuk M, Depaoliroach AA. Phosphoserine as a recognition determinant for glycogen synthase kinase-3: phosphorylation of a synthetic peptide based on the G-component of protein phosphatase-1. Arch. Biochem. Biophys. 1988; 267: 797-802.

[65]   Fiol CJ, Wang AQ, Roeske RW, Roach PJ. Ordered multisite protein phosphorylation. Analysis of glycogen synthase kinase 3 action using model peptide substrates. J. Biol. Chem., 1990; 265: 6061-6065.

[66]   Wang YH, Roach PJ. Inactivation of rabbit muscle glycogen synthase by glycogen synthase kinase-3. Dominant role of the phosphorylation of Ser-640 (site-3a). J. Biol. Chem., 1993; 268: 23876-23880.

[67]   Grimes CA, Jope RS. The multifaceted roles of glycogen synthase kinase 3beta in cellular signaling. Prog. Neurobiol. 2001; 65: 391-426.

[68]   Frame S, Cohen P. GSK3 takes centre stage more than 20 years after its discovery. Biochem. J., 2001; 359: 1-16.

[69]   Hughes K, Nikolakaki E, Plyte SE, Totty NF, Woodgett JR. Modulation of the glycogen synthase kinase-3 family by tyrosine phosphorylation. EMBO J. 1993; 12: 803-808.

[70]   Hongisto V, Vainio JC, Thompson R, Courtney MJ, Coffey ET. The Wnt pool of glycogen synthase kinase 3beta is critical for trophic-deprivation-induced neuronal death. Mol. Cell. Biol. 2008; 28(5): 1515-1527.

[71]   Aberle H, Bauer A, Stappert J, Kispert A. beta-catenin is a target for the ubiquitin-proteasome pathway, EMBO J. 1997; 16: 3797-3804.

[72]   Jope RS, Roh MS. Glycogen synthase kinase-3 (GSK3) in psychiatric diseases and therapeutic interventions. Curr. Drug Targets. 2006; 7(11):1421-1434.

[73]   Jope RS. Anti-bipolar therapy: mechanism of action of lithium, Mol. Psychiat., 1999; 4: 117–128.

[74]   Phiel CJ, Klein PS. Molecular targets of lithium action. Annu. Rev. Pharmacol. Toxicol. 2001; 41: 789–813.

[75]   Klein PS, Melton DA. A molecular mechanism for the effect of lithium on development. Proc. Natl. Acad. Sci. USA. 1996; 93: 8455–8459.

[76]   Stambolic V, Ruel L, Woodgett JR. Lithium inhibits glycogen synthase kinase-3 activity and mimics wingless signalling in intact cells. Curr. Biol. 1996; 6: 1664–1668.

[77]   Lovestone S, Davis DR, Webster MT, Kaech S, Brion JP, Matus A, Anderton BH. Lithium reduces tau phosphorylation: effects in living cells and in neurons at therapeutic concentrations. Biol. Psychiatry 1999; 45: 995–1003.

[78]   Alvarez G, Munõz-Montanõ JR, Satrustegui J, Avila J. Lithium protects cultured neurons against beta-amyloid-induced neurodegeneration. FEBS Lett. 1999; 453: 260–264.

[79]   Ilouz R, Kaidanovich O, Gurwitz D, Eldar-Finkelman H. Inhibition of glycogen synthase kinase-3beta by bivalent zinc ions: insight into the insulin-mimetic action of zinc. Biochem. Biophys. Res. Commun. 2002; 295: 102-106.

[80]   Martinez A, Alonso M, Castro A, Pérez C, Moreno FJ. First non-ATP competitive glycogen synthase kinase 3 beta (GSK-3beta) inhibitors: thiadiazolidinones (TDZD) as potential drugs for the treatment of Alzheimer's disease. J. Med. Chem. 2002; 45: 1292–1299.

[81] Conde S, Pérez DI, Martínez A, Perez C, Moreno FJ. Thienyl and phenyl alpha-halomethyl ketones: new inhibitors of glycogen synthase kinase (GSK-3beta) from a library of compound searching. J. Med. Chem., 2003; 46: 4631–4633.

[82] Bertrand JA, Thieffine S, Vulpetti A, Cristiani C, Valsasina B, Knapp S, Kalisz HM, Flocco M. Structural characterization of the GSK-3beta active site using selective and non-selective ATP-mimetic inhibitors. J. Mol. Biol., 2003; 333: 393–407.

[83] Bhat R, Xue Y, Berg S, Hellberg S, Ormö M, Nilsson Y, Radesäter AC, Jerning E, Markgren PO, Borgegård T, Nylöf M, Giménez-Cassina A, Hernández F, Lucas JJ, Díaz-Nido J, Avila J. Structural insights and biological effects of glycogen synthase kinase 3-specific inhibitor AR-A014418 J. Biol. Chem. 2003; 278:45937-45945

[84] Meijer L, Skaltsounis AL, Magiatis P, Polychronopoulos P, Knockaert M, Leost M, Ryan XP, Vonica C. A, Brivanlou A, Dajani R, Crovace C, Tarricone C, Musacchio A, Roe SM, Pearl L, Greengard P. GSK-3-selective inhibitors derived from Tyrian purple indirubins. Chem. Biol., 2003; 10: 1255–1266.

[85] Polychronopoulos P, Magiatis P, Skaltsounis AL, Myrianthopoulos V, Mikros E, Tarricone A, Musacchio A, Roe SM, Pearl L, Leost M, Greengard P, Meijer L. Structural basis for the synthesis of indirubins as potent and selective inhibitors of glycogen synthase kinase-3 and cyclin-dependent kinases, J. Med. Chem. 2004; 47: 935–946.

[86] Witherington J, Bordas V, Haigh D, Hickey DM, Ife RJ, Rawlings AD, Slingsby BP, Smith DG, Ward R W. 5-aryl-pyrazolo[3,4-b]pyridazines: potent inhibitors of glycogen synthase kinase-3 (GSK-3). Bioorg. Med. Chem. Lett. 2003; 13, 1581–1584.

[87] Fischer PM. CDK versus GSK-3 inhibition: a purple haze no longer? Chem. Biol. 2003; 10, 1144–1146.

[88] Meijer L, Thunnissen AM, White AW, Garnier M, Nikolic M, Tsai LH, Walter J, Cleverley KE, Salinas P C, Wu YZ, Biernat J, Mandelkow EM, Kim SH, Pettit GR. Inhibition of cyclin-dependent kinases, GSK-3beta and CK1 by hymenialdisine, a marine sponge constituent. Chem. Biol. 2000; 7: 51–63.

[89] Leclerc S, Garnier M, Hoessel R, Marko D, Bibb JA, Snyder GL, Greengard P, Biernat J, Wu YZ, Mandelkow EM, Eisenbrand G, Meijer L. Indirubins inhibit glycogen synthase kinase-3 beta and CDK5/p25, two protein kinases involved in abnormal tau phosphorylation in Alzheimer's disease. A property common to most cyclin-dependent kinase inhibitors? J. Biol. Chem. 2001; 276: 251–260.

[90] Bain J, McLauchlan H, Elliott M, Cohen P. The specificities of protein kinase inhibitors: an update. Biochem. J. 2003; 371: 199–204.

[91] Leost M, Schultz C, Link A, Wu YZ, Biernat J, Mandelkow EM, Bibb JA, Snyder GL, Greengard P, Zaharevitz DW, Gussio R, Senderowicz AM, Sausville EA, Kunick C, Meijer L. Paullones are potent inhibitors of glycogen synthase kinase-3beta and cyclin-dependent kinase 5/p25. Eur. J. Biochem., 2000; 267: 5983–5994.

[92] Kunick C, Lauenroth K, Leost M, Meijer L, Lemcke T. 1-Azakenpaullone is a selective inhibitor of glycogen synthase kinase-3 beta. Bioorg. Med. Chem. Lett. 2004; 14: 413–416.

[93] Mettey Y, Gompel M, Thomas V, Garnier M, Leost M, Ceballos-Picot I, Noble M, Endicott J, Vierfond J M, Meijer L. Aloisines, a new family of CDK/GSK-3 inhibitors. SAR study, crystal structure in complex with CDK2, enzyme selectivity, and cellular effects. J. Med. Chem. 2003; 46, 222–236.

[94] Naerum L, Nørskov-Lauritsen L, Olesen PH. Scaffold hopping and optimization towards libraries of glycogen synthase kinase-3 inhibitors. Bioorg.Med. Chem. Lett. 2002; 12, 1525–1528.

[95] Ring DB, Johnson KW, Henriksen EJ, Nuss JM, Goff D, Kinnick TR, Ma ST, ReederJW, Samuels I, Slabiak T, Wagman AS, Hammond ME, Harrison SD. Selective glycogen synthase kinase 3 inhibitors potentiate insulin activation of glucose transport and utilization *in vitro* and in vivo. Diabetes 2003; 52: 588–595.

[96] Wagman AS, Johnson KW, Bussiere DE. Discovery and development of GSK3 inhibitors for the treatment of type 2 diabetes. Curr. Pharmacol. Des. 2004; 10: 1105–1137.

[97] Ortega MA, Montoya ME, Zarranz B, Jaso A, Aldana I, Leclerc S, Meijer L, Monge A. Pyrazolo[3,4-b]quinoxalines. A new class of cyclin-dependent kinases inhibitors. Bioorg. Med. Chem. 2002; 10: 2177–2184.

[98] Lane ME, Yu B, Rice A, Lipson KE, Liang C, Sun L, Tang C, McMahon G, Pestell RG, Wadler SA. Novel cdk2-selective inhibitor, SU9516, induces apoptosis in colon carcinoma cells. Cancer Res. 2001; 61: 6170–6177.

[99] Zhang HC, White KB, Ye H, McComsey DF, Derian CK, Addo MF, Andrade-Gordon P, Eckardt AJ, Conway BR, Westover L, Xu JZ, Look R, Demarest KT, Emanuel S, Maryanoff BE. Macrocyclic bisindolylmaleimides as inhibitors of protein kinase C and glycogen synthase kinase-3. Bioorg. Med. Chem. Lett. 2003; 13, 3049–3053.

[100] Kuo GH, Prouty C, DeAngelis A, Shen L, O'Neill DJ, Shah C, Connolly PJ, Murray WV, Conway BR, Cheung P, Westover L, Xu JZ, Look RA, Demarest KT, Emanuel S, Middleton SA, Jolliffe L, Beavers MP, Chen X. Synthesis and discovery of macrocyclic polyoxygenated bis-7-azaindolylmaleimides as a novel series of potent and highly selective glycogen synthase kinase-3beta inhibitors. J. Med. Chem. 2003; 46, 4021–4031.

[101] Shen L, Prouty C, Conway BR, Westover L, Xu JZ, Look RA. Chen X, Beavers MP, Roberts J, Murray WV, Demarest KT, Kuo GH. Synthesis and biological evaluation of novel macrocyclic bis-7-azaindolylmaleimides as potent and highly selective glycogen synthase kinase-3 beta (GSK-3 beta) inhibitors. Bioorg.Med. Chem. 2004; 12: 1239–1255.

[102] Hers I, Tavaré JM, Denton RM. The protein kinase C inhibitors bisindolylmaleimide I (GF 109203x) and IX (Ro 31-8220) are potent inhibitors of glycogen synthase kinase-3 activity. FEBS Lett. 1999; 460: 433–436.

[103] Davies SP, Reddy H, Caivano M, Cohen P. Specificity and mechanism of action of some commonly used protein kinase inhibitors. Biochem. J. 2000; 351: 95–105.

[104] Coghlan MP, Culbert AA, Cross DA, Corcoran SL, Yates JW, Pearce NJ, Rausch OL, Murphy GJ, Carter PS, Roxbee CL, Mills D, Brown MJ, Haigh D, Ward RW, Smith DG, Murray KJ, Reith AD, Holder JC. Selective small molecule inhibitors of glycogen synthase kinase-3 modulate glycogen metabolism and gene transcription. Chem. Biol. 2000; 7: 793–803.

[105] Smith DG, Buffet M, Fenwick AE, Haigh D, Ife RJ, Saunders M, Slingsby BP, Stacey R, Ward RW. 3-Anilino-4-arylmaleimides: potent and selective inhibitors of glycogen synthase kinase-3 (GSK-3). Bioorg. Med. Chem. Lett. 2001; 11: 635–639.

[106] Ruetz S, Fabbro D, Zimmermann J, Meyer T, Gray N. Chemical and biological profile of dual Cdk1 and Cdk2 inhibitors. Curr. Med. Chem. AntiCanc. Agents. 2003; 3: 1–14.

[107] Olesen PH, Sørensen AR, Ursø B, Kurtzhals P, Bowler AN, Ehrbar U, Hansen BF. Synthesis and *in vitro* characterization of 1-(4-aminofurazan-3-yl)-5-dialkylaminomethyl-1H-[1,2,3]triazole-4-carboxylic acid derivatives. A new class of selective GSK-3 inhibitors. J. Med. Chem. 2003; 46: 3333–3341.

[108] Ding S, Wu TY, Brinker A, Peters EC, Hur W, Gray NS, Schultz, P. G., Synthetic small molecules that control stem cell fate. Proc. Natl. Acad. Sci. USA, 2003; 100: 7632–7637.

[109] Peat AJ, Garrido D, Boucheron JA, Schweiker SL, Dickerson SH, Wilson JR, Wang TY, Thomson SA, Novel GSK-3 inhibitors with improved cellular activity, Bioorg. Med. Chem. Lett. 2004; 14: 2127–2130.

[110] Dessalew N, Patel DS, Bharatam PV. 3D-QSAR and molecular docking studies n pyrazolopyrimidine derivatives as glycogen synthase kinase-3beta inhibitors. J. Mol. Graph. Model. 2006; 25: 885-895.

[111] Gadakar P, Phukan S, Dattatreya P, Balaji VN. Pose prediction accuracy in docking studies and enrichment of actives in the active site of GSK-3beta. J. Chem. Inf. Model. 2007; 47: 1446-1459.

[112] Lather V, Kristam R, Saini JS, Karthikeyan NA, Balaji VN. QSAR Models for Prediction of Glycogen Synthase Kinase-3beta Inhibitory Activity of Indirubin Derivatives. QSAR Comb. Sci., 2008; 27(6): 718-728.

[113] Dessalew N, Bharatam PV. Investigation of potential glycogen synthase kinase 3 inhibitors using pharmacophore mapping and virtual screening. Chem. Biol. Drug Des. 2006; 68: 154-165.

[114] Dessalew N, Bharatam PV. Retraction notice to "Colon-specific, mutual azo prodrug of 5-aminosalicylic acid with L-tryptophan: synthesis, kinetic studies and evaluation of its mitigating effect in trinitrobenzenesulfonic acid-induced colitis in rats. Bioorg. Med. Chem. 2007; 15: 3728-3736.

[115] Kim HJ, Choo H, Cho YS, No KT, Pae AN. Novel GSK-3beta inhibitors from sequential virtual screening. Bioorg. Med. Chem. 2008; 16: 636-643.

[116] Gund P. Pharmacophoric pattern searching and receptor mapping, Annu. Rep. Med. Chem., 1977; 4: 299–308.

[117] van Drie JH. Pharmacophore discovery-lessons learned. Curr. Pharm. Des., 2003; 9: 1649–1664.

[118] Engels MF, Thielemans T, Verbinnen D, Tollenaere JP, Verbeeck RJ. CerBeruS: a system supporting the sequential screening process. J. Chem. Inf. Comput. Sci. 2000; 40: 241–245.

[119] CATALYST 4.11 User Guide, Accelrys, San Diego, CA, USA, 2006.

[120] Rarey M, Kramer B, Lengauer T, Klebe G. A fast flexible docking method using an incremental construction algorithm. J. Mol. Biol. 1996; 261: 470-489.

[121] Liu T, Lin Y, Wen X, Jorrisen RN, Gilson MK. BindingDB: a web-accessible database of experimentally determined protein-ligand binding affinities. Nucleic Acids Research. 2007, 35: D198-D201.

[122] Chen X, Lin Y, Gilson M K. The Binding Database: Overview and User's Guide, Biopolymers Nucleic Acid Sci. 2002; 61: 127-141.

[123] Chen X, Lin Y, Liu M, Gilson MK. The Binding Database: data management and interface design. Bioinformatics. 2002; 18: 130-139.

[124] Chen X, Liu M, Gilson MK. BindingDB: A web-accessible molecular recognition database. J. Combi. Chem. High-Throughput Screen. 2001; 4: 719-725.

CHAPTER 3

General Aspects of Molecular Interaction Fields in Drug Design

Vinicius Barreto da Silva, Jonathan Resende de Almeida and Carlos Henrique Tomich de Paula da Silva

School of Pharmaceutical Sciences of Ribeirão Preto, University of São Paulo, Av. do Café, s/n, Monte Alegre, 14040-903, Ribeirão Preto, São Paulo, Brazil

Abstract: Computational techniques are effective tools for aiding the drug design process. Computational chemistry can be used to predict physicochemical properties, energies, biding modes, interactions and a wide amount of helpful data in lead discovery and optimization. The interactions formed between a ligand and a molecular target structure can be represented by molecular interaction fields (MIF). The MIF identify regions of a molecule where specific chemical groups can interact favorably, suggesting interaction sites with other molecules. In this context the MIF theory has been extensively used in drug discovery projects with a variety of applications, including QSAR, virtual screening, prediction of pharmacokinetic properties and determination of ligand binding sites in protein target structures.

INTRODUCTION

One of the challenges for the health sciences scientific community is the search for new and effective drugs in order to provide better treatments for patients that are suffering from diseases that affect mankind. Today, the field of drug development deals with a large amount of data generated from information provided by new genomic and proteomic techniques. In this way, new attractive and potential pharmacological targets are discovered and there is a need to rationalize the application of methods to transform these data to knowledge and introduce new drugs in clinical protocols for effective treatments.

A fundamental postulate in the classical drug design paradigm is the fact that the effect of a drug in the human body is a consequence of the molecular recognition between a ligand (the drug) and a macromolecule (the target). Structure-based drug design plays a central role in this field of research since the pharmacological activity of the ligand at its site of action is related to the spatial arrangement and electronic nature of the atoms of the ligands as well as how these atoms interact with their biological counterparts. Computational chemistry can be used to characterize the dynamics and energetics of such interactions and yield insights in molecular recognition processes in order to better rationalize drug design [1-9].

The available drugs available interact with their molecular targets via non-covalent interactions. Under this assumption, one of the main interests of computational chemistry is to develop methods, applying molecular recognition concepts, that could predict protein-ligand interactions in order to predict conformation and affinity of small molecules with molecular targets [10]. In this way new ligands can be obtained guiding the search for effective drugs. Computational chemistry can be applied to help in the other stages of drug design as well, i.e optimization of pharmacokinetic properties and prediction of toxicity data [11-16].

Molecular recognition is of central importance in biological processes. H-bonding, stacking, ionic and hydrophobic interactions are normally observed in ligand-protein complexes [17]. In order to understand the contribution of each interaction and the basis of biological functions in a particular biological or pharmacological process, the knowledge of molecular electrostatic potentials is critically important. In principle, interaction forces are composed of three components: electrostatic, inductive and dispersive [18].

The electrostatic interaction is characteristic of polar molecules, which carry a charge or a permanent dipole moment. The inductive forces are relevant when a polar molecule interacts with a non-polar molecule. In this way, the dipole of the polar molecule produces an electric field that changes the electronic distribution of the non-polar molecule inducing a dipole moment. When the interacting molecules are non-polar there are dispersion forces, whereas the permanent fluctuations in the electron distribution of one molecular entity can induce a temporary dipole in the neighboring molecule [18].

Molecular Interaction Fields (MIFs) are appropriate tools for investigating the energetic conditions between a drug target and a ligand and to help in understanding the interaction forces in the complexes. A MIF describes the variation of the interaction energy between a 3D molecular structure and a specific chemical probe. The 3D molecular structure can be represented by a protein drug receptor, an enzyme, a DNA polymer, an organic compound, *etc.* The chemical probe represents an atom or a small group of atoms (molecular fragment). The objective is to predict where ligands can bind to a biological target and understand the factors that interfere with binding in order to design ligands with improved biological activity [19,20]. The MIF theory is extensively applied in drug discovery projects, including structure-based drug design, QSAR and prediction of pharmacokinetic properties of ligands.

MOLECULAR INTERACTION FIELDS THEORY

Goodford [20] described a method to assess the fit of ligands within the active site of its molecular target by determining energetically favorable binding sites on biologically important macromolecules. The pioneer computational method was able to display energy contour surfaces in three dimensions in phase with the macromolecular chemical structure representation, leading in this way to the design of ligands considering simultaneously energy and shape.

The calculation of MIFs can translate the ability of a giving molecule to interact with others. The interaction of a molecule with a chemical probe, which represents any kind of functional group, located at any x, y, z coordinate around the molecule is the basic idea behind the MIF concept. Computing the measurement of this interaction at sample positions, a giving set of energy values are obtained and can be displayed graphically as energy contours. These contours represent specific areas in space where molecules holding a probe-like group could perform energetically favorable interactions, describing the potential of two molecules approaching each other to interact [18].

The calculations of MIFs for an attractive drug target structure can lead to identification of relevant regions of the biomacromolecule where potential ligands could establish intermolecular interactions. This is particularly important to guide the design and evaluation of potent and selective ligands. In the same way, the MIFs can be computed for a group of known ligands, without the prior knowledge of the drug receptor structure, in order to help the discrimination of the molecular characteristics, regarding the ability to establish interactions, which are important to maintain or improve biological activity. [21]

When performing calculations a regular array of GRID nodes are established throughout and around the molecular structure. In this way, a potential energy function is calculated for a specific chemical probe located at the first point of the GRID. Successive probe positions are sampled until the potential energy is computed for each GRID node (Fig. **1**). Considering a drug target macromolecule, the dimensions of the array are determined so that the first GRID node is positioned outside the protein structure leading to small energy values. Nevertheless, some subsequent points can intersect the macromolecule leading to large positive energies. The points which are located in the proteins interatomic spaces allow the determination of favorable ligand interaction sites where negative interaction energies are assigned [20]. These favorable regions represent promising locations where a ligand can place a functional group similar to the probe. When computed for a ligand molecule, these represent potential groups of the drug target binding site where noncovalent bonding interactions could be established [21].

The energy function used to compute the nonbonded interactions of the chemical probe with the molecule studied in a given node is composed, basically, of a sum of the Lennard-Jones and electrostatic functions. The Lennard-Jones function is used to explain the attractive van der Waals force by a combination of the dispersion and repulsion energies in order to detect the zone of mutual attraction between nonbonded atom pair interactions.

Considering Equation 1 and the calculation of van der Waals energy, r_{ij} represents the distance between a pair of nonbonded atoms. A_{ij} and C_{ij} are parameters representing the repulsion term and the attraction term, respectively.

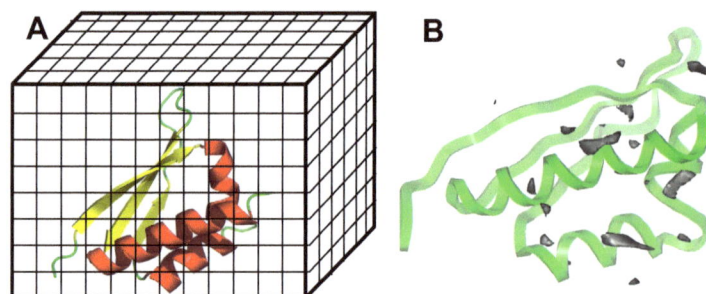

Figure 1: (A) Definition of the nodes where a chemical probe is positioned to compute the MIFs in relation to a protein structure. (B) Virtual interaction sites for water probe at -5.0 kcal/mol calculated for a biological protein.

When r_{ij} is small, a repulsion energy is generated, corresponding to a large value of E_{vdW}. Once the minimum distance between two atoms to generate a attraction force is defined and the threshold step function established, it is possible to determine a molecular surface representing the MIFs computed for interacting atoms [20].

$$E_{vdW} = \sum_{i=1}^{n} (A_{ij} r_{ij}^{-12} - C_{ij} r_{ij}^{-6})$$

(Eq. 1)

The electrostatic term can be computed based on the charge of the probe and the charge of the extended target atom, represented by the Coulomb potential. The magnitude of the energy is critically sensitive to the spatial dielectric behavior of the environment and the individual terms are evaluated pairwise between the chemical probe and every atom of the molecular target. In Equation 2, q_i and q_j represent the charge of the pairwise atoms, r_{ij} the distance between them and D the electrostatic constant.

$$E_C = \sum_{i=1}^{n} \frac{q_i q_j}{D r_{ij}}$$

(Eq. 2)

CoMFA

Comparative molecular field analysis (CoMFA) describes 3D structure-activity relationships quantitatively, correlating biological differences of ligands with changes in shape and in the intensity of non-covalent interaction fields around the molecule. In order to perform such analysis a set of molecules are first selected. All molecules should interact with the same macromolecular target in the same manner. The next step is to select a certain subgroup of molecules representing a training set in order to derive the CoMFA model. The residual ones can be used for further analysis as a test set to validate the reliability of the model derived [22].

For the molecules analyzed, atomic partial charges and low energy conformations can be generated to derive a pharmacophore hypothesis, based on the superposition of all individual aligned molecules. After superposition of all molecules, the MIFs are calculated for different chemical probes encoding the forces responsible for ligand-protein intermolecular interactions, including steric, hydrogen bonding, electrostatic and hydrophobic molecular fields [23]. The objective is to sample the interaction between the individual molecules of the aligned set of molecules and the molecular probes. The calculated energy values are arranged in a very large X matrix, which is then correlated to the Y vector of pharmacological activity. The fields correspond to tables, often including several thousands columns, which must be correlated with binding affinity values, usually on a log scale (pKi, pIC_{50}). PLS (Partial Least Squares) analysis is the most appropriate method for this purpose. Normally cross-validation is used to check the internal predictive potential of the derived model [22, 23].

The final CoMFA model is derived using the optimum number of components selected. The results are usually displayed as coefficient contour maps. A satisfactory CoMFA model should present statistical significance, explain the difference in activity of the training set of compounds and show predictive power for new compounds.

CoMSIA

CoMSIA (Comparative Molecular Similarity Indices Analysis) is one of the 3D QSAR methods where the steric and electrostatic features, hydrogen bond donor, hydrogen bond acceptor and hydrophobic fields are considered. This technique is often used in drug discovery to find the common features that are important in binding to relevant biological receptors [24,25].

The powerful CoMSIA approach calculates similarity indices in the space surrounding each of the aligned molecules in the data set [26]. In this way, probes are used to calculate the similarity indices of the investigated molecules at different grid points. The theory of CoMSIA is based on the bioactivity of a series of compounds with the same mechanisms and depends on the variance of nonbonding interacting forces between ligands and receptors [27].

MOLECULAR PROBES

The virtual molecular probes used to compute MIFs can be a small molecule or even a molecular fragment. Using different probes to compute MIFs for a particular molecular target it is possible to obtain the most relevant interaction positions in 3D space, defining specific virtual interaction sites that reflects ideal complementary sites for certain chemical compounds presenting functional groups with the same characteristics as the molecular probes used [19].

In order to obtain relevant virtual interaction sites, the probes used should represent the most important groups responsible for maintaining biomolecule-ligand intermolecular interactions. For example, considering a protein molecular target it seems reasonable to use at least three molecular probes to represent interactions with a potential ligand: carbonyl oxygen, amide nitrogen and a hydrophobic probe. The carbonyl oxygen and amide nitrogen probes are useful to find hydrogen bonding interaction sites, representing hydrogen bond acceptor and hydrogen bond donor groups, respectively. In the same way, a hydrophobic probe should be used to map virtual interaction sites that favors hydrophobic interactions [19].

Considering the GRID software, most probes are spheres parameterized to represent a specific atom or ion type. Usually, hydrogen atoms are treated implicitly. For example, a carbonyl carbon atom and a methyl are both treated as spherical entities, however the methyl probe presents a larger radius explained by the hydrogen atoms that are bonded to the carbon atom [28].

Nonspherical probes can be used as well. A carboxylate group, for example, is treated as a 3-point probe, where one of the oxygen atoms is centered at the grid point. In order to solve the problem of the asymmetric placement of the probe regarding the grid point, the probe is rotated around the "anchored" oxygen to optimize its orientation. A carbonyl oxygen probe, usually used to find hydrogen bond virtual interaction sites as discussed above, is represented by one oxygen atom with a couple of sp2 lone pairs. Each lone pair can accept one hydrogen bond, in this way the center of the oxygen is placed at each grid point in order to search for hydrogen bond donor atoms in the neighboring molecular target structure. The probe can be also rotated to find the best possible hydrogen bonds [28].

MAPPING BINDING SITES

The original computations of MIFs were intended to identify favorable interaction sites on a drug target in order to design ligands with enhanced biological activity [20]. The application of MIFs has been extremely important in drug design projects, especially when a ligand for a particular protein target is known and compounds with improved activity are desired. In this case, the computation of MIFs together with other molecular modeling techniques can be helpful in identifying regions where new substituents can be added or replaced in the structure of the ligands, exploring thus the chemical space to derive new chemical entities as promising drug candidates.

Kastenholz *et al.* [29] presented a computational tool based on GRID MIFs computations of target proteins (serine proteases of the chymotrypsin family), where consensus principal component analysis was used to analyze the GRID descriptors. The method is able to help in the design of selective ligands by highlighting the favored interaction sites and the type of interaction associated with the 3D structure of the molecular targets. This detailed analysis of a family of target proteins allows determination of structural differences, considering the receptor, important to selectivity, without the dependence on appropriate ligands for a QSAR analysis.

An interesting method based on MIFs developed to predict protein-ligands binding sites is implemented in the Q-SiteFinder server [30]. Q-SiteFinder uses the interaction energy values between a protein 3D structure and a simple van der Waals probe (methyl probe) within a 3D grid to determine binding clefts. The probe sites with the most favorable binding energies are retained and clustered according to their spatial proximity. The probe clusters are ranked according to their total interaction energies whereas binding sites can be identified and predicted. According to the results presented in the validation of the method at least one successful prediction in the top three predicted binding sites is accomplished in 90% of proteins complexes from the PDB dataset used. In Fig. **2** we observe a successful prediction of the most favorable binding site region in the active site of β-secretase enzyme

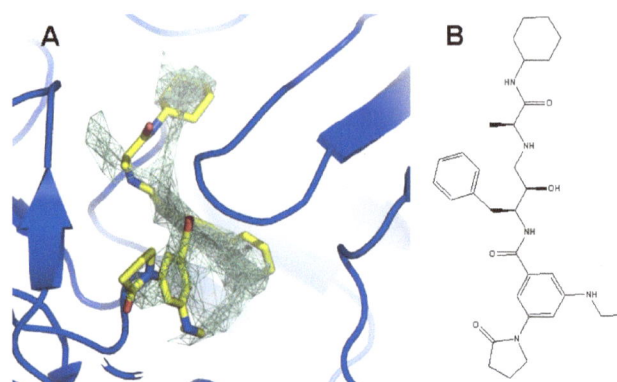

Figure 2: (A) Complex between human β-secretase and a potent inhibitor (PDB code: 2VJ6) in phase with the most favorable virtual binding site predicted with Q-SiteFinder. (B) Structure of the inhibitor in complex with β-secretase.

GRIND DESCRIPTORS

Pastor *et al.* [19] described the development of a mathematical description of molecules known as GRIND (Grid-INdependent Descriptors). The innovation of this approach was based on the computation of descriptors with independence regarding the orientation of the molecular structures in the space. The initial alignment of the series compounds is widely recognized as one of the most difficult and time-consuming steps in 3D-QSAR . Hence, considering that the GRIND approach does not require this step, the GRIND descriptors can be obtained easily, even for a large series of compounds.

The GRIND descriptors have been widely applied in drug Discovery projects usually in 3D-QSAR. The GRIND descriptors represent the most important GRID-interactions as a function of the distance [31-36]. GRIND encodes the geometrical relationships between the virtual receptor sites in such a way that they are no longer dependent upon their positions in the 3D space. The encoding is an auto- and cross-correlation transformation. The GRIND can be used in chemometric analysis performed with standard analysis methods such as PCA (Principal Component Analysis) and PLS [19].

Another applicability of GRIND descriptors was described by Li *et al.* [37] combining the use of GRIND descriptors and support vector machine in order to study a library of 495 compounds with the objective of discriminating between hERG blockers and nonblockers, since compounds that can inhibit the hERG channel are prone to develop cardiac toxicity. In this case the GRIND descriptors were used to assess toxicity of compounds in the early stages of drug discovery.

VIRTUAL SCREENING

Virtual screening (VS) is a strategy for computationally screening a database in search for novel drug leads and has become a new branch of medicinal chemistry. The basic goal of the virtual screening is the reduction of the enormous virtual chemical space of small organic molecules, to synthesize and screen against a specific target protein a number of compounds that inhibits and leads to the highest probability of being a good drug candidate [38].

Virtual screening can either be performed by the docking of potentials ligands into a protein binding site or by a similarity-based method. A similarity-based approach can be performed using a pharmacophore searching procedure, where the distances between GRID MIFs derived from the protein structure binding site can be used to drive a search for molecules with desired pharmacophore profile. In this way, the distance-based description of the protein is compared to the distances between structural properties in the potential ligand. This procedure could be taken as a preliminary task, enabling the analysis of large datasets, of which interesting hits should be further analyzed by more accurate methods [39].

Virtual screening tools grow with the knowledge available for a particular drug target and pharmacophore data. New developments indicate that progress can be made by combining pharmacophore filtering, docking methods and using several scoring functions in parallel [40]. Many methodologies are used for analyses within 3D constraints of an active target site. However, pharmacophore approaches have proven to be one of the widely applied methods in virtual screening [39].

Ahlstrm *et al.* [39] studied a set of strategies for structure-based design using GRID molecular interaction fields (MIFs) to derive a pharmacophoric representation of a protein. Thrombin was chosen as the model system. A pharmacophore representation of the thrombin protein based on GRID MIFs was used for the virtual screening methodology. A new procedure to perform a bioisosteric substitution of one scaffold for another, called scaffold hopping was used in this study. The starting point of the procedure was the selection of a template scaffold, which could be used during the search. When the scaffold is chosen, the number and positions of anchor points (atomic positions where the scaffold can be chemically modified) is decided.

Neves *et al.* [41] studied the development of a new ligand-based strategy combining important pharmacophoric and structural features according to the postulated aromatase binding mode, useful for the virtual screening of new potent non-steroid inhibitors. A small subset of promising drug candidates was identified from the large NCI database. The screening was based on the common features of a training set of second and third generation aromatase inhibitors combined with heme coordinating fragments inclusion volumes, and several druglikeness filters.

ADME PREDICTION

There are many methods and technologies that have been improved in the last years and are currently used to help in the drug discovery process. Many potent lead compounds for particular drug targets have been discovered; nevertheless the number of drugs being introduced in the market is much smaller. Most lead compounds fail in pre-clinical assays, because they present inadequate ADME properties (absorption, distribution, metabolism and excretion) and/or are toxic to humans [42].

It is now recognized that the definition of a successful drug is an appropriate balance of potency, safety and favorable pharmacokinetics. In order to reduce time, costs and the distance between the discovery of a new lead and the clinical approval, new computational techniques have being developed with the intent to predict pharmacokinetic properties and select compounds with suitable pharmacokinetic profiles, helping in guiding the drug discovery process and evaluation of drug candidates. [42-44].

In parallel with the experimental ADME field of research, *in silico* methods have been developed for specific *in vitro* assays or specific pathways in systems. These computational models are built based on experimental data. It is clear that a combination of *in silico* methods with selected *in vitro* tests can provide a cost-effective complement to exhaustive *in vitro* screening and animal experiments. [28].

The molecular interaction fields are useful tools employed computationally which can lead to models for studying ADME parameters. The interaction of a molecule with a hydrophobic probe can be used to highlight the hydrophobic surface exposed by the compound to the environment that is related to the lipophilicity. This is a parameter that can be used to predict solubility and membrane permeation, for example [28].

Another approach based on 3D molecular fields is the Volsurf procedure. The method produces 2D molecular descriptors from 3D molecular field maps. Volsurf descriptors are specifically designed to optimize pharmacokinetic properties. The Volsurf descriptors encode physico-chemical parameters allowing the study of quantitative structure-property relationships (QSPR), which are developed in the physical-chemical property space intending to modulate pharmacokinetic profiles [45]. These descriptors can be quantitatively compared and used to build multivariate models correlating 3D molecular structures with pharmacokinetic profiles, including structure-permeation relationships [46], renal clearance [47], metabolic stability [48] and volume of distribution [28].

Milleti *et al.* [49] described a method based on GRID descriptors of molecular interaction fields to predict the pKa of organic compounds. The pKa is a physical-chemical parameter closely related to lipophilicity and solubility, two of the most important properties used in pharmaceutical research to study absorption and distribution. The procedure is based on 4 steps: (1) building of a database of fragments to compute energy minima using the GRID force field; (2) Describing every atom of the molecule using the MIFs obtained from the database fragments; (3) Describing the molecular structure around each ionizable site by using binned MIFs summed at each topological distance; (4) building tables with statistical data containing molecular descriptors and experimental pKa values for different classes of ionizable sites.

CONCLUSION

The concept and theory of MIFs can be applied as appropriate tools of great importance in the discovery and development of drugs. These tools have extensive applications and contributions towards determining the energetic conditions involved in the binding between a ligand and its target via the molecular interaction of a molecule with a chemical probe. These tools can be used to improve the design of new ligands with enhanced biological activity based on interaction fields. This strategy can be used in biomacromolecules in order to indentify favorable interaction regions yielding new proposals for chemical entities which can fit properly in the binding site. MIFs can also be used with known ligands in order to determine molecular descriptors related with interaction and, consequently, with biological activity based on the pharmacophore concept. Once inhibitors of a particular molecular target are available, the derived pharmacophore can be useful in building QSAR models or in screening virtual databases of drug-like molecules in order to search for potential inhibitors with desired pharmacophore properties. Nowadays, the MIFs are not only used to find inhibitors but have been extensively used to predict pharmacokinetic properties of promising drug candidates and help in the proposal of compounds with suitable pharmacokinetics. One of the major problems in drug candidates failures is due to poor pharmacokinetics and toxicity. Taking into consideration that the pharmacokinetic profile and toxicity of drugs is governed by molecular interactions in the human body some descriptors computed by MIFs studies are able to provide information in this respect and help researchers propose more effective drugs, reducing financial costs.

REFERENCES

[1]   Taft CA, Silva CHTP. Eds. 2007. Current Methods in Medicinal Chemistry and Biological Physics 2007, Research Signpost, Kerala.

[2]   Taft CA. Eds. 2006. Modern Biotechnology in Medicinal Chemistry and Industry, Research Signpost, Kerala.

[3]   Taft CA, Silva CHTP. Current topics in computer-aided drug design. Curr. Computer-Aided Drug Des. 2006;2: 307-324.

[4]   Silva CHTP, Sanches SM, Taft CA. A molecular modeling and QSAR study of suppressors of the growth of Trypanosoma cruzi epimastigotes.;. J. Mol. Graph. Model. 2004; 23: 89-97.

[5]   Silva CHTP, Del Ponte G, Neto AF, Taft CA. Rational design of novel diketoacid-containing ferrocene inhibitors of HIV-1 integrase. Bioorg. Chem. 2005; 33: 274-284.

[6]   Silva CHTP, Taft CA. ADMET properties, database screening, molecular dynamics, density functional, and docking studies of novel potential anti-cancer compounds. J. Biomol. Struc. Dyn. 2006; 24: 236-268.

[7]   Silva CHTP, Carvalho I, Taft CA. Molecular dynamics, docking, density functional, and ADMET studies of HTV-1 reverse transcriptase inhibitors. J. Theor. Comput. Chem. 2006; 5: 579-586.

[8]   Silva CHTP, Carvalho I, Taft CA. Virtual screening, molecular interaction field, molecular dynamics, docking, density functional, and ADMET properties of novel AChE inhibitors in Alzheimer's disease. 2007; J. Biomol. Struc. Dyn. 24: 515-523.

[9]   Taft CA, Silva VB, Silva CHTP. Topics in Computer-Aided Drug Design. J. Pharm. Sci. 2008; 97: 1089-1098.

[10]   Böhm, HJ, Schneider G. 2003. Protein-Ligand Interactions, WILEY-VCH, Weinheim.

[11]   Guerra A, Paez JA, Campillo NE. Artificial Neural Networks in Medicinal Chemistry: Establishment of a Neural Network Model for the Prediction of Blood-Brain-Barrier Passage. QSAR & Combinat. Scien. 2008; 27, 586-594.

[12]   Clark DE, *In silico* ADMET tools: the dawn of a new generation? Exp. Opin. Drug Discov. 2007 ; 2, 1423-1429.

[13]   Norinder U Bergstroem CAS. Prediction of ADMET properties. ChemMedChem., 2006; 1: 920-937.

[14]   Lill MA. Computational Pharmaceutical Chemistry: Novel Technologies for Lead Optimization and the Prediction of ADMET Properties. Chimia, 2006; 60: 33-36.

[15]   Ekins S, Andreyev S, Ryabov A, Kirillov E. Rakhmatulin EA, Sorokina S, Bugrim A, Nikolskaya T. A combined approach to drug metabolism and toxicity assessment. Drug Metabol. Disposit. 2006.; 4: 495-503.

[16]   Bidault Y. A flexible approach for optimising in silico ADME/Tox characterisation of lead candidates. Exp. Opin. Drug Metabol. Toxicol. 2006; 2: 157-168.

[17]   Tewari AK, Dubey R. Emerging Trends in Molecular Recognition: Utility of Weak Aromatic Interactions. Bioorg. Med. Chem. 2008; 16: 126-143.

[18]   Höltje HD, Sippl W, Rognan D, Folkers G. Molecular Modeling: Basic Principles and Applications, 2003; WILEY-VCH, Weinheim.

[19]   Pastor M, Cruciani G, Mclay I, Pickett S, Clementi S. GRid-INdependent descriptors (GRIND): a novel class of alignment- independent three-dimensional molecular descriptors. J. Med. Chem. 2000; 43: 3233-3243.

[20]   Goodford PJ. A computational procedure for determining energetically favorable binding sites on biologically important macromolecules.. J. Med. Chem. 1985; 28: 849-857.

[21]   Duran A, Martinez GC, Pastor M. Development and Validation of AMANDA, a New Algorithm for Selecting Highly Relevant Regions in Molecular Interaction Fields. J. Chem. Inf. Model. 2008; 48: 1813-1823.

[22]   Mor M, Rivara S, Lodola A, Lorenzi S, Bordi F, Plazzi PV, Spadoni G, Bedini A, Duranti A, Tontini A, Tarzia G. Application of 3D-QSAR in the rational design of receptor ligands and enzyme inhibitors. Chem. Biodivers. 2005; 2: 1438-1451.

[23]   Mittal RR, Mckinnon RA, Sorich MJ. Effect of steric molecular field settings on CoMFA predictivity. J. Mol. Model. 2008; 14: 59-67.

[24]   Klebe G, Abraham U, Mietzner T. Molecular similarity indexes in a comparative-analysis (CoMSIA) of drug molecules to correlate and predict their biological-activity. . J. Med. Chem. 1994; 37: 4130-4146.

[25]   Suh ME, Park SY, Lee HJ. Three-Dimensional QSAR Using the k-Nearest Neighbor Method and Its Interpretation.. Bull. Korean Chem. Soc. 2002; 23: 417-422.

[26]   Ul-Haq, Z., Wadood, A., Uddin, R., CoMFA and CoMSIA 3D-QSAR analysis on hydroxamic acid derivatives as urease inhibitors. 2009. J. Enz. Inhib. Med. Chem., 24, 272-278.

[27]   Yang XS, Wang XD, Ji L, Li R, Sun C, Wang LS. Combining docking and comparative molecular similarity indices analysis (COMSIA) to predict estrogen activity and probe molecular mechanisms of estrogen activity for estrogen compounds.. Chinese Sci Bull. 2008; 53: 3626-3633.

[28]   Cruciani G; 2006. Molecular Interaction Fields: Applications in Drug Discovery and ADME Prediction, WILEY-VCH, Weinheim.

[29]   Kastenholz MA, Pastor M, Cruciani G, Haaksma EEJ, Fox T. GRID/CPCA: A New Computational Tool to Design Selective Ligands.. J. Med. Chem. 2000; 43: 3033-3044.

[30]   Laurie ATR, Jackson RM. Q-SiteFinder: an energy-based method for the prediction of protein–ligand binding sites. Struct. Bioinf. 2005; 21: 1908-1916.

[31]   Afzelius L, Masimirembwa CM, Karlén A, Andersson TB, Zamora I.. Discriminant and quantitative PLS analysis of competitive CYP2C9 inhibitors versus non-inhibitors using alignment independent GRIND descriptors.. J. Computer-Aided Mol. Design. 2002; 16: 433-458.

[32]   Carosati E, Lemoine H, Spogli R, Grittner D, Mannhold R, Tabarrini O, Sabatini S, Cecchetti V. Binding studies and GRIND/ALMOND-based 3D QSAR analysis of benzothiazine type K(ATP)-channel openers.. Bioorg. Med. Chem. 2005; 13:5581-5591.

[33]   Benedetti P, Mannhold R, Cruciani G, Ottaviani G. GRIND/ALMOND investigations on CysLT(1) receptor antagonists of the quinolinyl(bridged)aryl type. . Bioorg. Med. Chem. 2004; 12: 3607-3617.

[34]   Sciabola S, Carosati E, Baroni M, Mannhold R. Comparison of Ligand-Based and Structure-Based 3D-QSAR: A Case Study on (Aryl-)Bridged 2-Aminobenzonitriles Inhibiting HIV-1 Reverse Transcriptase. J. Med. Chem. 2005; 48: 3756-3767.

[35]   Cianchetta G, Singleton RW, Zhang M, Wildgoose M, Giesing D, Fravolini A, Cruciani G, Vaz RJ. A pharmacophore hypothesis for P-glycoprotein substrate recognition using GRIND-based 3D-QSAR. J. Med. Chem. 2005; 48: 2927-2935.

[36]   Fontaine F, Pastor M, Zamora I, Sanz F. Anchor-GRIND: Filling the gap between standard 3D-QSAR and the GRid-INdependent Descriptors. J. Med. Chem. 2005; 48: 2687-2694.

[37]   Li Q, Jørgensen FS, Oprea T, Brunak S, Taboureau O. hERG classification model based on a combination of support vector machine method and GRIND descriptors.. Mol. Pharm. 2008 ; 5: 117-127.

[38]   Vyas V, Jain A, Jain A, Gupta A. Virtual Screening: A Fast Tool for Drug Design. Sci Pharm. 2008; 76: 333-360.

[39]   Ahlstrm MM, Ridderstrm M, Luthman K, Zamora I. Virtual Screening and Scaffold Hopping Based on GRID Molecular Interaction Fields. J. Chem. Inf. Model. 2005; 45: 1313-1323.

[40]   Schneider G, Böhm H. Virtual screening and fast automated docking methods. Drug Discov. Today. 2002;7:64-70.

[41]   Neves MAC, Dinis TCP, Colombo G, Sa ML, Fast M. Fast Three Dimensional Pharmacophore Virtual Screening of New Potent Non-Steroid Aromatase Inhibitors J. Med. Chem. 2009; 52: 143-150.

[42]   Wolohan PRN, Clark RD. Predicting drug pharmacokinetic properties using molecular interaction fields and SIMCA. J. Computer-Aided Mol. Design 2003;17: 65-76.

[43]   MODI S. Computational approaches to the understanding of ADMET properties and problems.. Drug Discov. Today. 2003; 8: 621-623.

[44]   O'Brien SE, Groot MJ. Greater than the sum of its parts: combining models for useful ADMET prediction.. J. Med. Chem. 2005; 48: 1287-1291.

[45]. Cruciani G., Pastor M, Guba W. VolSurf: a new tool for the pharmacokonetic optimization of lead compounds. . Eur. J. Pharm. Sci. 2000; 2: S29-S39.

[46]   Cruciani G, Crivori P, Carrupt PA, Testa B. Cruciani G, Crivori P, Carrupt PA, Testa B. J. Mol. Struct., 503, 17. 2000. J. Mol. Struct. 2000; 503: 17-30.

[47]   Doddareddy MR, Cho YS, Koh HY, Kim DH, Pae AN. In silico renal clearance model using classical Volsurf approach. J. Chem. Inf. Model. 2006; 46: 1312-1320.

[48]   Van de Waterbeemd H, Lennernäs H, Artursson P. Drug Bioavailability: Estimation of Solubility, Permeability, Absorption and Bioavailability, 2003; WILEY-VCH, Weinheim.

[49]   Milletti F, Storchi L, Sforna G, Cruciani G, New and Original pK_a Prediction Method Using Grid Molecular Interaction Fields. J. Chem. Inf. Model. 2007; 47: 2172-2181.

New Developments in Medicinal Chemistry Vol. 1, 2010, 79-94

CHAPTER 4

2D-QSAR: The Mathematics behind the Drug Design Methodology

Ana Conejo-García, Miguel A. Gallo, Antonio Espinosa and Joaquín María Campos

Department of Pharmaceutical Chemistry, School of Pharmacy, Campus Cartuja, Granada, Spain

Abstract: The development of quantitative structure-activity relationships (QSARs or 2D-QSARs) is a science that has developed without a defined framework, series of rules, or guidelines for methodology. It has been more than 40 years since the QSAR paradigm first found its way into the practice of agrochemistry, pharmaceutical chemistry, toxicology, and eventually most facets of chemistry. Its staying power may be attributed to the strength of its initial postulate that activity is a function of structure as described by electronic attributes, hydrophobicity, and steric properties as well as rapid and extensive development in methodologies and computational techniques that have ensued to delineate and refine the many variables and approaches that define the paradigm. The overall goals of QSAR retain their original essence and remain focused on the predictive ability of the approach and its receptiveness to mechanistic or diagnostic interpretations. Our intention with this chapter is to offer the basis of the QSAR approach in a clear and intuitive way, with maximum simplification and trying to close the gap that exists between maths and students of pharmacy. Moreover, the interpretation of the equations is even more important than statistically obtaining significant and robust relationships. We will show our results on Choline Kinase (ChoK) inhibitors as antiproliferative agents to demonstrate the possibilities of the Hansch model in the drug design process.

INTRODUCTION

The development of quantitative structure-activity relationships (QSARs or 2D-QSARs) is a science that has developed without a defined framework, series of rules, or guidelines for methodology. It has been more than 40 years since the QSAR paradigm first found its way into the practice of agrochemistry, pharmaceutical chemistry, toxicology, and eventually most facets of chemistry [1].

Its staying power may be attributed to the strength of its initial postulate that activity is a function of structure as described by electronic attributes, hydrophobicity, and steric properties as well as rapid and extensive development in methodologies and computational techniques that have ensued to delineate and refine the many variables and approaches that define the paradigm.

The overall goals of QSAR retain their original essence and remain focused on the predictive ability of the approach and its receptiveness to mechanistic or diagnostic interpretations (Fig. **1**).

We do not intend to be exhaustive in this chapter. There are excellent reviews [2] and books [3, 4] on the QSAR subject and we invite the advanced reader to consult these publications for a more complete overview.

Our intention is to offer the basis of the QSAR approach in a clear and intuitive way, with maximum simplification, trying to close the gap that exists between maths and students of pharmacy.

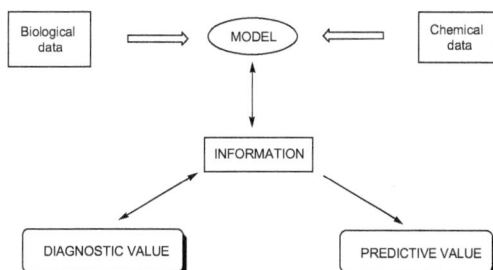

Figure 1: Elements of a QSAR study

Moreover, the interpretation of the equations is even more important than statistically obtaining significant and robust relationships. We will show our results on Choline Kinase (ChoK) inhibitors as antiproliferative agents to demonstrate the possibilities of the Hansch model in the drug design process.

ELECTRONIC EFFECTS

Louis Hammett (1894-1987) correlated the electronic properties of organic acids with their equilibrium constants and reactivity. Consider the dissociation of benzoic acid:

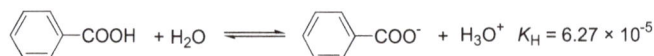

$$\text{C}_6\text{H}_5\text{-COOH} + \text{H}_2\text{O} \rightleftharpoons \text{C}_6\text{H}_5\text{-COO}^- + \text{H}_3\text{O}^+ \quad K_H = 6.27 \times 10^{-5}$$

Hammett observed that adding substituents to the aromatic ring of benzoic acid had a quantitative effect on the dissociation constant. For example:

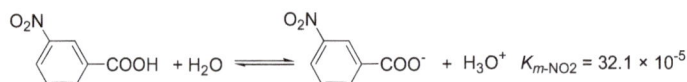

$$\text{O}_2\text{N-C}_6\text{H}_4\text{-COOH} + \text{H}_2\text{O} \rightleftharpoons \text{O}_2\text{N-C}_6\text{H}_4\text{-COO}^- + \text{H}_3\text{O}^+ \quad K_{m\text{-NO2}} = 32.1 \times 10^{-5}$$

A nitro group in the *meta* position increases the dissociation constant, because the nitro group is electron-withdrawing, thereby stabilizing the negative charge that develops. Now consider the effect of a nitro group in the *para* position.

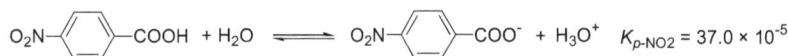

$$\text{O}_2\text{N-C}_6\text{H}_4\text{-COOH} + \text{H}_2\text{O} \rightleftharpoons \text{O}_2\text{N-C}_6\text{H}_4\text{-COO}^- + \text{H}_3\text{O}^+ \quad K_{p\text{-NO2}} = 37.0 \times 10^{-5}$$

The equilibrium constant is even larger than for the nitro group in the *meta* position, indicating even greater electron-withdrawal.

Now consider the case in which an ethyl group is in the *para* position:

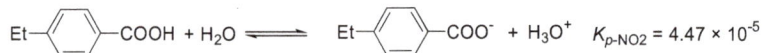

$$\text{Et-C}_6\text{H}_4\text{-COOH} + \text{H}_2\text{O} \rightleftharpoons \text{Et-C}_6\text{H}_4\text{-COO}^- + \text{H}_3\text{O}^+ \quad K_{p\text{-NO2}} = 4.47 \times 10^{-5}$$

In this case, the dissociation constant is lower than for the unsubstituted compound, indicating that the ethyl group is electron-donating, thereby destabilizing the negative charge that arises upon dissociation.

Hammett also observed that substituents have a similar effect on the dissociation of other organic acids. Consider the dissociation of phenylacetic acids:

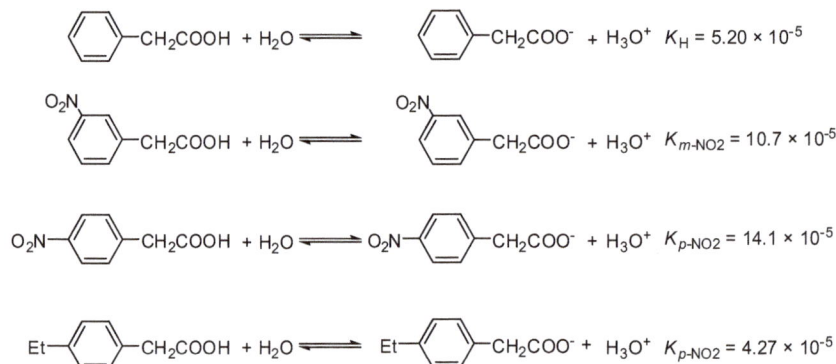

$$\text{C}_6\text{H}_5\text{-CH}_2\text{COOH} + \text{H}_2\text{O} \rightleftharpoons \text{C}_6\text{H}_5\text{-CH}_2\text{COO}^- + \text{H}_3\text{O}^+ \quad K_H = 5.20 \times 10^{-5}$$

$$\text{O}_2\text{N-C}_6\text{H}_4\text{-CH}_2\text{COOH} + \text{H}_2\text{O} \rightleftharpoons \text{O}_2\text{N-C}_6\text{H}_4\text{-CH}_2\text{COO}^- + \text{H}_3\text{O}^+ \quad K_{m\text{-NO2}} = 10.7 \times 10^{-5}$$

$$\text{O}_2\text{N-C}_6\text{H}_4\text{-CH}_2\text{COOH} + \text{H}_2\text{O} \rightleftharpoons \text{O}_2\text{N-C}_6\text{H}_4\text{-CH}_2\text{COO}^- + \text{H}_3\text{O}^+ \quad K_{p\text{-NO2}} = 14.1 \times 10^{-5}$$

$$\text{Et-C}_6\text{H}_4\text{-CH}_2\text{COOH} + \text{H}_2\text{O} \rightleftharpoons \text{Et-C}_6\text{H}_4\text{-CH}_2\text{COO}^- + \text{H}_3\text{O}^+ \quad K_{p\text{-NO2}} = 4.27 \times 10^{-5}$$

Electron-withdrawal by the nitro group increases dissociation, with the effect being less for the *meta* than for the *para* substituent, just as is observed for benzoic acid. The electron-donating ethyl group decreases the equilibrium constant, as is to be expected.

Data are typically graphed as illustrated in Fig. **2**:

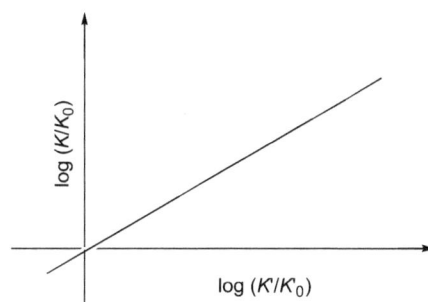

Figure 2: Example of a graph for a linear free energy relationship. K_0 and K'_0 represent equilibrium constants for unsubstituted compounds and K or K' for substituted derivatives. Values for the abscissa are calculated from the dissociation constants of unsubstituted and substituted benzoic acid. Values for the ordinate are obtained from phenylacetic acid with identical patterns of substitution.

Because this relationship is linear, equation (1) can be written:

$$\log (K/K_o) = \rho \log (K'/K'_o) \tag{1}$$

where ρ is the slope of the line. The values for the abscissa in Fig. **2** are always those for benzoic acid and are given via the symbol σ. Therefore, the following can be written:

$$\log (K/K_o) = \rho\sigma \tag{2}$$

ρ, the slope of the line, is a proportionality constant pertaining to a given equilibrium. It relates the effect of substituents on that equilibrium to the effect of those substituents on the benzoic acid equilibrium. That is, if the effect of substituents is proportionally greater than on the benzoic acid equilibrium, then $\rho > 1$; if the effect is less than on the benzoic acid equilibrium, $\rho < 1$. By definition, ρ for benzoic acid is equal to 1.

σ is a descriptor of the substituents. The magnitude of σ gives the relative strength of the electron-withdrawing or – donating of the substituents. σ is positive if the substituent is electron-withdrawing and negative if it is electron-donating.

These relationships as developed by Hammett are termed linear free energy relationships. Recall the equation relating free energy to an equilibrium constant.

$$\Delta G = - RT \ln K \tag{3}$$

That is, the free energy is proportional to the logarithm of the equilibrium constant. These linear free energy relationships are termed "extrathermodynamic". Although they can be stated in terms of thermodynamic parameters, no thermodynamic principle states that the relationships should be true.

To develop a better understanding of these relationships, it is instructive to consider some values of ρ and σ. Values of ρ are provided below:

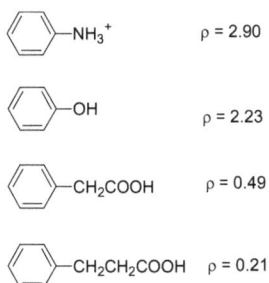

In the aniline and phenol equilibria, the dissociating hydrogen ion is one atom away from the phenyl ring, whereas in the benzoic acid equilibrium it is two atoms. Thus, substituents are able to exert a greater effect on the dissociation in aniline and phenol than in benzoic acid and the value is $\rho > 1$. In phenylacetic and phenyopropionic acids, the hydrogen ion that dissociates is three and four atoms away, respectively, from the phenyl ring.

Substituents are able to exert a lesser effect on the equilibrium than on the benzoic acid equilibrium and $\rho < 1$.

Some illustrative values of σ for substituents in the *meta* and *para* positions are given in Table **1**.

Table 1: σ values for some groups.

Substituent	σ_m	σ_p
-H	0.0	0.0
-NO$_2$	0.71	0.78
-Cl	0.37	0.23
-OMe	0.12	-0.27

By definition, σ for hydrogen is 0. The positive values of σ for the nitro goup indicates that it is electron-withdrawing. In order to understand the magnitudes of the σ values for the nitro group in *meta* versus *para* positions, the mechanisms of electron withdrawal or donation have to be considered. For a nitro group in the *meta* position, electron-withdrawal is due to an inductive effect produced by the electronegativity of the constituent atoms.

If only induction were operative, one would expect the electron-withdrawing effect of a nitro group in the *para* position to be less than in the *meta* position. The larger value for a *para*-substituted nitro group results from the combination of both inductive and resonance effects. For chlorine, the electronegativity of the atom produces an inductive electron-withdrawing effect, with the magnitude of the effect in the *para* position being less than in the *meta* position. For chlorine, only the inductive effect is possible.

The methoxy group can be electron-donating or –withdrawing, depending on the position of substitution. In the *meta* position, the electronegativity of the oxygen atom produces an inductive electron-withdrawing effect. In the *para* position, only a small inductive effect would be expected. Moreover, an electron-donating resonance effect occurs for the methoxy group in the *para* position, giving an overall electron-donating effect.

There are some limitations to these electronic parameters. For example, Hammet substituent constants cannot be measured for the *ortho* position since the substituents in this position have an important steric, as well as electronic, effect.

HYDROPHOBICITY

The formulation of the Hansch model was a real breakthrough in QSARs. First, Hansch recognized that *n*-octanol/water partition coefficients are, like some other molecular properties, an additive constitutive molecular property, *i.e.* they can be estimated from additive increments. The choice of *n*-octanol as reference solvent is justified by several reasons. *n*-Octanol is comparable to a biological membrane.

It is overall lipophilic, but its hydroxyl group can act as a hydrogen donor as well as a hydrogen acceptor. Thus, it may be considered to be "lipophilic but not hydrophobic", as biological membranes are. Lipophilicity is considered to be the ratio between the solubility of a substance in *n*-octanol and its solubility in water. It is usually expressed as the logarithm of the partition coefficient P, where P is equal to the ratio: drug in the *n*-octanol phase/drug in the aqueous phase. The determination of the partition coefficient P by the "shake flask" method with presaturated solvents is generally used, and extensive experimental details for this method have been published [5].

$$\log P = \log ([\text{drug}]_{org}/[\text{drug}]_{aq}) \qquad (4)$$

Secondly, Hansch formulated a parabolic equation to describe non-linear lipophilicity-activity relationships in a quantitative manner. Such non-linear relationships generally arise from the fact that the distribution of an organic compound in a biological multi-compartment system is determined by its lipophilicity. While hydrophilic compounds tend to remain in the aqueous phases, hydrophobic compounds get lost in membrane and lipid phases. Only compounds of intermediate lipophilicity have a good chance of crossing several aqueous and lipid barriers to arrive at their receptor site in reasonable time and concentration [6].

The binding of small molecules to biological macromolecules closely parallels the hydrophobicity factor as measured by the partition coefficient P [7]. Both linear [equation (5)] and non-linear [equation (6)] relationships between biological response and partition coefficients have been published [7] (Fig. **3**).

$$\log (1/C) = k_1 \log P + k_2 \tag{5}$$

$$\log (1/C) = -k_1 (\log P)^2 + k_2 \log P + k_3 \tag{6}$$

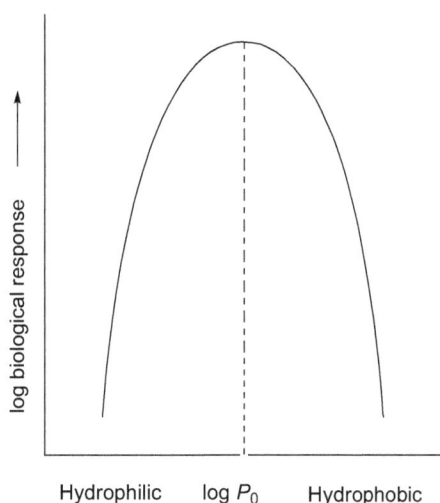

Figure 3: Parabolic dependency of biological response on *n*-octanol/water partition coefficient [equation (6)].

$\log (1/C)$ = logarithm of the inverse molar dose that produces a certain biological response in a fixed-time period. A logarithmic plot of partition coefficients against the corresponding activities resulted in a parabolic curve with the most active drugs located at the apex of the curve [6, 8, 9]. A theoretically plausible bilinear model was also proposed [10].

Partition coefficients can be calculated by knowing the contribution that various substituents make to hydrophobicity. This contribution is known as the substituent hydrophobicity constant (π).

The substituent hydrophobicity constant is a measure of how hydrophobic a substituent is, relative to hydrogen. The value can be obtained as follows. Partition coefficients are measured experimentally for a standard compound with and without a substituent (X). The hydrophobicity constant (π_X) for a substituent (X) is then obtained using equation (7):

$$\pi_X = \log P_X - \log P_H \tag{7}$$

where P_H is the partition coefficient for the standard compound, and P_X is the partition coefficient for the standard compound with the substituent. A positive value of π indicates that the substituent is more hydrophobic than hydrogen. A negative value indicates that the substituent is less hydrophobic. π_H is set to zero. π values are characteristic for the substituent and can be used to calculate how the partition coefficient of a drug would be affected by adding these substituents. The π-value for a nitro substituent is calculated from the log P of nitrobenzene and benzene.

$$\pi_{NO2} = \log P_{\text{nitrobenzene}} - \log P_{\text{benzene}} = 1.85 - 2.13 = -0.28 \qquad (8)$$

The partition coefficient P is a measure of the overall hydrophobicity of the drug and is therefore an important measure of how efficiently a drug is transported to its target site and bound to its receptor or enzyme. The π factor measures the hydrophobicity of a specific region on the skeleton of the drug. Thus, any hydrophobic bonding to a receptor involving that region will be more significant to the equation than the overall transport process. If the substituent is involved in hydrophobic bonding to a receptor or enzyme, then the QSAR equation using the π factor will emphasize that contribution to biological activity more dramatically than the equation using P.

STERIC FACTORS

The bulk, size, and shape of a drug may have an influence on the interaction with its receptor. Quantifying steric properties is more difficult than quantifying hydrophobic or electronic properties. Attempts have been made to quantify the steric features of subtituents by using Taft's steric factor (E_S). Taft in 1952 [11], as a modification to the Hammett equation, used the relative rate constants of the acid-catalysed hydrolysis of α-substituted methyl acetates to define the steric parameter because it had been shown that the rates of these hydrolyses were almost entirely dependent on steric factors. He used methyl acetate as his standard and defined E_S as:

$$E_S = \log [k_{(XCH2COOR)}/k_{(CH3COOR)}] \qquad (9)$$

where k is the rate constant of the appropriate hydrolysis and $E_S = 0$ when X = H. It is assumed that the values of E_S obtained for a group using the hydrolysis data are applicable to other structures containing that group. The methyl-based E_S values can be converted to H-based values by adding -1.24 to the corresponding methyl-based values.

Molar refractivity (MR) is the chameleon amongst the physicochemical parameters, despite its broad application in QSAR studies.

$$MR = MV \cdot (n^2 - 1)/(n^2 + 2) \qquad (10)$$

where MV = molecular volume, and n = refractive index. MR is generally scaled by 0.1.

It has been correlated with lipophilicity, molar volume, and steric bulk. Of course, due to its MV component [MV = MW/d (MW = molecular weight, d = density)], it is indeed related to volume and size of a substituent. The refractive index-related correction term in MR accounts for the polarizability and thus for the size and the polarity of a certain group [12, 13]. Since the refractive index n varies only slightly for most organic compounds, molar volume (MV) is usually highly interrelated with MR. For other steric parameters and more detailed information, refer to books and chapters by Hansch and Leo, Silipo and Vittoria, and Franke [3, 14-16].

Another approach to measuring the steric factor involves a computer programme called sterimol which calculates steric substituent values from standard bond angles, Van der Waals radii, bond lengths, and possible conformations for the substituent.

HANSCH EQUATION

The third and most important contribution was to add several different physicochemical parameters, like lipophilicity, electronic properties, and steric properties of substituents into one equation. These equations are known as Hansch equations and they usually relate biological activity to the most commonly used physicochemical properties [P and/or π, σ, and a steric factor (E_S)]. If the hydrophobicity values are limited to a small range then the equation will be linear, as follows [equation (11)]:

$$\log (1/C) = k_1 \log P + k_2 \sigma + k_3 E_S + k_4 \qquad (11)$$

If the P values are spread over a large range, then the equation will be parabolic [equation 12)]:

$$\log (1/C) = -k_1 (\log P)^2 + k_2 \log P + k_3 \sigma + k_4 E_S + k_5 \qquad (12)$$

The method of least squares may be used to estimate the regression coefficients (k_1-k_5) for the independent variables [$(\log P)^2$, $\log P$, σ, and E_S), and the value of the constant term (k_5) are determined by computer to obtain the best fitting line. The accuracy of fit of the equation to the data can be obtained by calculation of the correlation coefficient (r^2). If the regression equation is a perfect fit to the data ($r^2 = 1$), then a plot of the predicted versus observed should give a straight line with a slope of one and intercept of zero.

A guide to the overall significance of a regression model can be obtained by calculation of a quantity called the F statistic. An F statistic is used by looking up a standard value for F from a table of F statistics and comparing the calculated value with the tabulated one. If the calculated value is greater than the tabulated value, the equation is significant at that particular confidence level. Only the F values larger than the 95% significance limits prove the overall significance of a regression equation. As might be expected, the F values are greater for higher levels of significance.

$$F_{k,\,n-k-1} = r^2 \cdot (n-k-1)/k \cdot (1-r^2) \tag{13}$$

k is the number of independent variables in the equation, n is the number of data points. An F statistic is usually quoted as $F_{k,\,n-k-1}$.

The significance of the individual terms is assessed by calculation of the standard error of the regression coefficients, a measure of how much of the dependent variable prediction is contributed by that term. A statistic, the t statistic, may be calculated for each regression coefficient by division of the coefficient by its standard error (SE):

$$t = |\,b/\text{SE of } b\,| \quad t \text{ has to be taken as absolute value.} \tag{14}$$

Like the F statistic, the significance of t statistics is assessed by looking up a standard value in a table; the calculated value should exceed the tabulated one. As a rule of thumb, the regression coefficient should be at least twice as large as its standard error if it is to be considered significant. Several t- and F-distribution tables can be found [17].

Another useful statistics that can be calculated to characterize the fit of a regression model to a set of data is the standard error of prediction. This gives a measure of how well one might expect to be able to make individual predictions. The model will be useful if the prediction standard error is less than ten per cent of the range of measurements. The probability level is invariably 0.05 for QSAR.

Modern validation techniques are called bootstrapping or cross-validation. Cross-validation (CV) evaluates a model not by how well it fits the data but by how well it predicts data. The data set consisting of n compounds is divided into groups. Leaving out one group according to a fixed or random pattern, the multiple linear regression for the reduced set of data is recalculated and the missing values are predicted. This is repeated until every compound is left out once and only once. When each time only one compound is left out, this is referred to as the leave-one-out (LOO) method. A recommendation is to divide the data set into seven groups. Using the predicted values the PRESS (predictive residual sum of squares) and SD values are obtained as:

$$\text{PRESS} = \sum (\text{property}_{\text{observed}} - \text{property}_{\text{predicted}})^2 \tag{15}$$

$$\text{SD} = \sum (\text{property}_{\text{observed}} - \text{property}_{\text{mean}})^2 \tag{16}$$

and the cross-validated correlation coefficient is calculated as:

$$q^2 = r^2_{\text{CV}} = (\text{SD} - \text{PRESS})/\text{SD} \tag{17}$$

q^2 will always be smaller than r^2. When $q^2 > 0.3$, a model is considered significant [18].

To avoid statistically non-significant relationships or chance correlations, one should always apply the following rules of thumb [18]:

1. The ratio of compounds to descriptors should be > 5.

2. The descriptors should not be intercorrelated (interdescriptor correlation coefficient should be less than <
    0.5).

CHOLINE KINASE

The rational design of novel antiproliferative and antitumour strategies is based on the recognition of novel
intracellular targets for the modifications produced by the activity of different oncogenes and the changes in tumour
suppressor genes [19].

The development of human cancer is thought to be the result of mutations in multiple genes that control normal cell
proliferation, differentiation and apoptosis. Genes that are often found mutated in malignancies are referred to as
proto-oncogenes. Activation of these proto-oncogenes to oncogenes and/or the loss of function of tumour suppressor
genes may cause deranged intracellular signalling. The *ras* gene encodes 21-kDa proteins, which play an important
role in signal transduction. One of the most commonly altered gene products in human solid tumours includes Ras
proteins. Ras mutations, which are found in approximately 30% of all human malignancies, lead to an increase in
cell proliferation and tumour formation [20].

Choline kinase (ChoK), a cytosolic enzyme presents in various tissues, catalyses the phosphorylation of choline to
form phosphorylcholine (*P*Cho). Choline is not synthesized by the cells and either a high-affinity transport system in
nerve terminals, or an ubiquitous low-affinity transport system is responsible for its uptake. Free choline can also be
generated from phosphatidylcoholine (PC) by phopholipase D (PLD), an enzyme that is regulated by growth factors
and activated by oncogenes. More recently, PC hydrolysis has been implicated in cell signalling. PC is the most
abundant phospholipid in eukaryotic cell membranes and is hydrolyzed by phophatidylcholine-specific
phospholipase D (PC-PLD) to give choline and phosphatidic acid (PA).

ChoK has recently gained attention as a relevant component in signalling pathways involved in the regulation of cell
growth. This latter function was noticed by the discovery of elevated levels of *P*Cho in cells transformed by *ras*
oncogenes. Finally, some carcinogens, such as polycyclic aromatic hydrocarbons and 1,2-dimethylhydrazine,
induced rat liver and colon cancers with increased ChoK activity, further supporting the possible role of ChoK in
cancer generation.

The analysis of the inhibition of the structures was tested using a purified ChoK preparation from yeast as a target.
This assay allows us to evaluate the effect on compound activities without considering the possible passage through
membranes.

The antiproliferative assays was carried out on the HT-29 cell line. This cell line was established from a colon
adenocarcinoma, one of the most frequent solid cancers in humans that is also mainly resistant to chemotherapy,
making these cells appropriate for the search of new antitumour drugs.

The substituents at position 4 of the pyridinium moiety were electron-releasing, neutral or electron-withdrawing
groups (negative values of σ_R denote the electron-donating character and positive value, the electron-withdrawing
character of the substituent). To start with, the selection of the substituents to be introduced in position 4 of the
pyridinium nucleus was dictated by criteria of minimum effort and maximum informative content. Following this
line, the smallest number was chosen from easily synthetically accessible compounds which could give the
maximum spread and orthogonality of the main physicochemical properties, *i.e.*, the electronic and hydrophobic
ones. From the results obtained it is clear that the presence of electron-withdrawing groups (-COOH, **5** and -CN, **6**)
leads to inactive compounds as ChoK inhibitors.

Table **2** shows the structure, biological results and clog *P* values for compounds **1-10**. clog *P* values were calculated
by using the Ghose-Crippen modified atomic contribution system (ATOMIC5 option) of the PALLAS 2.0
programme [21].

Table 2: Structure, biological results[a] and parameter values for compounds 1-10.

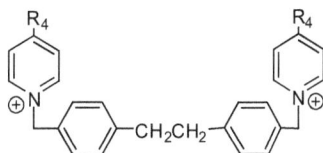

Comp	R_4	$(IC_{50})_{ChoK}$[a] (μM)	$(IC_{50})_{HT-29}$[a] (μM)	σ_R[b]	clog P[c]
1	-NMe$_2$	17.0	2.00	-0.88	-2.83
2	-NH$_2$	23.0	4.00	-0.80	-4.67
3	-CH$_2$OH	100.0	> 100.0	-0.07	-4.25
4	-CH$_3$	100.0	20.0	-0.16	-1.82
5	-COOH	136.7	> 1000	0.11	-3.50
6	-CN	> 1000	200	0.08	-3.15
7	-N(Allyl)$_2$	17.0	0.55	-0.80[d]	-0.44
8	-NC$_4$H$_8$[e]	20.0	1.00	-0.85[d]	-1.94
9	-NC$_5$H$_{10}$[f]	9.60	0.40	-0.89[d]	-0.93
10	-NC$_6$H$_{12}$[g]	15.0	0.40	-0.86[d]	0.09

[a]All values are the mean of two independent determinations performed in duplicate. [b]σ_R: Electronic parameter for resonance effects [22]. [c]Predicted by using the Ghose-Crippen modified atomic contribution system (opción ATOMIC5) of the PALLAS 2.0 programme [21]. [d]This value have been estimated by ^{13}C NMR spectroscopy [23]. [e]Pirrolidino. [f]Piperidino. [g]Perhydroazepino.

The inhibitory potency of the compounds correlates with the resonance effect of R_4. This is consistent with conventional chemical concepts. R_4 is in direct conjugation with the positively charged ring nitrogen. The greater resonance effect of R_4 would obviously cause better delocalization of the positive charge. This trend can be quantified using the resonance electronic effect of R_4, σ_R:

$$p(IC_{50})_{ChoK} = 3.92 \ (\pm 0.00) - 0.92 \ (\pm 0.06) \ \sigma_R \ n = 5, \ r = 0.994, \ s = 0.052 \ \textbf{(18)}$$

where $pIC_{50} = - \log IC_{50}$, bearing in mind that the higher the value of pIC_{50} the more potent is the compound. This equation presents highly significant correlation. Though the number of data points is small, the high correlation coefficients establish the importance of electronic characters (σ_R) of the substituents. Accordingly, substituents with higher or similar electron-releasing effects than the -NH$_2$ and -NMe$_2$ groups were sought. In principle the results found seem contradictory. The essential positive charge on the nitrogen is increased by the electron withdrawal by the substituents and thus, the interaction of the positive nitrogen atom with a putative anionic site of the enzyme is increased. This apparent inconsistency will be explained afterwards.

Endocyclic amino groups, such as the diallylamino, pyrrolidino, piperidino, and perhydroazepino moieties and an acyclic amino group such as the diallylamino one, could exert a favourable electron-releasing effect. Moreover their higher lipophilicities compared with those of the -NH$_2$ and -NMe$_2$ groups could help in the antiproliferative activities of even more potent compounds if lipophilicity plays a leading role. In a recent publication we have estimated by ^{13}C NMR spectroscopy the previously unknown σ_R descriptors for the diallylamino, pyrrolidino, piperidino and perhydroazepino groups in a simple, fast and reproducible manner [23].

Diagnostic Aspect

The electronic influence of R_4 on **1-10** alters its charge distribution and molecular orbital (MO) energies. The Hammett constants do not reflect which portion of the drug would actually be involved in the interaction with the enzyme. A quantum chemical treatment of electronic effects does provide some help in this direction and is potentially more powerful than the Hammett-type approach since it allows greater flexibility in the construction of the data set. Thus, MO calculations were made. To simplify the computational problem, the calculations were made on model compounds consisting of only one of the two substituted pyridinium moieties and in which the linker between the two charged nitrogen atoms was replaced by a methyl group (Table **3**) [24].

The inhibitory potency of ChoK of the analogues correlates well with the energy of the lowest unoccupied molecular orbital (E_{LUMO}) [equation (19)] and with the energy of the highest occupied molecular orbital (E_{HOMO}) [equation (20)]:

$$p(IC_{50})_{ChoK} = 5.33\ (\pm 0.17) + 0.02\ (\pm 0.00)\ E_{LUMO}\ n = 10,\ r = 0.878,\ s = 0.207,\ F_{1,8} = 26.83,\ \alpha < 0.001 \quad \textbf{(19)}$$

$$p(IC_{50})_{ChoK} = 8.83\ (\pm 0.85) + 0.01\ (\pm 0.00)\ E_{HOMO}\ n = 10,\ r = 0.874,\ s = 0.210,\ F_{1,8} = 25.81,\ \alpha < 0.001 \quad \textbf{(20)}$$

E_{LUMO} and E_{HOMO} are given in Kcal/mol. When $p(IC_{50})_{ChoK}$ was related with the energy of the frontier orbitals, it was found that the higher the energies of the HOMO or the LUMO are (*i.e.* closer to zero), the more potent the compound. If HOMO is considered to contribute at the level of interaction of the compound with ChoK, it follows that the compound acts as an electron donor, with the enzyme acting as an "electron sink".

Table 3: Structures for the model compounds mod 1-11, and biological data for the symmetrical bispyridinium compounds 1-11.[a]

$$R_4\text{---}\langle\bigcirc\rangle\overset{\oplus}{N}\text{---Me}$$

Comp	R$_4$	E_{HOMO} (kcal/mol)	E_{LUMO} (kcal/mol)	$p(IC_{50})_{ChoK}$[b]
mod 1	-NMe$_2$	-296.7	-30.62	4.77
mod 2	-NH$_2$	-315.4	-36.77	4.64
mod 3	-CH$_2$OH	-338.4	-55.03	4.00
mod 4	-Me	-341.0	-56.41	4.00
mod 5	-COOH	-346.4	-78.69	3.86
mod 6	-CN	-357.7	-88.26	-[c]
mod 7	-N(Allyl)$_2$	-285.1	-27.92	4.77
mod 8	-NC$_4$H$_8$[d]	-293.2	-28.61	4.70
mod 9	-NC$_5$H$_{10}$[e]	-290.0	-26.17	5.02
mod 10	-NC$_6$H$_{12}$[f]	-290.8	-27.36	4.82
mod 11	-H	-344.6	-63.50	4.51

[a]Model compound numbers (**mod 1-10**) correspond to the compound numbers of Table **2** (**1-10**); in addition, the R$_4$-unsubstituted model compound has been included; [b]All values are the means of two independent determinations performed in duplicate; pIC_{50} = -log IC$_{50}$; the pIC_{50} of the corresponding bispyridinium compound of table **2** is given for simplicity; [c]It cannot be accurately calculated because IC$_{50}$ > 1000 μM; [d]pirrolidino; [e]piperidino; [f]perhydroazepino.

Fundamental chemical concepts are in discordance with this because these compounds are electron deficient and cannot act as electron donors. It is therefore difficult to attribute a chemical meaning to the E_{HOMO} correlation. In any thorough investigation of substituent effects, it is essential to prove that one's conclusions are *both* statistically valid *and* make chemical sense. Neither approach is sufficient alone [24].

Solvation of the Model Compounds

However, if LUMO is assumed to contribute at the level of interaction of the compound with ChoK, it is necessary to consider the possibility of the formation of a charge transfer interaction of the HOMO of ChoK with the LUMO of the compound (Fig. **4**).

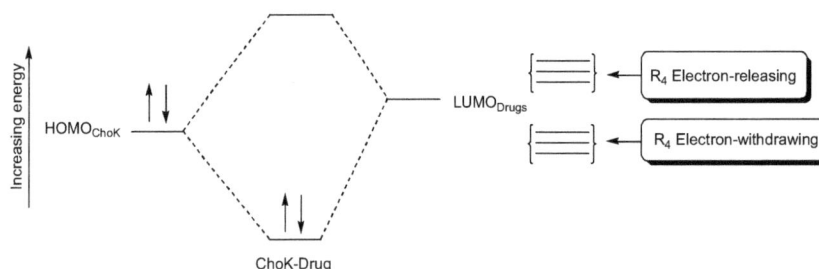

Figure 4: Interaction between HOMO of ChoK and LUMO of drugs.

With the solvent (H_2O) molecules acting as electron donors, the bispyridinium compounds **1-11** behave as electron acceptors. The increase of the E_{LUMO} of the molecule would result in its weaker solvation, and thus, a stronger interaction with ChoK. A possible chemical meaning for the E_{LUMO} correlation is therefore offered by the hypothesis that a higher value for E_{LUMO} indicates a weaker solvation of the compound (Fig. **5**) [24].

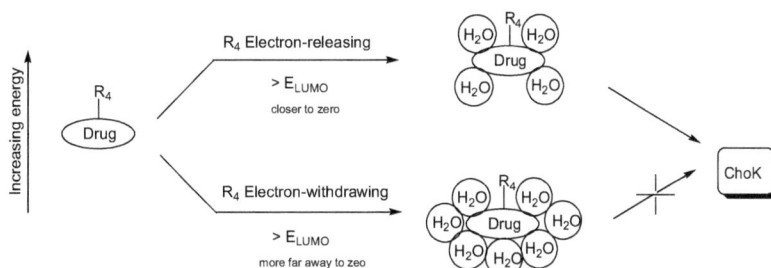

Figure 5: Solvation of model compounds.

QSAR Studies on the ChoK Inhibition and clog P

In order to study the possible influence of lipophilicity on the inhibition of ChoK under *ex vivo* conditions, we selected structures with the following characteristics:

1.   Cationic heads that allow the dispersion to a great extent of the positive charge with a "zero electronic effect", *i. e.*, with no substituents at position 4. To this end unsubstituted quinolinium and isoquinolinium rings have been used.

2.   Aralkyl spacers with different number of methylene groups.

Table 4: Structures, activity data and parameters used for deriving equation (21).

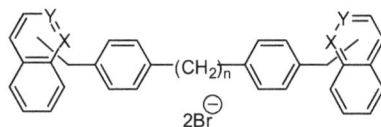

Comp	X	Y	n	$(IC_{50})_{ChoK}$[a] (μM)	$(IC_{50})_{HT-29}$[a] (μM)	clog P[b]
12	=N$^+$-	=CH-	0	50	10	-0.71
13	=N$^+$-	=CH-	1	100	6.02	-0.86
14	=N$^+$-	=CH-	2	34	4	-0.43
15	=N$^+$-	=CH-	3	9	2.5	0.08
16	=CH-	=N$^+$-	0	>100	ND[c]	-0.85
17	=CH-	=N$^+$-	1	60	20	-1.00
18	=CH-	=N$^+$-	2	60	20	-0.57
19	=CH-	=N$^+$-	3	20	2	-0.06

[a]All values are the means of two independent determinations performed in duplicate. [b]Predicted by using the Ghose-Crippen modified atomic contribution system (option ATOMIC5) of the PALLAS 2.0 programme [21]. [c]ND: Not determined.

For these compounds, the ChoK inhibition activity is found to be correlated with lipophilicity as shown in equation (21):

$$p(IC_{50})_{ChoK} = 4.83 \, (\pm 0.09) + 0.81 \, (\pm 0.15) \text{ clog } P \; n = 7, r = 0.922, s = 0.151, F_{1,5} = 28.57 \text{ (significance at } \alpha < 0.005)$$

$$(21)$$

On the basis of this equation (21), we suggest that hydrophobic interactions may occur between the bissalts **12-19** and ChoK. Hydrophobicity is not only related to absorption and distribution phenomena but also to the interactions with the active site of ChoK. Besides the electrostatic interactions, the cationic heads and the spacers between the two positive nitrogen atoms appear to hydrophobically bind more strongly to the enzyme. It must be kept in mind that all compounds have been tested in an *ex vivo* system using purified ChoK from yeast (in a test tube without cells) as a target. This assay has allowed the evaluation of the effect on **12-19** activities without considering the possible effects on other properties such as permeability into intact cells.

Table 5: Structure, biological data and values of parameters for compounds 20 and 21.

Comp	R$_4$	(IC$_{50}$)$_{ChoK}$[a] (μM)	(IC$_{50}$)$_{HT-29}$[a] (μM)	σ$_R$[b]	clog P[c]
20	-NH$_2$	10.0	2.00	-0.80	-2.13
21	-NHCOBu^f	10.5	4.74	-0.35^d	1.40

[a]All values are the means of two independent determinations performed in duplicate. [b]σ$_R$: Electronic parameter for resonance effects [22]. [c]Predicted by using the Ghose-Crippen modified atomic contribution system (option ATOMIC5) of the PALLAS 2.0 programme [21]. ^{d}Due to the fact that the σ$_R$ pivaloylamino group is not available, the σ$_R$ acetamido group has been used instead [22].

Due to the fact that both the electron-donating ability of the substituent at position 4 of the heteroaromatic cationic head (Table **2**) and the lipophilicity of the bissalts (Table **3**) play a very significant role in the inhibition of ChoK, we tried to put together these two features in the same molecule, and prepared compounds **20** and **21** (Table **5**) with the idea of obtaining even more potent ChoK inhibitors. It must be pointed out that the -NH$_2$ group is a strong electron-donating group while the pivaloylamino moiety should be a weak one. The results came up to our expectations and we next attempted to correlate the ChoK inhibitory potency with the two descriptors, obtaining equation (22), including all the compounds of Tables 2, 4 and 5:

$$p(IC_{50})_{ChoK} = 4.44 - 0.73\ (\pm 0.14)\ \sigma_R + 0.12\ (\pm 0.04)\ \text{clog}\ P\ n = 19, r = 0.836, s = 0.241, F_{2,16} = 18.61\ \text{(significance at}$$
$$\alpha < 0.001) \tag{22}$$

Interestingly, our QSAR studies showed that the potency of inhibitors does not necessarily depend on overall log P but on the substituent constant π at a specific site on the molecules. The symmetrical molecules present two clearly differentiated moieties: a linker of lipophylic nature and the cationic heads constituted by the chemical environment of quaternized nitrogen. The use of such site-specific π factors fits very well in equation (23):

$$p(IC_{50})_{ChoK} = 0.55 - 1.04\ (\pm 0.13)\ \sigma_R + 0.63\ (\pm 0.15)\ \pi_{linker} + 0.30\ (\pm 0.08)\ \pi_{cat\ head}\ n = 19, r = 0.917, s = 0.181, F_{3,15} =$$
$$26.46\ \text{(significance at}\ \alpha < 0.001) \tag{23}$$

In deriving equation (7) we must know that $\pi_{cat\ head}$ is zero (π_{2H} due to the H-2 and H-3 protons of the pyridinium moiety) for compounds **1-10**, while it is 1.27 ($\pi_{CH2=CH-CH2}$ is the contribution of the benzene ring fused to the pyridinium one) for the bisquinolinium and bisisoquinolinium structures **12-21**. π_{linker} is the substituent constant of the -CH$_2$-C$_6$H$_4$-(CH$_2$)$_n$-C$_6$H$_4$-CH$_2$- grouping, ranging from 5.14 (n = 0) and 6.28 (n = 3).

Both the higher coefficient and value of π_{linker} compared with those of $\pi_{cat\ head}$ lead to the conclusion that the former hydrophobicity component is far more important than the latter. In conclusion, the positive coefficients of the π terms means that hydrophobic moieties and electron-donating groups favour the ChoK inhibitory activity, at least within the spanned range of spacers and heteroaromatic rings used.

Antiproliferative Activities of Bisquinolinium Compounds

Studies have been aimed at the establishment of structure-activity relationships and the structural parameters that define Choline Kinase (ChoK) inhibitory and antiproliferative activities of a set of forty bisquinolinium compounds. These derivatives have electron-releasing groups at position 4. With the aim of obtaining new structure-activity relationships and the study in depth of the structural parameters that define the ChoK inhibitory and antiproliferative activities, the synthesis of a new set of compounds is proposed based on changing the pyridinium for quinolinium moieties of the biscationic acyclic compounds.

The aim of this section specifically focuses on studying the effect to be expected on the biological activities by a variation in the linker that connects the two quinolinium cations. These quinolinium moieties have electron-releasing groups at their position 4, with other different groups at positions 3, 7 and 8 of the heterocycle (Fig. **4**) [25].

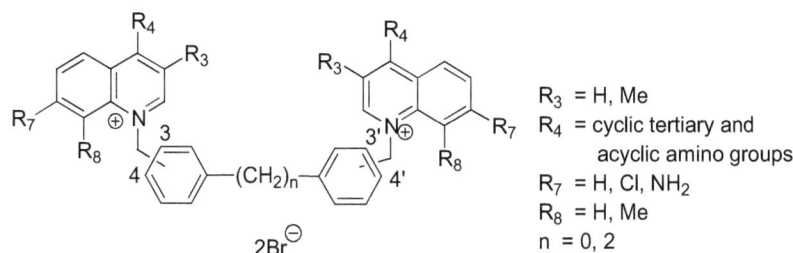

Figure 6: Bisquinolinium compounds.

There was a trial to correlate the human ChoK inhibitory activity for the whole set of compounds with the electronic and lipophilic parameters, but all the attempts turned out to be fruitless. In general it can be deduced that the activity against the HT-29 cell line is greater than the corresponding activity against ChoK, with which the symmetrical bisquaternized salts could act on another point of the pathway triggered by *ras* activation [25].

The octanol-water partition coefficient, used in its logarithmic form (log *P*), is the most widely accepted measure of lipophilicity. Reproducibility and accuracy of experimental log *P* determinations are not exact for extremely lipophilic and/or hydrophilic compounds such as the bisquinolinium structures (Fig. **4**). Fragmental methods make it possible to create data banks and to perform log *P* calculations by computer.

The clog *P* values of the bissalts were calculated by using the Ghose-Crippen modified atomic contribution system [26] (ATOMIC5 option) of the PALLAS 2.0 program [21]. π_{spacer} is the substituent constant for the linker calculated by using the Ghose-Crippen modified atomic contribution system [26] (ATOMIC5 option) of the PALLAS 2.0 program [21].

One of the most important chemico-physical properties used in QSAR studies is the molar refractivity (MR). The significance of MR in QSAR equations of some ligand-enzyme interactions has being interpreted with the help of 3D structures. These investigations showed that substituents modelled by MR bind in polar areas, while substituents modelled by a π bind in a hydrophobic space [27, 28]. Correspondingly, a positive sign of MR in a QSAR equation can be explained by binding the substituents to a polar surface, while a negative sign or a nonlinear relationship indicates a limited area or steric hindrance at this binding site [28].

The Hammett-type σ_R values for the amino, dimethylamino and anilino groups were taken from the Hansch and Leo tables [13], whilst we have previously published [23] such values for the pyrrolidino, perhydroazepino, and *N*-methylanilino groups. The same methodology [23] was used to estimate the unknown σ_R value for the 4-chloro-*N*-methylanilino group by using the ^{13}C chemical shifts of the previously reported compounds 1,1'-biphenyl-3,3'-diylmethylene)bis[4-(4-chloro-*N*-methylanilino)- pyridinium] dibromide and 1,1'-biphenyl-4,4'-diylmethylene)bis[4-(4-chloro-*N*-methylanilino)pyridinium] dibromide [29].

When the effect of the volume $(MR_8)^\S$, global lipophilicity (clog *P*), the substituent constant of the linker, and the electronic parameters $(\sigma_{R4})^\S$ of the R$_4$ substituent were taken into account for the antiproliferative activity, equation (23) was obtained:

$$p(IC_{50})_{HT-29} = -2.66 - 0.03 \ (\pm 0.00) \ MR_8^2 + 0.10 \ (\pm 0.02) \ clog P + 1.05 \ (\pm 0.31) \ \pi_{linker} - 3.73 \ (\pm 0.71) \ \sigma_R \ \textbf{(24)}$$

---

§ The subscript refers to the position of the substituent

$$n = 40, r = 0.920, s = 0.223, F_{4,35} = 47.9 \; \alpha < 0.001$$

Equation (24) gives a good cross-validated r^2_{CV} value (q^2) of 0.837. A most significant aspect of this study is that every data point was included in the formulation of equation (24). Such an outcome is rarely found and merits special consideration. We find this to be quite unusual since one usually finds some outliers in QSAR papers which must be omitted to obtain a high correlation.

From equation (24) the following aspects may be highlighted: (1) the coefficient of MR_8 is a squared negative term, and hence the presence of the methyl group at position 8 is detrimental in relation to the antiproliferative activity; accordingly, it is advisable that a hydrogen atom be in this position because this atom has a smaller value for MR; (2) there is no electronic contribution of the group located at position 7 of the quinolinium ring. This is most remarkable in the case of the 7-NH_2 group, which is located at the same relative position (although in the other aromatic ring) as the 4-substituent in relation to the N^+ atom, and its presence should have further facilitated the delocalization of the positive charge of the endocyclic N atom.

A plausible explanation is that the 7-methyl group exerts a steric hindrance making it impossible for that 7-NH_2 group to adopt a coplanar disposition in relation to the aromatic ring. This is necessary for the electronic delocalization to take place. Therefore, 7-substituent contributes only to the global lipophilicity of the molecules; (3) finally, lipophilicity contributes in two aspects to the antiproliferative activity: (a) on one hand, a global contribution (clog P) and on the other, a contribution at a specific site on the molecules (π_{linker}). Both descriptors are orthogonal and therefore the participation of both is justified in the QSAR equation.

The relative contribution of π_{linker} in equation (1) is higher than that of log P and, it can be hypothesized that favourable hydrophobic interactions between the enzyme and the linker would modulate the coupling inhibitor-ChoK. Although according to equation (1) the increase in the global lipophilicity and in the lipophilicity of the linker would augment the antiproliferative activity, the solubility was the reason for limiting the spacers to the 3,3'-, 4,4'-biphenyl and 4,4' bibenzyl moieties.

When the experimental $p(IC_{50})_{HT-29}$ values are correlated with the theoretical ones calculated by equation (24), equation (25) is obtained corresponding to the straight line represented in Fig. **5**:

$$p(IC_{50})_{HT-29 \; experimental} = -0.35 + 1.05 \; (\pm 0.08) \; p(IC_{50})_{HT-29 \; theoretical} \qquad \textbf{(25)}$$

$$n = 40, r = 0.916, s = 0.220, F_{1,38} = 199, \alpha < 0.001$$

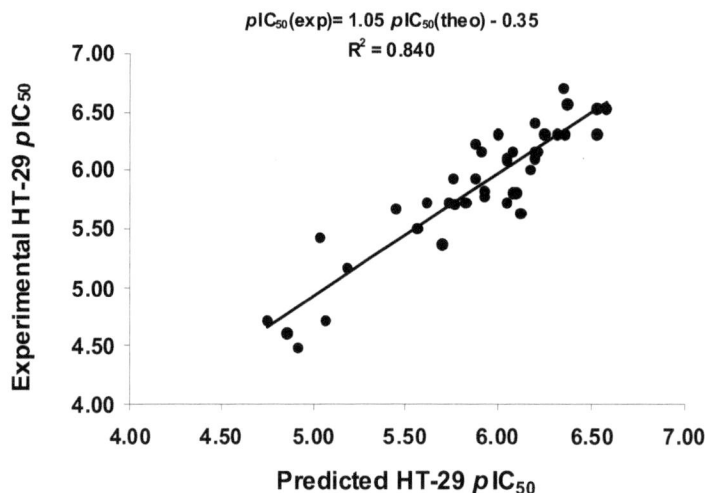

Figure 7: Graph between experimental and predicted antiproliferative activities for the test set.

CONCLUSIONS

Classical 2D-QSAR methods still play an important role in drug design, despite the progress in protein crystallography, molecular modelling, and structure-based drug design. QSAR methods are cheap and efficient tools to derive and prove hypotheses on structure-activity relationships in a quantitative manner, especially in those cases where the 3D structure of the biological target is not known. We have the ability to intuitively extract high-level information from facts at different levels, without being programmed like a computer. QSAR cannot and will never substitute the creativity and intuition of an experienced medicinal chemist. But our logical reasoning is limited to one or two, at most, three dimensions. QSAR aims at giving an objective interpretation of multidimensional results in medicinal chemistry and at deriving new hypotheses to an extent which is far beyond the intellectual capacity of the human mind.

REFERENCES

[1]   Hansch C, Leo A. Substituent Constants for Correlation Analysis in Chemistry and Biology. New York: John Wiley & Sons; 1979.

[2]   Kubinyi H, Wolff M. Burger's Medicinal Chemistry and Drug Discovery, Volume 1: Principles and Practice. New York: John Wiley & Sons; 1995.

[3]   Hansch C, Leo A, Heller SR. Exploring QSAR. Fundamentals and Applications in Chemistry and Biology. Washington, DC: American Chemical Society; 1995.

[4]   Kubinyi H, Mannhold R, Krogsgaard-Larsen, P, Timmerman, H. QSAR: Hansch Analysis and Related Approaches. New York: VCH; 1993.

[5]   Purcell WP, Bass, BE, Clayton, JM. Strategy of Drug Design. A Guide to Biological Activity. New York: John Wiley & Sons; 1973.

[6]   Hansch, C, Clayton, JM. Lipophilic character and biological activity of drugs. II: the parabolic case. J Pharm Sci 1973;62:1-21.

[7]   Hansch, C. Quantitative approach to biochemical structure-activity relationships. Acc Chem Res 1969;2:232-239 and references therein.

[8]   Hansch, C, Smith, N, Engle, R, Wood, H. Quantitative structure-activity relation of antineoplastic drugs. Nitrosoureas and triazenoimidazoles. Cancer Chemother Rep. 1972;56:443-456.

[9]   Montgomery, JA, Mayo, JG, Hansch, C. Quantitative structure-activity relations in anticancer agents. Activity of selected nitrosoureas against a solid tumour, the Lewis lung carcinoma. J Med Chem. 1974;17:477-480.

[10]   Kubinyi, H. Quantitative structure-activity relations. 7. The bilinear model, a new model for nonlinear dependence of biological activity on hydrophobic character. J Med Chem. 1977;20:625-629.

[11]   (a) Taft, RW. Linear Free Energy Relationships from Rates of Esterification and Hydrolysis of Aliphatic and Ortho-substituted Benzoate Esters. J Am Chem Soc. 1952;74:2729-2732; (b) Taft, RW. Polar and Steric Substituent Constants for Aliphatic and o-Benzoate Groups from Rates of Esterification and Hydrolysis of Esters. J Am Chem Soc. 1952;74:3120-3128; (c) Taft, RW. Linear Steric Energy Relationships. J Am Chem Soc. 1953;75:4538-4539.

[12]   van de Waterbeemd, H, Testa, B. The parametrization of lipophilicity and other structural properties in drug design. Adv Drug Res. 1987;16:85-225.

[13]   Dunn III, WJ. Molar refractivity as an independent variable in quantitative structure-activity studies. Eur J Med Chem 1977;12:109-112.

[14]   Hansch, C, Leo, A. Substituent Constants for Correlation Analysis in Chemistry and Biology. New York: Wiley; 1979.

[15]   Silipo, C, Vittoria, A. Principles and Usage of Steric Parameters in Correlation Analysis of Pesticides. Rational Approaches to Structure, Activity and Ecotoxicology of Agrochemicals. Draber, W, Fujita, T, Eds. Boca Raton, Florida: CRC Press; 1992.

[16.   Franke, R. Theoretical Drug Design Methods. Amsterdam: Elsevier; 1984.

[17]   Sachs, L. Applied Statistics. A Handbook of Techniques. New York: Springer-Verlag New York Inc; 1984.

[18]   van de Waterbeemd, H, Rose, S. Wermuth, CG. (Ed.). Quantitative Approaches to Structure-Activity Relationships. The Practice of Medicinal Chemistry. Amsterdam: Elsevier Academic Press; 2003.

[19]   Kerr, DJ, Workman, P. New Molecular Targets for Cancer Chemotherapy. Boca Raton, Florida: CRC Press; 1994.

[20]   Campos, J, Núñez, MC, Rodríguez, V, Gallo, MA, Espinosa, A. QSAR of 1,1'-(1,2-ethylenebisbenzyl)bis(4-substitutedpyridinium) Dibromides as Choline Kinase Inhibitors: a Different Approach for Antiproliferative Drug Design. Bioorg & Med Chem Lett 2000;10:767-770 and references therein.

[21]   PALLAS FRAME MODULE, a prediction tool of physicochemical parameters, is supplied by CompuDrug Chemistry, Ltd, PO Box 23196, Rochester, NY 14692.

[22]   Charton, M. Electrical effect substituent constants for correlation analysis. Prog Phys Org Chem 1981;13:119-251.

[23]   Campos, JM, Núñez, MC, Sánchez, RM, Gómez-Vidal, JÁ, Rodríguez-González, A, Báñez, M, Gallo, MA, Lacal, JC, Espinosa, A. Quantitative Structure-Activity Relationships for a Series of Symmetrical Bisquaternary Anticancer Compounds. Bioorg Med Chem 2002;10:2215-2231.

[24]   Campos, J, Núñez, MC, Rodríguez, V, Entrena, A, Hernández-Alcoceba, R, Fernández, F, Lacal, JC, Gallo, MA, Espinosa, A. LUMO energy of model compounds of bispyridinium compounds as an index for the inhibition of choline kinase. Eur J Med Chem 2001;36:215-225.

[25]   Sánchez-Martín, R, Campos, JM, Conejo-García, A, Cruz-López, O, Báñez-Coronel, M, Rodríguez-González, A, Gallo, MA, Lacal, JC, Espinosa, A. Symmetrical Bis-Quinolinium Compounds: New Human Choline Kinase Inhibitors with Antiproliferative Activity against the HT-29 Cell Line. J Med. Chem 2005;48:3354-3363.

[26]   Viswanadhan, VN, Ghose, AK, Revankar, GR, Robins, PK. Atomic physicochemical parameters for three-dimensional structure directed quantitative structure-activity relationships. 4. Additional parameters for hydrophobic and dispersive interactions and their application for an automated superposition of certain naturally occurring nucleoside antibiotics. J Chem Inf Comput Sci 1989;29:163-172.

[27]   Blaney, JM, Hansch, C. Quantitative Drug Design. Ramsden, CA, Ed. Comprehensive Medicinal Chemistry. The Rational Design, Mechanistic Study & Therapeutic Application of Chemical Compounds. Hansch, C, Sammes, PG, Taylor, JB, Eds. Oxford: Pergamon Press; 1990.

[28]   Hansch, C, Blaney, JM. Chemische Struktur und biologische Aktivität von Wirkstoffen. Methoden der Quantitativen Struckutr-Wirkung-Analyse, Seydel, JK, Schaper, K-J, Eds. Weinheim: Verlag Chemie; 1979.

[29]   Conejo-García, A, Báñez-Coronel, M, Sánchez-Martín, RM, Rodríguez-González, A, Ramos, A, Ramírez de Molina, A, Espinosa, A, Gallo, MA, Campos, JM, Lacal, JC. Influence of the linker in bispyridinium compounds on the inhibition of human choline kinase. J Med Chem 2004;47:5433-5440.

New Developments in Medicinal Chemistry Vol. 1, 2010, 95-113

CHAPTER 5

Rapid Development of Chiral Drugs in the Pharmaceutical Industry

María del C. Núñez, Miguel A. Gallo, Antonio Espinosa and Joaquín M. Campos

Department of Pharmaceutical Chemistry, School of Pharmacy, Campus Cartuja, Granada, Spain

Abstract: The issue of drug chirality is now a major theme in the design and development of new drugs, underpinned by a new understanding of the role of molecular recognition in many pharmacologically relevant events. In general, three methods are used for the production of a chiral drug: the chiral pool, separation of racemates, and asymmetric synthesis. Although the use of chiral drugs predates modern medicine, only since the 1980's has there been a significant increase in the development of chiral pharmaceutical drugs. The thalidomide tragedy increased awareness of stereochemistry in the action of drugs, and as a result the number of drugs administered as racemic compounds has steadily decreased. In 2001, more than 70% of the new chiral drugs approved were single enantiomers. Approximately 1 in 4 therapeutic agents are marked as racemic mixtures, the individual enantiomers of which frequently differ in both their pharmacodynamic and pharmacokinetic profiles. The use of racemates has become the subject of considerable discussion in recent years, and an area of concern for both the pharmaceutical industry and regulatory authorities. Pharmaceutical companies are required to justify each decision to manufacture a racemic drug in preference to its homochiral version. Moreover, the use of single enantiomers has a number of potential clinical advantages, including an improved therapeutic/pharmacological profile, a reduction in complex drug interactions, and simplified pharmacokinetics. In a number of instances stereochemical considerations have contributed to an understanding of the pharmacological effects observed of a drug administered as a racemate. However, relatively little is known of the influence of patient factors (e.g. disease state, age, gender and genetics) on drug enantiomer disposition and action in man. Examples may also be cited where the use of a single enantiomer, non-racemic mixtures and racemates of currently used agents may offer clinical advantages. The issues associated with drug chirality are complex and depend upon the relative merits of the individual agent. In the future it is likely that a number of existing racemates will be re-marketed as single enantiomer products with potentially improved clinical profiles and possible novel therapeutic indications.

INTRODUCTION

The importance of obtaining optically pure materials hardly requires restatement. The manufacture of chemical products applied either for the promotion of human health or to combat pests which otherwise adversely impact human food supply is now increasingly concerned with enantiomeric purity. A large proportion of such products contain at least one chiral centre. The desirable reasons for producing optically pure materials include the following:

1. Biological activity often associated with only one enantiomer.

2. Enantiomers may exhibit different types of activity, both of which may be beneficial, or one may be beneficial and the other undesirable; the production of only one enantiomer allows the separation of the effects.

3. The unwanted isomer is at least an "isomeric ballast" applied to the environment.

4. Registration considerations: production of material as the required enantiomer is now a question of law in certain countries, the unwanted enantiomer being considered as an impurity.

5. When the switch from racemate to enantiomer is feasible, there is the possibility to double the capacity of an industrial process.

6. The physical characteristics of enantiomers versus racemates may confer processing or formulation advantages [1].

It has been recognized for a long time that the shape of a molecule has considerable influence on its physiological action. Examples of property differentiation within enantiomer pairs are numerous and often dramatic. A selection is given in Table **1**.

Carlton A. Taft and Carlos H. T. P. Silva (Eds)

Table 1: Differences in the properties of enantiomers.

(S) Bitter taste	Asparagine	(R) Sweet taste
(S) Caraway odor	Carvone	(R) Spearmint odor
(R) Orange odor	Limonene	(S) Lemon odor
(R,R) Antibacterial	Chloramphenicol	(S,S) Inactive
(S) 5-6 More potent hypoprothrombinaemic agent than (R) [2]	Warfarin	(R) Less active

The Thalidomide Tragedy

The thalidomide tragedy of 1961 in Europe is a landmark in drug regulation. The sedative-hypnotic drug thalidomide exhibited irreversible neurotoxicity and teratological (mutagenic) effects as a result of which babies were born deformed. The drug was prescribed to pregnant women to counter morning sickness. Thalidomide is a racemate – of a glutamic-acid derivative – and in 1984, in the foreword of a book on X-ray crystallography [3], the following statement appeared: "The thalidomide tragedy would probably never have occurred if, instead of using the racemate, the (R)-isomer had been brought on to the market. In studies..... it was shown that after i.p. administration only the (S)-(-)-enantiomer exerts an embryotoxic and teratogenic effect.

The (R)-(+)-enantiomer is devoid of any of those effects under the same experimental conditions". This quote has been widely used subsequently, and was even alluded to in the citation for the 2001 Nobel Prize in Chemistry, which was awarded to Knowles, Noyori and Sharpless for the development of catalytic asymmetric synthesis, and has had a great impact on the development of new drugs [4]. Regrettably, the proposal that the thalidomide tragedy could have been avoided if the single enantiomer had been used is misleading, for two reasons:

1. First, it is based on unreliable biological data: the studies purported to show that (S)-(-)-thalidomide, was in the mouse – a species that is generally regarded as unresponsive – and involved very high doses [5]. However, earlier work in the rabbit, the species that is most sensitive to thalidomide, clearly showed the equal teratogenic potency of its enantiomers [6].

2. Second, the chiral centre in thalidomide is unstable in protonated media and undergoes a rapid configurational inversion [7]. So, the individual enantiomers of thalidomide are both inverted rapidly to the racemic mixture, process that occurs faster *in vivo* than *in vitro* [8].

Therefore, even if there were differences in the toxicity of the enantiomers of thalidomide, their rapid racemization *in vivo* would blunt them so that they could not be exploited. This case shows the importance of considering data in full and not leaping to conclusions, however tempting these may be [9].

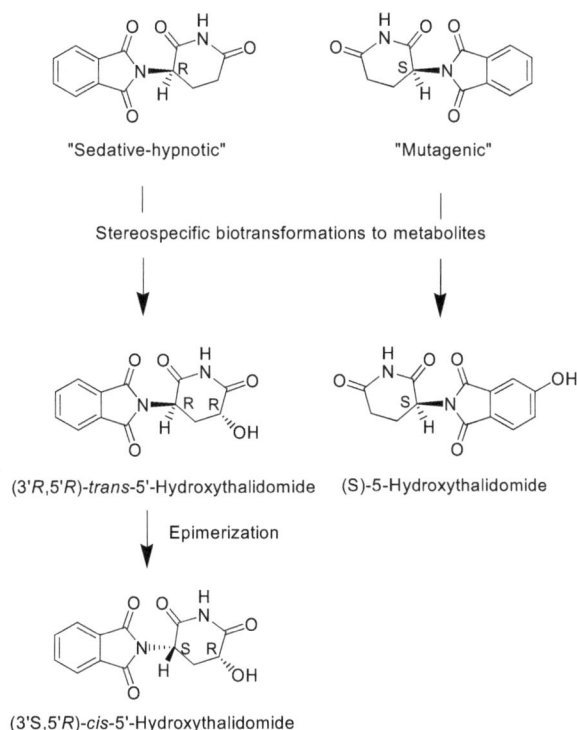

"Sedative-hypnotic"   "Mutagenic"

Stereospecific biotransformations to metabolites

(3'R,5'R)-*trans*-5'-Hydroxythalidomide   (S)-5-Hydroxythalidomide

Epimerization

(3'S,5'R)-*cis*-5'-Hydroxythalidomide

Figure 1: Thalidomide and stereospecific biotransformation to its metabolites.

The metabolic elimination of thalidomide (Fig. **1**) is mainly by pH-dependent spontaneous hydrolysis in all body fluids with an apparent mean clearance of 10 L/h for the (R)-(+)- and 21 L/h for the (S)-(-)-enantiomer in adult subjects. Blood concentrations of the (R)-(+)-enantiomer are consequently higher than those of the (S)-(-)-enantiomer at pseudoequilibrium. The metabolites in humans have been studied both from the incubation of thalidomide with human liver homogenates and *in vivo* in healthy volunteers. The *in vitro* studies demonstrated the hydrolysis products 5-hydroxythalidomide and 5'-hydroxythalidomide while *in vivo* only the 5'-hydroxy metabolite was found, in low concentrations, in plasma samples from eight healthy male volunteers who had received thalidomide orally. The hydrolysis of the thalidomide enantiomers by *in vitro* incubation was shown by Meyring *et al.*, to be stereospecific [10a].

The chiral centre of the thalidomide enantiomers is unaffected by the stereoselective biotransformation process. (3'R,5'R)-*trans*-5'-Hydroxythalidomide is the main metabolite of (R)-(+)-thalidomide, which epimerizes spontaneously to give the more stable (3'S,5'R)-*cis* isomer. On the contrary, (S)-(-)-thalidomide is preferentially metabolized by hydroxylation in the phthalimide moiety, resulting in the formation of (S)-5-hydroxythalidomide [10] (Fig. **1**).

It seems that a multitude of its pharmacological activities could be due not only to the mother molecule but also to its numerous chiral and achiral metabolites. Because of this *in vivo* interconversion of thalidomide, it is difficult to determine exactly the pharmacological effect of each enantiomer.

Thalidomide has been a subject of numerous studies, although the former is tainted from its past history. In 1998 the U.S. Food and Drug Administration approved thalidomide for use in treating leprosy symptoms and studies indicate some promising results for use in treating symptoms associated with AIDS, Behchet disease, lupus, Sjogren syndrome, rheumatoid arthritis, inflammatory bowel disease, macular degeneration, and some cancers [11].

PHARMACOLOGY

The body with its numerous homochiral compounds being amazingly chiral selective, will interact with each racemic drug differently and metabolize each enantiomer by a separate pathway to generate different pharmacological activities.

Racemic Drugs with one Major Bioactive Enantiomer

In this group, there are a number of cardiovascular drugs, agents widely used for the treatment of hypertension, heart failure, arrhytmias, and other diseases. Among these are the β-adrenergic blocking agents, calcium channel antagonists and angiotensin-converting enzyme (ACE) inhibitors. The majority of racemic pharmaceuticals have one major bioactive enantiomer (called eutomer), the other is inactive or less active (called distomer) or toxic or can exert other desired or undesired pharmacological properties.

Levorotary-isomer of all β-blockers is more potent in blocking β-adrenoceptors than their dextrorotary-isomer, such as (*S*)-(-)-propranolol (Fig. **2**) 100 times more active than its (*R*)-(+)-antipode [12,13]. A number of β-blockers are still marketed as racemic forms such as acebutolol, atenolol, alprenolol, betaxolol, carvedilol, metoprolol, labetalol, pindolol, etc., except timolol and penbutolol (Fig. **2**) that are used as single (S)-(-)-isomers.

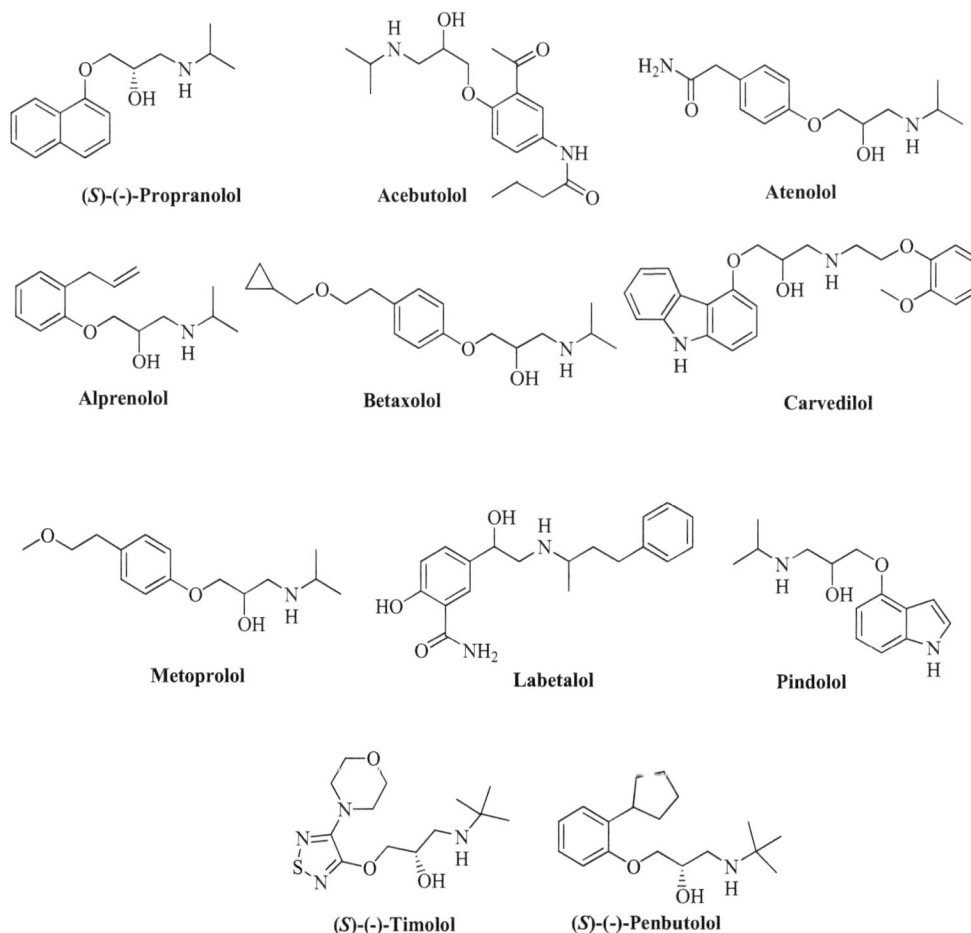

Figure 2: Racemic drugs with one major bioactive enantiomer (β-blockers).

Many calcium channel antagonists are used under racemic form such as verapamil, nicardipine, nimodipine, nisoldipine, felodipine, manidipine…, except diltiazem (Fig. **3**) that is a single (*S*,*S*)-(+)-isomer.

For example, the pharmacological potency of (*S*)-(-)-verapamil is 10-20 times greater than its (*R*)-(+)-antipode in terms of negative chromotropic effect on auricoventricular (AV) conduction and vasodilatator in man and animals [14,15].

All ACE inhibitors such as captopril, benazepril, enalapril, imidapril (Fig. **3**) are diastereoisomeric compounds and most of them are marketed as single isomers. Valsartan, an angiotensin II receptor antagonist, is used as its (*S*)-enantiomer and the activity of the (*R*)-enantiomer is clearly lower than the (*S*)-enantiomer (Fig. **4**) [16].

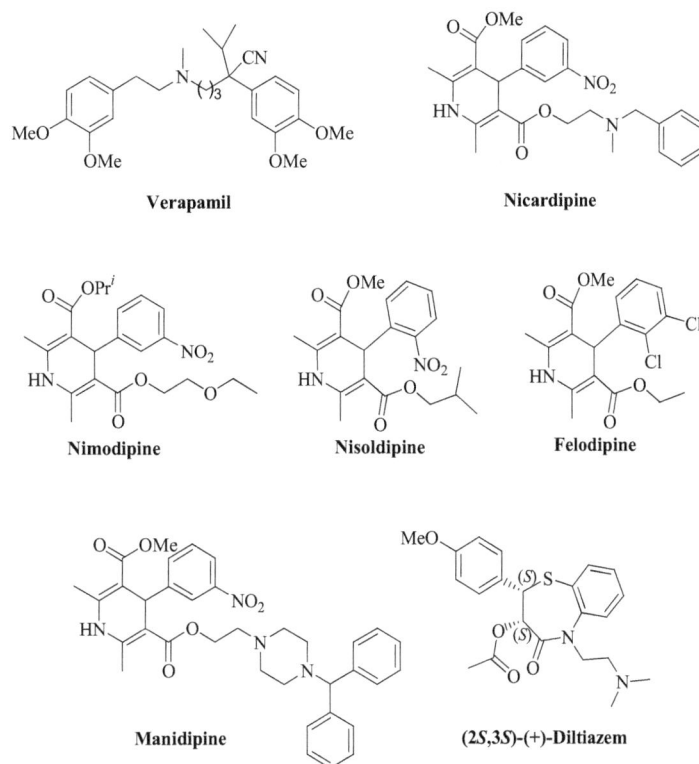

Figure 3: Racemic drugs with one major bioactive enantiomer (calcium-channel antagonists).

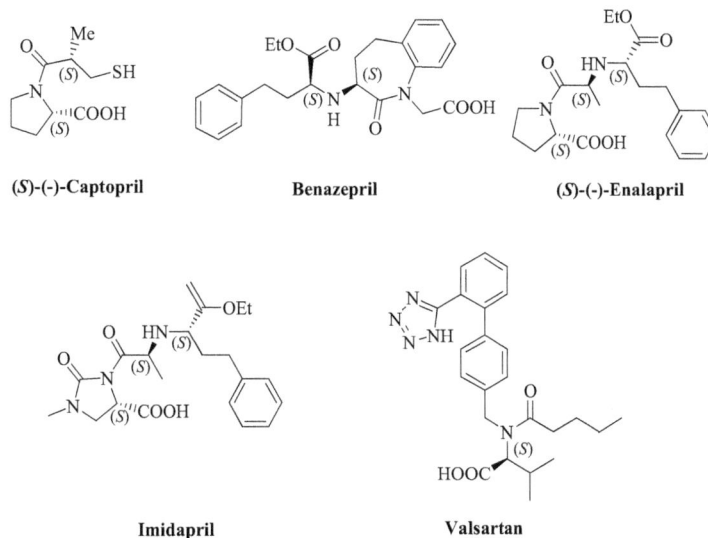

Figure 4: Racemic drugs with one major bioactive enantiomer (ACE).

Albuterol (salbutamol) is the racemate of 4-[2-(*tert*-butylamino)-1-hydroxyethyl]-2-(hydroxymethyl)phenol and is the leading bronchodilator, an adrenoceptor agonist that can increase the bronchial airway diameter without increasing heart rate. The bronchodilator activity resides in (*R*)-(-)-albuterol [Levalbuterol] (Fig. **5**). (*S*)-(+)-Albuterol, however, is not inert, as it indirectly antagonizes the benefits of (*R*)-(-)-albuterol and may have proinflammatory effects. There are pharmacokinetic differences between the enantiomers with (*S*)-(+)-albuterol being cleared more slowly.

The (*S*)-(+)-enantiomer tends to accumulate in preference to the therapeutically effective (*R*)-(-)-enantiomer. FDA approved a chiral switch drug, levalbuterol as a preservative-free nebulizer solution. However, some clinical studies have reported that it is neither safer nor more effective than the same dose of racemic albuterol. In contrast, levalbuterol may cost as much as 5 times more than its racemate [17,18].

In neurology and psychiatry, many pharmaceuticals used are chiral compounds and most of them are marketed as racemates. For example, (S)-(-)-secobarbital is more potent as an anaesthetic agent than (R)-(+)-secobarbital (Fig. **5**), *i.e.* it causes a smoother more rapid anaesthetic effect [19,20]. Ketamine (Fig. **5**) is an intravenous anaesthetic.

The (R)-(+)-isomer is more potent and less toxic than its (S)-(-)-antipode, but unfortunately, ketamine is still used as a racemic drug [21,22]. In the treatment of depression, (S)-(+)-citalopram [Escitalopram] (Fig. **5**) is over 100-fold more potent as a selective serotonin reuptake inhibitor than the (R)-(-)-enantiomer [23].

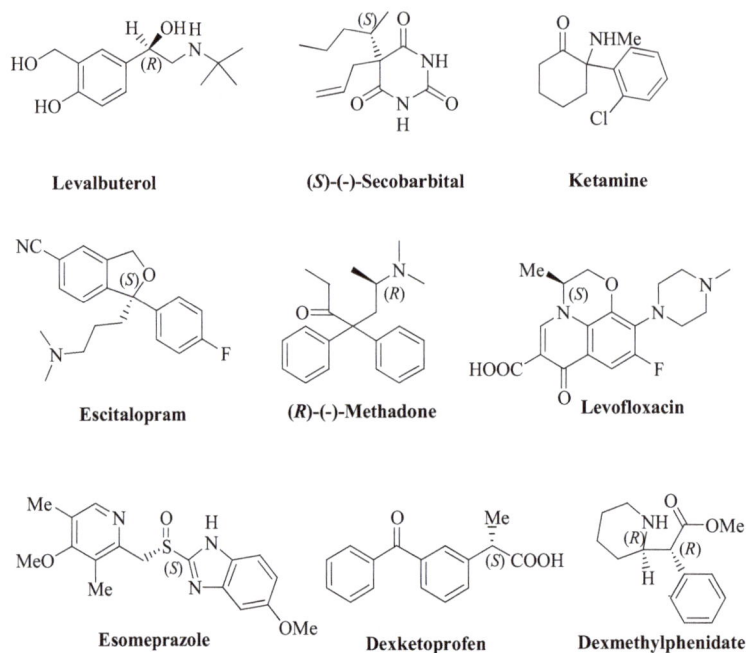

Figure 5: Racemic drugs with one major bioactive enantiomer.

Methadone, a central-acting analgesic with high affinity for μ-opiod receptors, has been used to treat opiate dependence and cancer pain. Methadone is a chiral synthetic compound used in therapy under a racemic mixture. In humans, (R)-(-)-methadone (Fig. **2**) is about 25-50 fold more potent as an analgesic than its (S)-(+) antipode [23,24].

The list of racemic drugs with one eutomer is long in the fields of anticonvulsants, antibiotics, antihistamics, proton pump inhibitors [25-27]. Some of these racemates recently undergo chiral switch to single enantiomer such as levofloxacin (from ofloxacin), levalbuterol (from albuterol), escitalopram (from citalopram), esomeprazole (from omeprazole), dexketoprofen (from ketoprofen), dexmethylphenidate (from methylphenidate).

Racemic Drugs with Equally Bioactive Enantiomers

There are few racemic drugs that could belong to this group such as cyclophosphamide (antineoplastic), flecainide (antiarrhythmic), and fluoxetine (antidepressant) [25] (Fig. **6**).

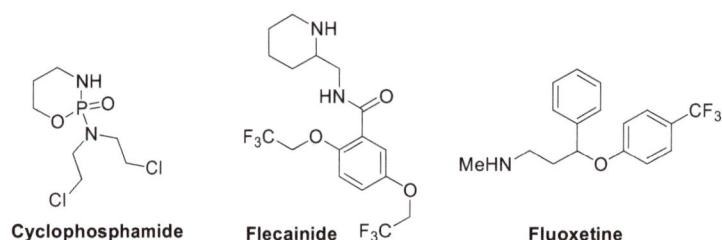

Figure 6: Racemic drugs with equally bioactive enantiomers.

Racemic Drugs with Chiral Inversion

The largest group of non-steroidal anti-inflammatory drugs (NSAID) that are currently in use is the 2-arylpropionic acids or "profens". These are widely used for the treatment of inflammatory diseases, such as rheumatoid arthritis, as both analgesics and antipyretics. However, the racemates are responsible for many adverse reactions reported each year. These adverse reactions affect a range of organs, including the gastrointestinal tract, kidney, bone marrow, the respiratory system and the liver. Unidirectional enzyme-mediated inversion was previously described only with profens, namely ibuprofen, ketoprofen, fenoprofen, benoxaprofen, *etc.* (Fig. **7**).

For example, the activities of the two enantiomers of ibuprofen and ketoprofen are essentially undistinguishable *in vivo*, owing to a unidirectional metabolic bioconversion of the (*R*)-enantiomers to the (*S*)-enantiomers. The combination of the stereospecificity of action, together with the configurational inversion reaction provided drug companies with a rationale for the use of the (*S*)-enantiomers of these drugs in therapy. The treatment with (*S*)-enantiomers reduces the total dose and also the toxicity associated with the (*R*)-enantiomer by removing the rate (and extent) of inversion as a source of variation in metabolism and pharmacological effects.

In the ketoprofen case, the (*S*)-(+)-ketoprofen [dexketoprofen] (Fig. **5**) is several times more potent than the racemate. The presentation of dexketoprofen as the tromethamine salt provides three advantages: effective analgesia at lower doses, rapid onset, and reduced gastric irritation and improved tolerability (due to the novel salt form).

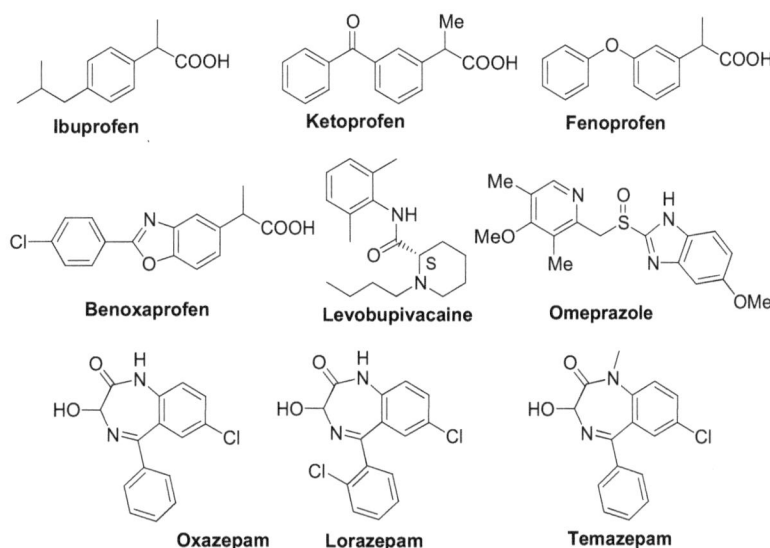

Figure 7: Racemic drugs with chiral inversion.

Similarly, racemic ibuprofen (Fig. **7**) undergoes rapid and substantial stereochemical inversion (about 50-60%), so that the metabolic exposure is mainly due to (*S*)-(+)-ibuprofen [dexibuprofen], with the presence of a little (*R*)-(-)-ibuprofen. The (*S*)-(+)-ibuprofen present is derived from both the 50% of the racemate in that form and the chiral inversion of the (*R*)-(-)-enantiomer. While racemic ibuprofen and (*S*)-(+)-ibuprofen are often viewed as being bioequivalent, the use of (*S*)-(+)-ibuprofen gives faster onset of action and reduces the variability in the stereochemical inversion as a source of variability in the pharmacological response [9].

Racemic bupivacaine is currently the most widely used long-acting local anaesthetic. Its usage include surgery and obstetrics; however, it has been associated with potentially fatal cardiotoxicity, particularly when given intravascularly by accident. (*S*)-(-)-Bupivacaine [levobupivacaine] (Fig. **7**) was introduced by Purdue Pharma LP under the tradename of Chirocaine® as a new long-acting local anaesthetic with a potentially reduced toxicity compared with bupivacaine. Numerous studies have compared levobupivacaine with bupivacaine and in most (but not all) studies there is evidence that levobupivacaine is less toxic [28]. Studies have also shown that, following i.v. administration, levobupivacaine produces significantly less effects on cardiovascular function than racemic bupivacaine does [29].

Omeprazole (Fig. **7**) presents one of the most interesting cases in drug development. Racemic omeprazole is a very potent inhibitor of gastric acid secretion, with a long-lasting action. In clinical studies, it proved superior to previous treatments for gastroesophageal reflux disease and peptic ulcers. Omeprazole is a gastric anti-secretory proton pump inhibitor [30] marketed under the tradenames of Losec® and Prilosec® by AstraZeneca. Launched in 1988 by Astra AB (in 1999, Astra AB merged with Zeneca PLC to create AstraZeneca PLC), omeprazole was a blockbuster commercial success and became the world's best-selling drug with sales of US $6.2 billion in 2000.

The first patents on omeprazole expired in the European Union in 1999 and in the United States of America in 2001. Based partly on the fact that omeprazole exhibits polymorphic metabolism, *i.e.* a few individuals (3% among the Caucasian populations and 15-20% among Orientals) metabolize omeprazole slowly (slow metabolizers) compared to the rest of the population (rapid metabolizers), AstraZeneca developed the chiral switch drug esomeprazole [which is the (*S*)-(-)-enantiomer of omeprazole] (Fig. **5**) based on the premise that the therapeutic benefit would be achieved by less inter-individual variation (slow versus rapid metabolizers), and that average higher plasma levels would provide higher dose efficiency in patients [31].

Esomeprazole was introduced as the magnesium trihydrate salt first in Europe (in 2000) and later in the USA (in 2001) under the trade name of Nexium®. Reflux oesophagitis was healed with a 40 mg per day dose of esomeprazole magnesium in ~ 78% of patients after four weeks of treatment and in 93% of patients after eight weeks, compared with 65% and 87% of patients respectively, treated daily with 20 mg of omeprazole. The benefits of esomeprazole have been extensively studied [32].

From inception, omeprazole has been described and claimed in its patents as 5-methoxy-2-(4-methoxy-3,5-dimethylpyridin-2-ylmethanesulfinyl)-1*H*-benzimidazole. But Jenkins *et al.* [33] confirmed that the synthetic methods did not yield a single compound having the methoxy group in the 5-position on the benzimidazole ring as previously thought, nor did all of the methods yield consistent results. In fact the presence of omeprazole as conventionally referred to as a bulk drug substance (in its solid state) was confirmed in the form of two pharmaceutically active compounds, having the methoxy group on the benzimidazole ring at the 6- and 5-positions.

3-Hydroxybenzodiazepines [oxazepam, lorazepam, temazepam (Fig. **7**)] can racemize *in vitro* by aqueous solutions. For the first time some authors [34] have found the difference in (*R*)-(-)- and (*S*)-(+)-oxazepam concentrations in treated rabbit serum. They explained that the chiral inversion by tautomerization of oxazepam cannot occur *in vivo* because each enantiomer is transported by proteins (albumin) with different affinity. The binding affinities of the eantiomers to albumin may inhibit the attack of hydroxyl ions from water and thus retard the racemization *in vivo*. Therefore, (*R*)-(-)- and (*S*)-(+)-oxazepam concentrations are different in the serum of these treated rabbits.

On the other hand, He *et al.* [35] have also demonstrated that the *in vitro* chiral inversion of these benzodiazepine enantiomers was temperature-dependent and was inhibited by lowering the temperature of the aqueous solutions to about 10 °C [35,36]. The (*S*)-(+)-oxazepam enantiomer is 100-200 fold more potent as a tranquilizer and sedative than (*R*)-(-)-oxazepam [36].

METHODS FOR OBTAINING OPTICALLY ACTIVE COMPOUNDS

This section is not concerned with detailed appraisal of the many and well known processes for obtaining pure enantiomers. Methodologies and principles of the techniques are described more fully in the corresponding references.

Separation of Racemates

The separation of enantiomers by chromatography has advanced over the past few decades [37-42], notably with the development of supercritical fluid chromatography (SFC) [38-42] and hybrid processes consisting of simulated moving bed (SMB) chromatography and crystallization [43,44]. However, the scale is often limited, and operational cost is high.

Racemic resolution by crystallization began in 1848 when Pasteur observed crystals of sodium ammonium tartrate that were mirror images with respect to each other. Until now, separation of enantiomers by crystallization can be classified in two main categories:

1. The use of a foreign chiral element to form diastereomers followed by fractional crystallization [45-49] or the formation of a diastereoselective host-guest inclusion complex [50]. The antituberculostatic drug ethambutol (Fig. **8**), and the cardiovascular drug diltiazem (Fig. **3**) are separated in this way. These methods of resolution are very widely used industrially.

2. The direct crystallization of one enantiomer from a racemic mixture, which includes the well-known "preferential crystallization" of pure enantiomers form conglomerate mixtures [45,51-53]. This unusual enantiomeric resolution is referred to as "preferential enrichment" [53-55], and the application of crystallization inhibitors to chiral separation in racemic compound-forming systems has been reported [56-58]. The anti-typhoid chloramphenicol (Fig. **8**) is separated in this way. This is widely used in the industry but hardly 20 per cent of racemates appear in this form of mechanical mixture or "conglomerates".

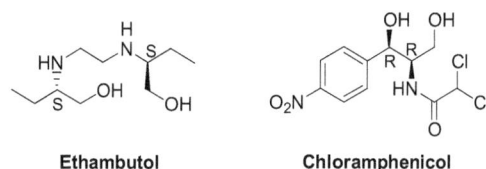

Figure 8: Separation of racemates.

Asymmetric Synthesis

The field of asymmetric synthesis has enjoyed tremendous progress over the last few decades with the advent of asymmetric reactions and enantioselective catalysts [1,62]. There are two possibilities: (1) Non-enzymatic methods, and (2) Enzymatic methods.

Non-Enzymatic Methods

Asymmetric Hydrogenation

The asymmetric hydrogenation, the Sharpless epoxidation amongst asymmetric oxidations, and cycloadditions are the most important non-enzymatic processes. Knowles and co-workers at Monsanto discovered that a cationic rhodium complex containing DIPAMP, a chelating diphosphine with two chiral phosphorus atoms, catalyzes highly enantioselective hydrogenations of enamides such as **1** (Fig. **9**). In the key step of the synthesis of L-DOPA, enamide **1** is hydrogenated in the presence of a catalytic amount of [Rh(*R*,*R*)-DIPAMP)COD]$^+$BF$_4^-$ affording the protected aminoacid **2** in quantitative yield and in 95% ee. A simple acid-catalyzed hydrolysis step completes the synthesis of L-DOPA [63].

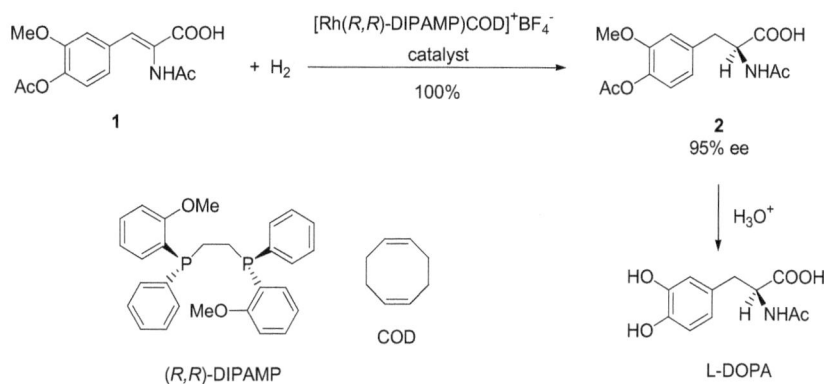

Figure 9: The Monsanto synthesis of L-DOPA using catalytic asymmetric hydrogenation.

The *Monsanto Process* was the first commercialized catalytic asymmetric synthesis employing a chiral transition metal complex and it has been in operation since 1974. The spectacular success of this L-DOPA synthesis has significantly contributed to the remarkable growth of research aimed at the development and application of other catalytic asymmetric reactions in ensuing years.

Mechanism of Catalytic Asymmetric Hydrogenation

The reaction mechanism of the phosphine Rh complex-catalyzed hydrogenation has been elucidated by Halpern [64], as also the mechanism of hydrogenation of an enamide, using a diphosphine yielding a phenylalanine derivative as shown in Fig. **10**.

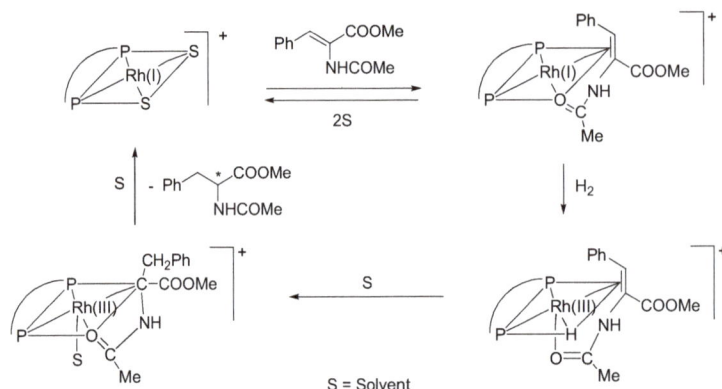

Figure 10: Mechanism of the Rh-diphosphine-catalyzed hydrogenation of an enamide.

First, solvent molecules (S) in the catalyst precursor are displaced by the olefinic substrate to form a chelate-Rh complex in which the olefinic bond and the carbonyl oxygen interact with the Rh(I) centre. Hydrogen is oxidatively added to the metal to form a Rh(III) dihydride intermediate. The two hydrogen atoms on the metal are successively transferred to the carbon atoms of the coordinated olefinic bond by way of a five-membered chelate alkyl-Rh(III) intermediate. The secondary binding of the carbonyl oxygen of the amide moiety results in a ring system that stabilizes the reactive intermediate. Kinetic data suggest that, at roomtemperature, the oxidative addition of H_2 is rate-limiting for the overall reaction. When an appropriate chiral phosphine ligand and proper reaction conditions are chosen, high eantioselectivity is achieved. If a diphosphine ligand of C_2 symmetry is used, two diastereoisomers of the enamide coordination complex can be produced, because the olefin interacts with either the *re* face or the *si* face. This interaction leads to enantiomeric phenylalanine products via diastereoisomeric Rh(III) complexes.

Noyori's General Hydrogenation Catalysts

Noyori's discovery of the BINAP-Ru(II) complex catalysts was a major advance in stereoselective organic synthesis [65]. The scope of the application of these catalysts is far reaching. These chiral Ru complexes serve as catalyst precursors for the highly enantioselective hydrogenation of a range α,β- and β,γ-unsaturated carboxylic acids [65]. An example is shown in Fig. **11**.

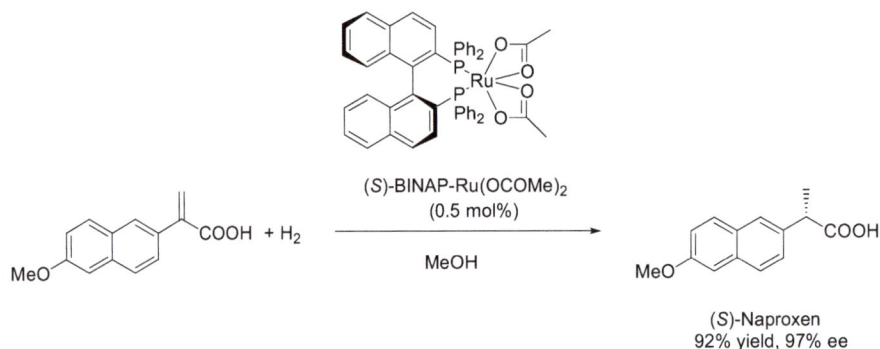

(*S*)-BINAP-Ru(OCOMe)$_2$
(0.5 mol%)

MeOH

(*S*)-Naproxen
92% yield, 97% ee

Figure 11: The anti-inflammatory agent (*S*)-naproxen is produced in high yield and high eantiomeric excess using the Noyori's catalyst.

This reaction, unlike Rh(I)-catalyzed olefin hydrogenation, proceeds via a metal monohydride mechanism. The enantioselectivity is much higher in the use of the Rh catalyst and the sense of asymmetric induction is the opposite.

Sharpless's Chirally Catalyzed Oxidations

Parallel to the progress in catalytic asymmetric hydrogenations Barry Sharpless has developed chiral catalysts for very important oxidation reactions. The epoxidation reaction discovered in 1980 by Sharpless and Kazuki is an example of a strategy of using a reagent to achieve stereochemical control. Using titanium(IV) tetraisopropoxide, *tert*-butyl hydroperoxide, and an enantiomerically pure dialkyl tartrate, the Sharpless reaction accomplished the epoxidation of allylic alcohols with excellent etereoselectivity. This powerful reaction is very predictable. If the D-(-)-tartrate ligand [D-(-)-DET] is used in epoxidation, the oxygen atom is delivered to the top face of the olefin where the allylic alcohol is depicted as in Fig. **12** (i.e. the OH group in the lower right hand corner).

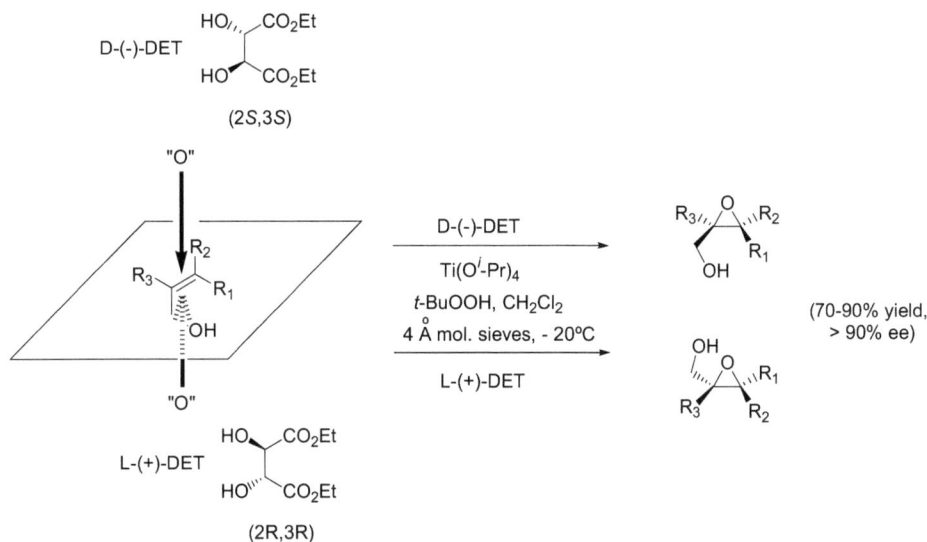

Figure 12: The predictive stereoselectivity of the Sharpless epoxidation.

The L-(+)-tartrate ligand [L-(+)-DET] allows the bottom face of the olefin to be epoxidised. When achiral allylic alcohols are employed, the Sharpless reaction exhibits exceptional enantiofacial selectivity (*ca.* 100:1) and provides convenient access to synthetically versatile epoxy alcohols.

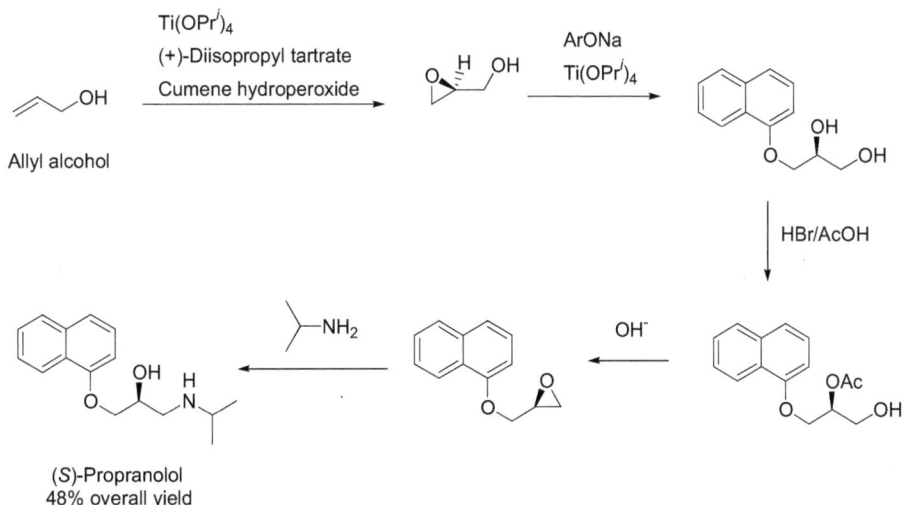

Figure 13: Routine synthesis of (*S*)-propranolol.

The emergence of the powerful Sharpless asymmetric epoxidation in the 1980s has stimulated major advances in both academic and industrial organic synthesis. Through the action of an eantiomerically pure titanium-tartrate complex, a myriad of achiral and chiral allylic alcohols can be epoxidised with exceptional stereoselectivity. Interest in the Sharpless epoxidation as a tool for industrial organic synthesis increased substantially after Sharpless *et al.* discovered that the asymmetric epoxidation process can be conducted with catalytic amounts of the enantiomerically pure titanium-tartrate complex simply by adding molecular sieves to the epoxidation reaction mixture [66].

Using this practical and reproducible catalytic variant, an industrial process for ton-scale productions of (*S*)- and (*R*)-glycidol and (*S*)- and (*R*)-methylglycidol has been developed. These low-molecular weight epoxy alcohols are versatile building blocks for the synthesis of a number of chiral molecules.

As far as drug synthesis is concerned, one of the most significant applications of the Sharpless method amongst the innumerable ones found in the past 20 years is the routine preparation (Fig. **13**) of antipodal pairs of known chirality of β-blockers such as propranolol [67].

Enzymatic Methods

Biocatalysis or biotransformation encompasses the use of biological systems, whether whole cells, cellular extracts or isolated enzymes, to catalyze the conversion of one compound to another. The potential of microorganisms and enzymes for the transformation of synthetic compounds with high chemo-, regio- and enantioselectivities has been demonstrated.

For thousands of years, mankind has used biological processes in an empirical way, e.g., to produce alcoholic beverages, bread, fermented foods and dairy products. Thanks to the investigations by Louis Pasteur and Robert Koch in the second half of the 19th century, we learned that these processes are in fact catalyzed by micro-organisms or by microbial enzymes, respectively. This knowledge opened the way for the more rational development of new microbial and enzymatic processes in the food and dairy sector and in the chemical and pharmaceutical industries. Early denominations of this new approach were "Zymotechnology" or "Technical Biology".

The term "Biotechnology" was first used in the year 1917. In these early times of industrial biotechnology, the leading representatives of the new science were already promoting the idea of using biological systems to create more efficient, more selective, and environmentally friendlier processes for the conversion of raw materials into industrial products, thereby substituting problematic chemical transformations. The concept of a more sustainable use of the limited resources was thus one of the driving forces for the political vision of sustainable development promoted by national and international conferences and organizations.

A report published by the OECD [68] analyzes the state of the art and the future development needs for industrial biotechnology. Some important conclusions in this report summarizing the state of the art are:

- Biotechnological operations are currently used in a wide range of major industrial processes.

- Economic competitiveness has been established for a variety of biotechnological applications to achieve cleanliness.

- Biotechnology-based processes have been successfully integrated into large-scale operations.

- Industrial penetration of biotechnology is increasing as a consequence of advances in recombinant DNA technologies.

- Biotechnological operations have led to cleaner processes with lowered production of wastes and in some cases lower energy consumption.

- The fine chemicals industry is one of the industrial segments where the impact of biotechnology is felt most strongly.

Preparation of L-DOPA by an Enzymatic Process

L-DOPA, a metabolic precursor of dopamine, is a very important drug for the treatment of parkinsonism. A very interesting industrialized bioprocess is the production of L-DOPA using β-tyrosinase (tyrosine phenol lyase) in a resting cell system. This enzyme catalyzes a variety of reactions: α,β-elimination (I), β-replacement (II) and the reverse of α,β-elimination (III) (R, R' = phenyl-, hydroxyphenyl-, dihydroxyphenyl-, trihydroxyphenyl-).

$$RCH_2CHNH_2COOH + H_2O \rightarrow RH + CH_3COCOOH + NH_3 \qquad \textbf{(I)}$$

$$RCH_2CHNH_2COOH + R'H \rightarrow RH + R'CH_2CHNH_2COOH + RH \qquad \textbf{(II)}$$

$$R'H + CH_3COCOOH + NH_3 \rightarrow R'CH_2CHNH_2COOH + H_2O \qquad \textbf{(III)}$$

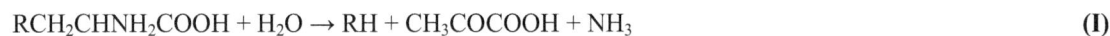

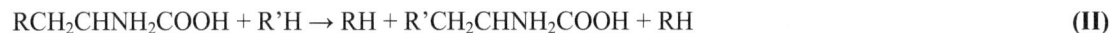

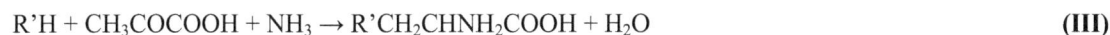

L-Tyrosine and related aminoacids can be synthesized in very high yields through the reverse of α,β-elimination (III). In the case of L-DOPA synthesis by the resting cells of *Erwinia herbicola*, high concentrations of L-DOPA are obtained in the reaction mixture (Fig. **14**). Ajinomoto Co. Ltd started the commercial production of L-DOPA via this new biological route [69]. The enzymatic process shows a fivefold improved productivity in comparison with the chemical process, and with a significant reduction in the time required to complete the process (Table **2**) [69].

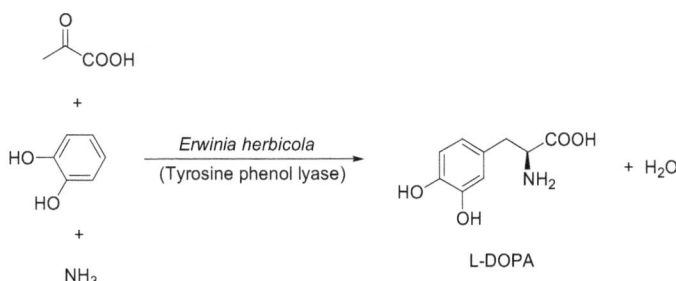

Figure 14: The new synthetic process for L-DOPA.

Table 2: Comparison between the enzymatic and the chemical processes for the production of L-DOPA [70].

	Enzymatic synthesis	**Chemical synthesis**
Main starting materials	Catechol, pyruvic acid, and ammonia	Vainillin, hydantoin, H_2, $(CH_3CO)_2O$
Number of individual reactions	1	8
Reaction by-products	H_2O	NH_3, CO_2, CH_3COOH
Optical separation	Not necessary	Separation of reaction intermediates (acetyl-D/L-veratroylglycine) with the enzyme acylase and racemisation of the D-compound
Production facilities (reaction and isolation)	Versatile equipment	Special plant is required
Time required for production	Approx. 3 days	Approx. 15 days

The Chiral Pool: Carbohydrates and Derivatives

Carbohydrates are renewable, often cheap and abundantly available, but as chiral building blocks they are generally available only in one enantiomeric form and rarely bear a close structural relationship to a target. They suffer from a profusion of chirality.

The carbon chains are generally too long, requiring costly transformation to smaller, more useful species. Mannitol is an exception; the symmetry of the molecule permits cleavage to two identical subunits, which are still chiral. This is utilized in the synthesis of (*S*)-solketal (**4**) [71] from D-mannitol (**3**) (Fig. **15**) and in the synthesis of 2,3-*O*-isopropylidene-D-glycerol in a convenient procedure reported by Emons *et al.* [72].

Utilization of D-glucose in the classical Reichstein-Grussner process for L-ascorbic acid (vitamin C) is a major, and one of the earliest, industrial examples of a chiral pool substance being used in synthesis (Fig. **16**), albeit for the production of further "pool" material. The process was developed in the 1920s. The C_2 and C_3 glucose stereogenic centers are changed into the C_4 and C_5 carbon atoms of ascorbic acid. In this way, none of the reactions of the synthetic pathway need to be stereoselective. The only important problem to be solved is the selective oxidation of one of the primary and secondary hydroxyl groups of D-sorbitol.

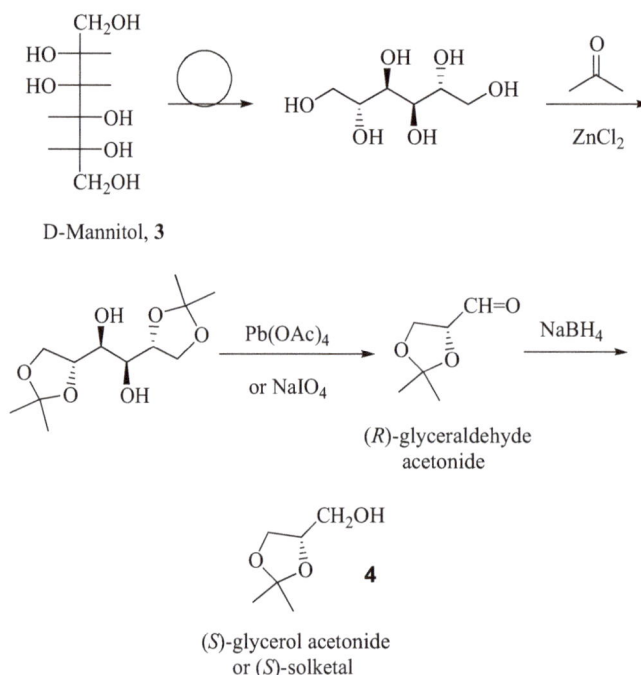

Figure 15: Synthesis of (S)-solketal from D-mannitol.

The sequence is initiated by means of an enzymatic oxidation with *Acetobacter suboxidans*, through which the second problem is solved with effectiveness difficult to be reached by means of the traditional chemical methods, because it avoids using protective groups. The remaining process is more conventional and is based on the treatment of L-sorbose with acetone in an acidic medium. In this way, the two *cis*-diol moieties are protected as ketals, with only the primary hydroxyl group remaining free, to be oxidized later on.

The two final steps of deprotection and cyclization finally lead to L-ascorbic acid (γ-lactone of the enolic form of the 2-oxo-L-gulonic acid). This pathway shows how the chemical oxidation requires the use of protective groups, whilst the enzymatic one allows direct transformations. Taking advantage of this feature, completely enzymatic pathways of vitamin C have been developed (Fig. **17**).

In one of them, D-glucose is transformed into the 2-oxo-L-gulonic acid through the initial oxidation by *Erwinia herbicola* to the 2,5-dioxo-L-gulonic acid, which is reduced subsequently by *Corynebacterium*. Genetic engineering techniques have been recently adjusted to incorporate into the *Erwinia herbicola* DNA the sequence of bases that codifies the biosynthesis of the enzyme *Corynebacterium* that carries out the final oxidation, giving rise to a new organism which allows the one-step transformation of D-glucose into the 2-oxo-L-gulonic acid (Fig. **17**).

CONCLUSIONS

The intrinsically chiral and non-racemic nature of the living world often results in different interactions with the enantiomers of a given substance. If this substance is a drug, it might well be that only one of the two isomers is capable of exerting the desired therapeutic effect. The other may be inert (but must still be metabolized by the organism), harmful (causing even dramatic biological damages), or responsible for difficult-to-predict (and possibly undesirable) side effects.

Well aware of this fact and stimulated by the new policy statements issued by the regulatory agencies, the pharmaceutical industry has, over the past decade or so, systematically begun to develop chiral drugs in eantiomerically enriched and possibly pure form. This new trend has caused a tremendous change in the industrial small- and large-scale production to enantiomerically pure drugs, leading to the revisiting and updating of old technologies (as the resolution of racemic mixtures), and to the development of new methodologies of their large-scale preparation (as the use of stereoselective syntheses and biocatalyzed reactions).

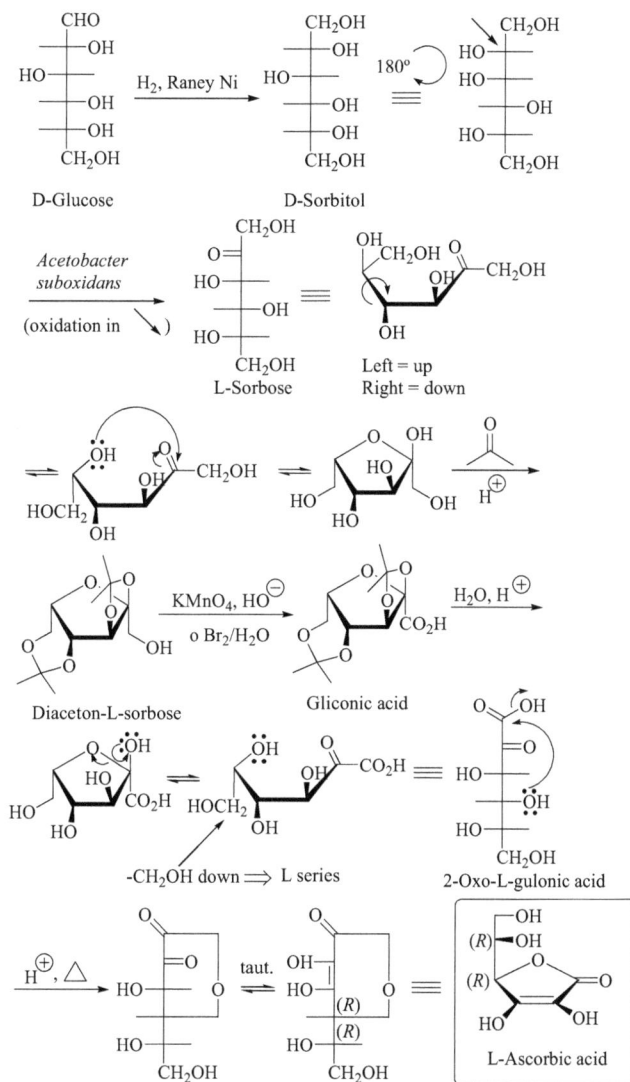

Figure 16: Synthesis of L-ascorbic acid from D-glucose (Reichstein-Grussner process).

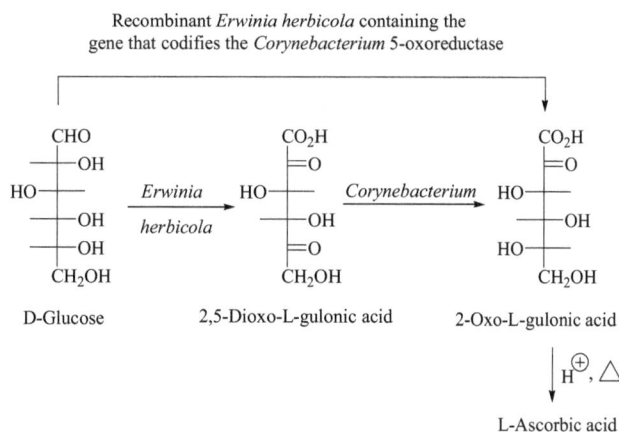

Figure 17: Enzymatic synthesis of vitamin C.

According to Agranat *et al.* [9] and contrary to popular belief, the thalidomide tragedies could not have been avoided by the use of single enantiomers, because both enantiomers have equal teratogenic potencies in the rabbit.

In addition, the enantiomers rapidly racemize in the body, so even if they had differed in teratogenicity, the use of single enantiomers would have been precluded. The thalidomide tragedy increased awareness of stereochemistry in the action of drugs, and as a result the number of drugs administered as racemic compounds has steadily decreased. In 2001, more than 70% of the new chiral drugs approved were single enantiomers [9].

Approximately 1 in 4 therapeutic agents are marked as racemic mixtures, the individual enantiomers frequently differ in both their pharmacodynamic and pharmacokinetic profiles. The use of racemates has become the subject of considerable discussion in recent years, and an area of concern for both the pharmaceutical industry and regulatory authorities. Pharmaceutical companies are required to justify each decision to manufacture a racemic drug in preference to its homochiral version. Moreover, the use of single enantiomers has a number of potential clinical advantages, including an improved therapeutic/pharmacological profile, a reduction in complex drug interactions, and simplified pharmacokinetics. In a number of instances stereochemical considerations have contributed to an understanding of the pharmacological effects observed of a drug administered as a racemate.

However, relatively little is known of the influence of patient factors (e.g. disease state, age, gender and genetics) on drug enantiomer disposition and action in man. Examples may also be cited where the use of a single enantiomer, non-racemic mixtures and racemates of currently used agents may offer clinical advantages.

The issues associated with drug chirality are complex and depend upon the relative merits of the individual agent. In the future it is likely that a number of existing racemates will be re-marketed as single enantiomer products with potentially improved clinical profiles and possible novel therapeutic indications.

The research pharmaceutical industry is currently facing a number of increasingly complex challenges, such as the regulatory constraints, the dramatic increase in development costs with the boost of the crude oil and the generalized economic crisis, the development time periods and the protection of innovation, and human resources and organization.

The development of innovative new drugs is a time-consuming, expensive and a risky process. Increasing the rate of innovation is a requirement to achieve much-needed advances in patient care, as well as to secure the future of the pharmaceutical industry.

Currently, there is a perception in the external environment that the pharmaceutical R&D is no longer innovative, fails to bring out new drugs or, at best, produces a rising number of "me-too" drugs with no advantage over existing treatments. In addition, the cost to discover and develop new medicines (*i.e.* cost per launch) has risen dramatically in recent years.

REFERENCES

[1]   Collins AN, Sheldrake GN, Crosby J. Chirality in industry. The commercial manufacture and applications of optically active compounds. New York: John Wiley & Sons; 1992.

[2]   Testa B, Trager WF. Racemates versus enantiomers in drug development: dogmatism or pragmatism. Chirality 1990;2:129-33, and references cited therein.

[3]   Horn AS, De Ranter CJ. X-Ray crystallography and drug action. Oxford: Clarendon; 1984.

[4]   Ahlberg P. The Nobel Prize in Chemistry 2001 – presentation speech. The Royal Swedish Academy of Science (cited August 26th 2002).

[5]   Blaschke G, Kraft HP, Fickentscher K, Köhler F. Chromatographic separation of racemic thalidomide and teratogenic activity of its enantiomers. Arzneimittelforschung 1979;29:1640-1642.

[6]   Fabro S, Smith RL, Williams RT. Toxicity and teratogenicity of optical isomers of thalidomide. Nature 1967;215:296-297.

[7]   Reist M, Carrupt PA, Francotte E, Testa B. Chiral inversion and hydrolysis of thalidomide: mechanisms and catalysis by bases and serum albumin, and chiral stability of teratogenic metabolites. Chem Res Toxicol 1998;11:1521-1528.

[8]   Eriksson T, Bjorkman S, Roth B, Fyge A, Höuglund P. Stereospecific determination, chiral inversion *in vitro* and pharmacokinetics in humans of the enantiomers of thalidomide. Chirality 1995;7:44-52.

[9]   Agranat I, Caner H, Caldwell J. Putting chirality to work: the strategy of chiral switches. Nat Rev Drug Discov 2002;10:753-768 and references therein.

[10]   (a) Meyring M, Muhlbacher J, Messer K, *et al. In vitro* biotransformation of (*R*)- and (*S*)-thalidomide: application of circular dichroism spectroscopy to the stereochemical characterization of the hydroxylated metabolites. Anal Chem 2002;74:3726-3735. (b) Eriksson T, Bjorkman S, Hoglund P. Clinical pharmacology of thalidomide. Eur J Clin Pharmacol 2001;57:365-376. (c) Eriksson T, Bjorkman S, Roth B, Hoglund P. Hydroxylated metabolites of thalidomide: formation in-vitro and in-vivo in man. J Pharm Pharmacol 1998;50: 1409-1416.

[11]   (a) Gordon JN, Goggin PM. Thalidomide and its derivatives: emerging from the wilderness. Postgrad Med J 2003;79:127-132. (b) Weeber M, Vos R, Klein H, de Jong-van den Berg L, Aronson AR, Molema G. Generating Hypotheses by Discovering Implicit Associations in the Literature: A Case Report of a Search for New Potential Therapeutic Uses of Thalidomide. J Am Med Inform Assoc 2003;10:252-259. (c) Weber D, Rankin K, Gavino M, Delasalle K, Alexanian R, Thalidomide Alone or With Dexamethasone for Previously Untreated Multiple Myeloma. J Clin Oncol 2003;21:16-19. (d) Friedrich MJ. Despite Checkered Past, Thalidomide and its Analogues Show Potential. J Natl Cancer Inst. 2002;94:1270-1272; (e) Lewis R. The Return of Thalidomide. The Scientist 2001;15:1.

[12]   Stoschitzky K, Lindner W, Zernig G, Racemic beta-blockers-fixed combinations of different drugs. J Clin Basic Cardiol 1998;1:15-19.

[13]   Barrett A, Cullum C. The biological properties of the optical isomers of propranolol and their own cardiac arrhytmias. Brit J Pharmacol 1968;34:43-55.

[14]   Echizen H, Manz M, Eichelbaum M. Electrophysiologic effects on dextro- and levo- verapamil on sinus node and AV node function in humans. J Cardiovasc Pharm 1988;12:543-546.

[15]   Satoh K, Yanagisawa T, Taira N. Coronary vasodilatator and cardiac effects of optical isomers of verapamil in the dog. J Cardiovasc Pharm 1980;2:309-318.

[16]   Patocka J, Dvorak, A. Biomedical aspects of chiral molecules. J Appl Medicine 2004;2:95-100.

[17]   Nowak R. Single-isomer Levalbuterol: A Review for the Acute Data. Curr Allergy Asthma Rep 2003;3:172-178.

[18]   Asmus MJ, Hendeles L. Levalbuterol nebulizer solution: Is it worth five times the cost of Albuterol? Pharmacotherapy 2000;20:123-129.

[19]   Drayer DE. Pharmacodynamic and pharmacokinetic differences between drug enantiomers in human: an overview. Clin Pharmacol Ther 1986;40:125-133.

[20]   Ho II, Harris RA. Mechanism of action of barbiturates. Annu Rev Pharmacol 1988;37:1919-1926.

[21]   Katzung BG. Basic and clinical pharmacology. New York: Lange Medical Books/McGraw Hill, 2004.

[22]   Lee EJD, Williams KM. Chirality. Clinical pharmacokinetic and pharmacodynamic considerations. Clin Pharmacokinet 1990;18:339-345.

[23]   Rentsch KM. The importance of stereoselective determination of drugs in the clinical laboratory. J Biochem Bioph Meth 2002;54:1-9.

[24]   Pham-Huy C, Chikhi-Chorfi N, Galons H, *et al.* Enantioselective high-performance liquid chromatography determination of methadone enantiomers and its major metabolite in human biologic fluids using a new derivatized cyclodextrin-bonded phase. J Chromatogr B 1997;700:155-163.

[25]   Davies NM, Teng XV. Importance of chirality in drug therapy and pharmacy practice. Implication for psychiatry. Adv Pharm 2003;1:242-252.

[26]   Marzo A, Heftman E. Enantioselective analytical methods in pharmacokinetics with specific reference to genetic polymorphic metabolism. J Biochem Bioph Meth 2002;54:57-70.

[27]   Jamali F, Mehver R, Pasutto FM. Enantioselective aspects of drug action and disposition: Therapeutic pitfalls. J Pharm Sci US 1989;78:695-715.

[28]   (a) Gristwood RW, Cardiac and CNS toxicity of levobupivacaine: strength of evidence for advantage over bupivacaine. Drugs Saf 2002;25:153-163. (b) Gristwood RW, Greaves JL. Levobupivacaine: a new safer long acting local anaesthetic agent. Expert Opin Inv Drugs 1999;8:861-876.

[29]   Bardsley H, Gristwood R, Baker H, Watson N, Nimmo W. A comparison of the cardiovascular effects of levobupivacaine and rac-bupivacaine following intravenous administration to healthy volunteers. Br J Clin Pharmacol 1998;46:245-249.

[30]   Lindberg P, Brandstrom A, Wallmark B, Mattsson H, Rikner L, Hoffmann KJ, Omeprazole: the first proton pump inhibitor. Med Res Rev 1990;10:1-60.

[31]   Lindberg P, Weidolf L. Method for the treatment of gastric acid-related diseases and production of medication using the (-)-enantiomer of omeprazole. U.S. Patent 5877192, 1999.

[32]   (a) Olbe L, Carlsson E, Lindberg P. A proton-pump inhibitor expedition: the case histories of omeprazole and esomeprazole. Nat Rev Drug Discov 2003;2:132-139; (b) Kale-Pradhan PB, Landry HK, Sypula WT. Esomeprazole for acid peptic disorders. Ann Pharmacother 2002;36:655-663. (c) Lindberg P, Keeling D, Frylund J, Andersson T, Lundborg P, Carlsson E. Esomeprazole-enhanced bio-availability, specificity for the proton pump and inhibition of acid secretion.

Aliment Pharmacol Ther 2003;17:481-488. (d) Chong E, Ensom MH. Pharmacogenetics of the proton pump inhibitors: a systematic review. Pharmacotherapy 2003;23:460-471.

[33]   (a) Jenkins DJ, Sancilio FD, Stowell GW, Whittall LB, Whittle RR. Alkoxy substituted benzimidazole compounds, pharmaceutical preparations containing the same, and methods of using the same, U.S. Patent 6,262,085, 2001. (b) Jenkins DJ, Sancilio FD, Stowell GW, Whittall LB, Whittle RR. Alkoxy substituted benzimidazole compounds, pharmaceutical preparations containing the same, and methods of using the same, U.S. Patent 6,369,087, 2002.

[34]   Pham-Huy C, Villain-Pautet G, He H, *et al.* Separation of oxazepam, lorazepam and temazepam enantiomers by HPLC on a derivatized cyclodextrin-bonded phase: Application to the determination in plasma. J Biochem Bioph Meth 2002;54:287-299.

[35]   He H, Liu Y, Sun C, Wang X, Pham-Huy C. Effect of temperature on enantiomer separation of oxazepam and lorazepam by HPLC on a β-cyclodextrin derivatized bonded chiral stationary phase. J Chromatogr Sc 2004;42:62-66.

[36]   Mohler H, Richards JC. The benzodiazepines. From molecular biology to clinical practice. New York: Raven Press; 1983.

[37]   Miller L, Orihuela C, Fronek R, Honda D, Dapremont O. Chromatographic resolution of the enantiomers of a pharmaceutical intermediate from the milligram to the kilogram scale. J Chromatogr A 1999;849:309-317.

[38]   Williams KL, Sander LC. Enantiomer separations on chiral stationary phases in supercritical fluid chromatography. J Chromatogr A 1997;785:149-158.

[39]   Liu Y, Lantz AW, Armstrong DW. High efficiency liquid and super-subcritical fluid-based enantiomeric separations: An overview. J Liq Chromatogr Relat Technol 2004;27:1121-1178.

[40]   Welch CJ, Leonard WR, DaSilva JO, *et al.* Preparative chiral SFC as a green technology for rapid access to enantiopurity in pharmaceutical process research. LC-GC Eur 2005;18:264-266, 270, 272.

[41]   Zhang Y, Wu D, Wang-Iverson DB, Tymiak AA. Enantioselective chromatography in drug discovery. Drug Discov Today 2005;10:571-757.

[42]   Maftouh M, Granier-Loyaux C, Chavana E, *et al.* Screening approach for chiral separation of pharmaceuticals. Part III. Supercritical fluid chromatography for analysis and purification in drug discovery. J Chromatogr A 2005;1088:67-81.

[43]   Amanullah M, Mazzotti M. Optimization of a hybrid chromatography-crystallization process for the separation of Troeger's base enantiomers. J Chromatogr A 2006;1107:36-45.

[44]   Lorenz H, Polenske D, Seidel-Morgenstern A. Application of preferential crystallization to resolve racemic compounds in a hybrid process. Chirality 2006;18:828-840.

[45]   Jacques J, Collet A, Wilen SH. Enantiomers, racemates and resolutions. New York: Wiley; 1981.

[46]   Kozma D. DRC Handbook of optical resolutions via diastereomeric salt formation. Florida: CRC Press; 2002.

[47]   Fogassy E, Nogradi M, Kozma D, Egri G, Pálovics E, Kiss V. Optical resolution methods. Org Biomol Chem 2006;4:3011-3030.

[48]   Kinbara K. Design of resolving agents based on crystal engineering. Synlett 2005;5:732-743.

[49]   Borghese A, Libert V, Zhang T, Alt CA. Efficient fast screening methodology for optical resolution agents: Solvent effects are used to affect the efficiency of the resolution process. Org Process Res Dev 2004;8,:532-534.

[50]   Toda, F. Isolation and optical resolution of materials utilizing inclusion crystallization. Top Curr Chem 1987;140:43-69.

[51]   Eliel E, Wilen SH, Mander LN. Stereochemistry of organic compounds. New York: Wiley; 1994.

[52]   Kinbara K, Hashimoto Y, Sukegawa M, Nohira H, Saigo K. Crystal structures of the salts of chiral primary amines with achiral carboxylic acids: Recognition of the commonly-occurring supramolecular assemblies of hydrogen-bond networks and their role in the formation of conglomerates. J Am Chem Soc 1996;118: 3441-3449.

[53]   Sakai K, Hirayama R, Tamura R. Novel optical resolution technologies. Heidelberg: Springer-Verlag Berlin; 2007.

[54]   Ushio T, Tamura R, Takahashi H, Azuma N, Yamamoto K. Unusual enantiomeric resolution phenomenon observed upon Recrystallization of a Racemic compound. Angew Chem Int Ed Engl 1996;35:2372-2374.

[55]   Tamura R, Fujimoto D, Lepp Z, *et al.* Mechanism of preferential enrichment, an unusual enantiomeric resolution phenomenon caused by polymorphic transition during crystallization of mixed crystals composed of two enantiomers. J Am Chem Soc 2002;124:13139-13153.

[56]   Yokota M, Doki N, Shimizu K. Chiral separation of a racemic compound induced by transformation of racemic crystal structures: DL-glutamic acid. Cryst Growth Des 2006;6:1588-1590.

[57]   Mughal RK, Davey RJ, Blanden N. Application of crystallization inhibitors to chiral separations. 1. Design of additives to discriminate between the racemic compound and the pure enantiomer of mandelic acid. Cryst Growth Des 2007;7:218-224.

[58]   Mughal RK, Davey RJ, Blagden N. Application of crystallization inhibitors to chiral separations. 2. Enhancing the chiral purity of mandelic acid by crystallization. Cryst Growth Des 2007;7:225-228.

[59]   Collins AN, Sheldrake GN, Crosby J. Chirality in industry II: Developments in the manufacture and applications of optically active compounds. New York: John Wiley & Sons; 1997.

[60] Patel RN. Biocatalysis and biotechnology for functional foods and industrial products. Boca Raton Florida: CRC Press LLC; 2007.

[61] Colonna S, Richelmi C. Organic biotransformations. Chimica e l'Industria, 2004;86:58-62.

[62] Eggert T. Industrial biotransformations. Weinheim: Wiley-VCH Verlag GmbH & Co. KGaA; 2006.

[63] Knowles WS. Aymmetric hydrogenation. Acc Chem Res 1983;16:106-112.

[64] Halpern J. Asymmetric Catalytic Hydrogenation: Mechanism and Origin of Enantioselection, in Morrison, J. D., ed., Asymmetric Synthesis, New York: Academic Press; 1985.

[65] Miyashita A, Yasuda A, Takaya H, Toriumi K, Souchi T, Noyori R. Synthesis of 2,2'-bis(diphenylphosphino)-1,1'-binaphthyl (BINAP), an atropisomeric chiral bis(triaryl)phosphine, and its use in the rhodium(I)-catalyzed asymmetric hydrogenation of α-(acylamino)acrylic acids. J Am Chem Soc 1980;102:7932-7934.

[66] Katsuki T, Sharpless KB. The first practical method for asymmetric epoxidation. J Am Chem Soc 1980;102:5974-5976.

[67] Klunder JM, Ko K, Sharpless KB. Asymmetric epoxidation of allyl alcohol: efficient routes to homochiral β-adrenergic blocking agents. J Org Chem 1986;51:3710-3712.

[68] Biotechnology for Clean Industrial Products and Processes – Towards Industrial Sustainability. Paris: OECD; 1998.

[69] Yamada H. Screening of Novel Enzymes for the Production of Useful Compounds. In: New Frontiers in Screening for Microbial Biocatalysts. Kieslich, K, van der Beek, CP, de Bont, JAM, van den Tweel, WJJ (Eds). Amsterdam: Elsevier; 1998.

[70] Ghisalba O. Biocatalyzed Reactions, in New Trends in Synthetic Medicinal Chemistry. Methods and Principles in Medicinal Chemistry, Volume 7; Mannhold, R, Kubinyi, H, Timmerman, H. (Eds.). Weinheim: Wiley-VCH: 2000.

[71] Baer E. L-α-Glycerophosphoric acid (barium salt). Biochem Prep 1952;2:31-38.

[72] Emmons CHH, Kuster BFM, Vekemans JAJM, Sheldon RAA, new convenient method for the synthesis of chiral C_3-synthons. Tetrahedron: Asymmetry 1991;2:359-362.

CHAPTER 6

General Aspects of the Microwave-Assisted Drug Development

Peterson de Andrade, Lílian Sibelle Campos Bernardes and Ivone Carvalho

School of Pharmaceutical Sciences of Ribeirão Preto, University of São Paulo, Av. do Café, s/n, Monte Alegre, 14040-903, Ribeirão Preto, São Paulo, Brazil

Abstract: Microwaves are a powerful and reliable energy sources that may be adapted to many applications. Since the introduction of microwave-assisted organic synthesis in 1986, the use of microwave irradiation has now introduced a completely new approach to drug discovery. The efficiency of microwave flash-heating chemistry in dramatically reducing reaction times has recently fascinated many pharmaceutical companies, which are incorporating microwave chemistry into their drug development efforts. Thereby, the time saved by using microwaves is important for accelerating traditional organic synthesis or high-speed medicinal chemistry.

INTRODUCTION

Dr. Percy Le Baron Spencer, a self-taught engineer of the Raytheon Corporation, was responsible for the invention of the microwave oven. He accidentally discovered that microwave energy could cook food when a candy bar in his pocket melted while he was testing a new magnetron (microwave generator), during a radar-related research project around 1945. The intrigued Dr. Spencer decided to place some popcorn kernels near the magnetron tube and watched them quickly transferred into popcorn. In another experiment, he put the tube near an egg and observed its heating and further explosion [1,2].

With the aim of studying the food heating effect, he created a metal box with an opening, which he fed microwave power, and continued to experiment with other foods. The results of his investigation showed that microwaves could increase the internal temperature of foods much faster than the conventional heating. Thus, Dr. Spencer had now invented what would become the microwave oven. In 1947, the Raytheon company built the first commercial microwave oven: the Radarange (about 0.8 m tall and 340 kg weight) [1,2].

Originally applied for heating foodstuffs, the microwave energy has found a variety of technical applications in the chemical and related industries since the 1950s. Its application range from analytical chemistry (microwave digestion, ashing, extraction) to biochemistry (protein hydrolysis, sterilization), pathology (histoprocessing, tissue fixation) and medical treatments (diathermy). In the 1970s, the construction of the magnetron was improved and simplified. As a direct result, the price of domestic microwave oven fell considerably and its use became more common [3,4].

During this decade, the microwave technology has been used in inorganic chemistry. It was implemented in organic chemistry since the mid-1980s. The main reasons for the slow uptake can be illustrated by (i) the lack of controllability and reproducibility, (ii) safety aspects concerning with flammability of organic solvents, (iii) low degree of understanding the basis of microwave heating and (iv) the lack of available systems for adequate temperature and pressure controls [4,5].

The first two reports on microwave-assisted organic chemistry were published in 1986. Richard Gedye studied four different types of organic reactions (acid hydrolysis of benzamide, benzoic acid esterification, permanganate oxidation of toluene and the SN_2 reaction between sodium 4-cyanophenoxide and benzyl chloride) which were done in sealed Teflon vessels heated by a domestic Toshiba model. He observed remarkable rate enhancements and dramatic savings in reaction times. Raymond J. Giguere and George Majetich reported results on reaction vessel design, safety precautions, and solvent choice in a study of thermal reactions and concluded that microwave thermolysis has considerable potential for rapid acceleration of chemical reactions [6,7].

Although most of the early pioneering experiments in Microwave-Assisted Organic Synthesis (MAOS) were performed in domestic microwave ovens, which have proven to be problematic, the companies began to address their efforts in the design of microwave ovens specifically for use in laboratories. The first custom-built commercial microwave synthesizer, to conduct chemical synthesis, was introduced in 2000. It was designed to produce a uniform microwave field and was equipped with technology that could control the temperature of the chemical reaction [8,9].

As a consequence, the amount of articles describing efficient rapid chemical synthesis promoted by microwave irradiation has grown quickly from ~200 in 1995 to ~1000 in 2001 and ~3300 in 2009. The efficiency of microwave flash-heating chemistry in reducing reaction times (from days or hours to minutes or seconds), reducing side reactions, increasing yields, and improving reproducibility has been responsible for attracting many academic and industrial research groups to microwave research projects. The current trend is that, in a few years, most chemists will probably use microwave energy to heat chemical reactions [5,10].

Microwave-assisted heating under controlled conditions is an important technology for both organic and medicinal chemistry. From a medicinal chemistry perspective, the competitive landscape of the pharmaceutical industry demands constant innovation and accelerated timelines for the development of nascent programs. MAOS have recently fascinated many pharmaceutical industries, not so much in terms of production of a large variety of compounds in a reduced time, but more with the synthesis of novel, complex and decorated scaffolds. Nowadays, the pharmaceutical companies have incorporated the microwave chemistry into their drug discovery process introducing novel approaches to drug discovery and development [8,11,12].

MICROWAVE RADIATION

Microwaves are generated by a cavity magnetron, which is a high-powered vacuum tube, and are useful for industrial, scientific and medical applications (e.g., microwave oven, radar, magnetic resonance etc).

Microwave is a form of electromagnetic energy (irradiation) in a frequency range of 0.3 to 300 GHz, corresponding to wavelengths ranging from 1 cm to 1 m. The microwave region of the eletromagnetic spectrum (Fig. **1**) lies between infrared and radio frequencies.

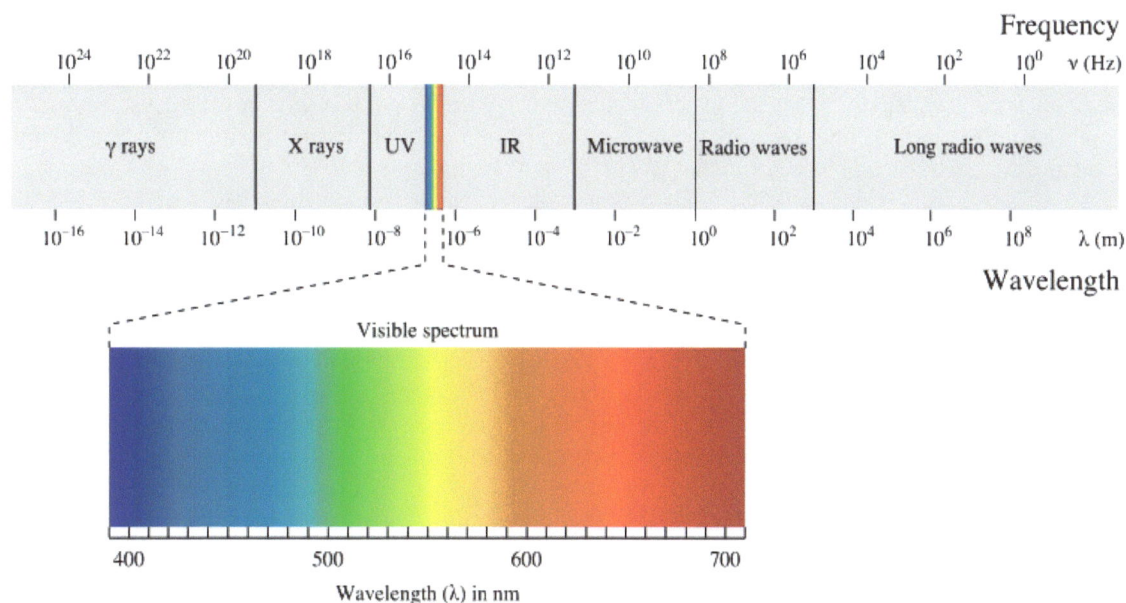

Figure 1: The electromagnetic spectrum. Figure adapted from http://en.wikipedia.org/wiki/File:EM_spectrum.svg

Whithin this region only molecular rotation is affected, not molecular structure. Microwaves move at the speed of light (300.000 Km/s) and the energy in microwave photons (0.037 Kcal/mol) is very low relative to the typical energy required to cleave molecular bonds (80-120 Kcal/mol). Thus, it is clear that microwaves cannot "induce" chemical reactions by direct absorption of electromagnetic energy, as occurs in photochemistry (ultraviolet and visible radiation) [3,8].

All domestic microwave ovens and all microwave reactors for chemical synthesis that are commercially available today operate at a frequency of 2.45 GHz (wavelength of 12.25 cm) in order to avoid interference with telecommunication and cellular phone frequencies. In addition, 2.45 GHz frequency is preferred because it has the right penetration depth to interact with laboratory reaction conditions. On the other hand, wavelengths between 1 cm and 25 cm are used for RADAR transmissions and the remaining wavelength range is used for telecommunications [3,8].

THE CONVENTIONAL HEATING

A very commom procedure in organic chemistry is the heating of reactions. During a long time, the heating was traditionally carried out through an external heat source. In 1855, Bunsen invented the burner whereas the energy from this heat source could be applied to the reaction vessel. However, fire is now rarely used and the Bunsen burner was later superseded by the hot plate, oil bath or heating mantle as sources of applying heat to a chemical reaction [13].

Although having proven successful for >150 years, heating chemical reactions using these traditional equipments creates a localized hot surface (local overheating) on the reaction vessel, where products, substrates and reagents often decompose over time. It can be explained because, in classical heating, the energy must first be transferred from the heat source to the wall of the reaction vessel in order to reach the solvent and reactants (Fig. **2**) [11,14].

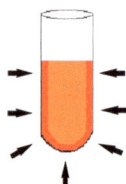

Figure 2: Schematic heating by conduction. Figure adapted from Hayes, 2002.

This method for transferring energy into a system is slow and inefficient, since it depends on convection currents and on the thermal conductivity of several materials that must be penetrated. It results in the higher temperature of the vessel (wall effect) when compared with the reaction mixture. In addition, longer reaction times and diminished yields are also typical of heating by conduction [3,11].

THE MICROWAVE HEATING

Microwave heating is a different process. The microwave irradiation produces efficient internal heating by direct coupling of microwave energy with the molecules (solvents, reagents, catalysts) that are present in the reaction mixture, leading to a rapid rise in temperature (Fig. **3**). The very efficient internal heat transfer results in minimized wall effects (no overheating), once this process is not dependent upon the thermal conductivity of the vessel materials. A properly designed vessel allows the temperature increase to be uniform throughout the sample, decreasing the amount of by-products and/or product decomposition [5,14].

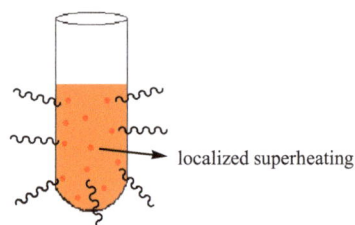

localized superheating

Figure 3: Schematic heating by microwaves. Figure adapted from Hayes, 2002.

Since the response of various materials to microwave radiation is diverse, they can be broadly classified based on their response to microwaves: i) materials that are transparent to microwaves (e.g., sulphur), ii) materials that reflect microwaves (e.g., copper) and iii) materials that absorb microwaves (e.g., water). These latter are called dielectric materials, comprising permanent or induced dipoles, which allow charge to be stored, but no conductivity is observed. Thereby, only materials that absorb microwave radiation are relevant for microwave chemistry [15].

The theory of microwave heating has been developed by many workers, amongst them Debye, Frohlich, Daniel, Cole and Cole, Hill and Hasted [16]. This theory is based on the efficient heating of materials by "microwave dielectric heating" effect, which drives chemical reactions by taking advantage of the ability of some liquids and solids to convert electromagnetic radiation into heat [5,14]. As microwave irradiation is a short electromagnetic wave, which consists of an electric and magnetic field component (Fig. **4**), several materials can be heated by applying it. However, only the electric field is responsible for transferring energy to heat substances and the magnetic field normally does not play any role in chemical synthesis [8].

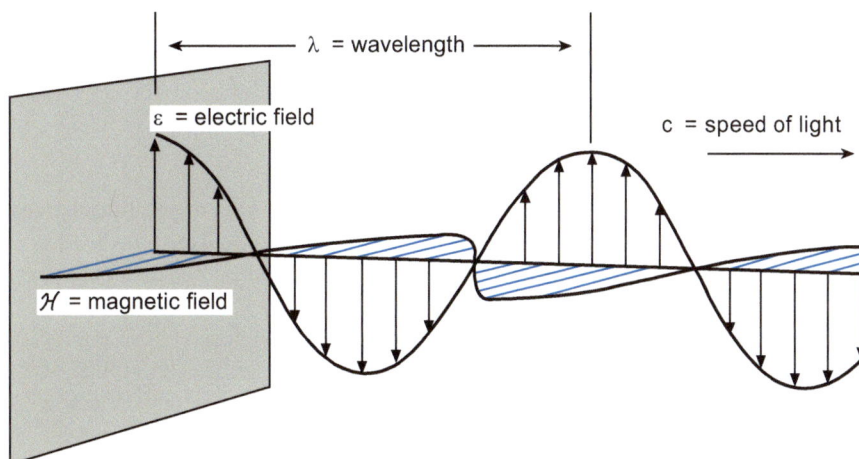

Figure 4: Electric and magnetic field components in microwaves. Figure adapted from Hayes, 2002.

The origin of the heating effect produced by the high frequency electromagnetic waves arises from the ability of an electric field to exert a force on polar molecules and ions. If the charge carriers are bound to certain regions they will move until a counter force balances them and the result is a dielectric polarization. However, if the particles present in the substance can move freely through it, then a current has been induced [16]. Thus, electric component of an electromagnetic field causes heating by two fundamental mechanisms: dipolar polarization (polarization of dielectrics) and ionic conduction. The dipoles in the reaction mixture (the polar solvent molecules) are involved in the dipolar polarization effect and the charged particles in a sample (ions) are affected by ionic conduction [17].

At the molecular level, the dipoles and ions are sensitive to external electric fields and will attempt to align themselves or be in phase with the field [4]. As the applied field oscillates, they try to realign themselves with the alternating electric field which results in a rotation of molecules and an oscillation of ions (Fig. **5**).

The existence of resisting forces (inter particle interaction and electric resistance) restricts the movement of these particles generating random motion. Therefore, the energy absorbed in this process is converted into kinetic energy, which is lost as heat through molecular friction and dielectric loss [18].

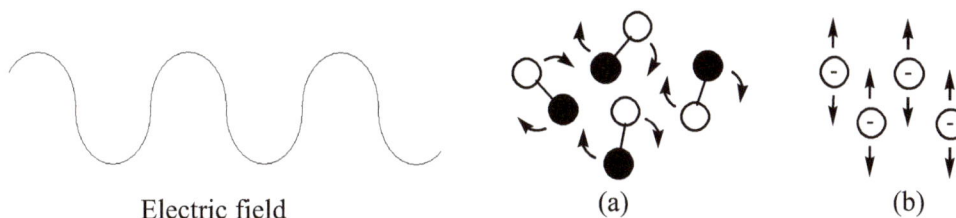

Electric field   (a)   (b)

Figure 5: Dipolar polarization (a) and ionic conduction mechanisms (b). Figure adapted from Lidström *et al.* 2001.

Dipolar polarization should not be confused with conduction, since the latter results from translational motion of the charges when the electric field is applied [15]. As the dipole re-orientates to align itself with the electric field, the field is already changing and generates a phase difference between the orientation of the field and that of the dipole. This phase difference causes energy to be lost from the dipole by molecular friction and collisions yielding dielectric heating [4].

Ionic conduction in the matrix by the interaction with microwave radiation is a much stronger heat generator than the corresponding motion of dipoles. Ionic species heat up very quickly when exposed to microwave irradiation. This property can be used to improve the heating ability of non-polar solvents [13].

It has to be emphasized that the microwave heating effect depends on the frequency as well as the power applied. The heat generated by this process is directly related to the ability of the matrix to align itself with the frequency of the field. If the particle does not have enough time to realign (high-frequency irradiation) or reorients too quickly (low-frequency irradiation) with the applied field, no heating occurs. The allocated frequency of 2.45 GHz used in all commercial systems lies between these two extremes and gives the particle time to respond (rotate) to the alternating electric field [17].

IMPORTANT PARAMETERS

One source of microwave dielectric heating lies in the ability of an electric field to polarize charges in a material and the inability of this polarization to follow quick reversals of an electric field[16]. Thus, the heating characteristics of a particular material (e.g., a solvent) under microwave irradiation are dependent on its dielectric properties [5].

Two parameters define the dielectric properties of materials and are used extensively in microwave chemistry. The first one is the dielectric constant or relative permittivity (ε'), which describes the ability of the molecule to be polarized or to store electric charge by the electric field. The second one is the dielectric loss or complexed permittivity (ε''), which is the amount of input microwave energy that is lost to the sample dissipated as heat, reflecting the conductance of the material [8,16].

The ability of a specific substance to convert energy of the electromagnetic radiation into thermal energy at a given frequency and temperature is determined by the following equation: $\tan \delta = \varepsilon'' / \varepsilon'$. Tangent delta ($\tan \delta$) or so-called loss factor is defined as the ratio of the dielectric loss to the dielectric constant. In summary, these three main dielectric parameters (tangent delta, dielectric constant and dielectric loss) are related to the ability of a solvent to absorb microwave energy [8].

Considering the importance of solvents in organic chemistry, as well as in microwave chemistry, Table **1** shows the dielectric parameters differences among some common organic solvents[8]. According to the loss factors ($\tan \delta$), these solvents can be classified as high ($\tan \delta > 0.5$), medium ($\tan \delta$ 0.1-0.5) and low ($\tan \delta < 0.1$) microwave absorbing. The dielectric loss (ε'') value is the most indicative parameter of how quickly a solvent will reach high temperatures and, in general, the higher this value, the more efficient the solvent converts microwave energy into thermal heat. Thus, a reaction medium with a high $\tan \delta$ value will present efficient absorption and, as a consequence, quick heating [3,8].

Table 1: The loss factors ($\tan \delta$) measured at 20 °C and 2.45 GHz of different solvents [8].

Solvent	tan δ	ε″	ε′
Ethylene Glycol	1.350	49.950	37.0
Ethanol	0.941	22.866	24.3
DMSO	0.825	37.125	45.0
2-Propanol	0.799	14.622	18.3
1-Propanol	0.757	15.216	20.1
Formic Acid	0.722	42.237	58.5
Methanol	0.659	21.483	32.6

			Table 1: cont....
Nitrobenzene	0.589	20.497	34.8
1-Butanol	0.571	9.764	17.1
Isobutanol	0.522	8.248	15.8
2-Butanol	0.447	7.063	15.8
2-Methoxyethanol	0.410	6.929	16.9
o-Dichlorobenzene	0.280	2.772	9.9
NMP	0.275	8.855	32.2
Acetic Acid	0.174	1.079	6.2
DMF	0.161	6.070	37.7
1,2 Dichloroethane	0.127	1.321	10.4
Water	0.123	9.889	80.4
Chlorobenzene	0.101	0.263	2.6
Chloroform	0.091	0.437	4.8
MEK	0.079	1.462	18.5
Nitromethane	0.064	2.304	36.0
Acetonitrile	0.062	2.325	37.5
Ethyl Acetate	0.059	0.354	6.0
Acetone	0.054	1.118	20.7
THF	0.047	0.348	7.4
Dichloromethane	0.042	0.382	9.1
Toluene	0.040	0.096	2.4
Hexane	0.020	0.038	1.9
o-Xylene	0.018	0.047	2.6

On the other hand, solvents without a permanent dipole (carbon tetrachloride, toluene, dioxane, hexane etc) are almost microwave transparent, but a low tan δ value does not preclude these solvents from being used in a microwave-heated reaction. Since either the substrates or some of the reagents/ catalysts are likely to be polar, the overall dielectric properties of the reaction medium will, in most cases, allow sufficient heating by microwave irradiaton [3].

EQUIPMENT

Most of the novel work is now performed in reactors constructed specifically for organic synthesis, i.e., most of today's commercially available microwave reactors feature built-in magnetic stirrers, direct temperature control of the reaction mixture with the aid of fiber-optic probes, shielded thermocouples or infrared sensors, and softwares that enables on-line temperature/pressure control by regulation of microwave power output [18,22].

Currently, there are two different approaches with respect to microwave reactor design: multimode and single-mode (or monomode) reactors. When microwaves enter a cavity, they are reflected by the walls. The reflections of the waves eventually generate a three dimensional stationary pattern of standing waves within the cavity, called modes [4,22].

In the so-called multimode instruments (Fig. **6**), also known as the kitchen microwave oven, the essential characteristic is the deliberate avoidance and/or disruption of any standing wave pattern inside the cavity. Thus, the engineering goal is to produce as much chaos inside the cavity as possible. In addition, the multimode systems rotate samples to ensure that the field distribution is as homogeneous as possible [8,22,23].

Despite being a good solution to provide a uniform heating pattern of general food items, the multimode cavities have different levels of energy intensity (multiple pockets of energy = hot and cold spots) dispersed throughout the cavity volume due to the physics of their design. It means that the final result is the drastic variation of the heating efficiency between different positions of the load when small samples are heated [4,8]. In addition, the magnetrons are optimized to give high efficiency for a 1 Kg standard test load and consequently they operate less reliably for small loads [4].

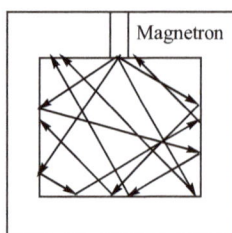

Figure 6: Scheme of a multimode reactor. Figure adapted from Lew *et al.* 2002.

On the other hand, the essential characteristic of single-mode cavities (Fig. **7**) is the deliberate creation of a standing wave pattern inside the cavity. In this case, the electromagnetic irradiation is directed through an accurately designed rectangular or circular wave guide onto the reaction vessel mounted at a fixed distance from the radiation source. The dimensions of the cavity must be carefully controlled to correspond in some systematic way to the characteristic wavelength of the microwaves, leading to a homogeneous distribution of energy inside the reaction cavity [5,23,24].

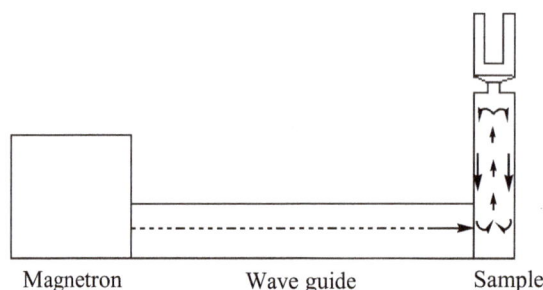

Magnetron   Wave guide   Sample

Figure 7: Scheme of a single-mode reactor. Figure adapted from Lew *et al.* 2002.

The key difference between these reactor systems is that in multimode cavities several reaction vessels can be irradiated simultaneously whereas only one vessel can be irradiated at a time in monomode cavities. In the latter case, high throughput can be achieved by integrated robotics that move individual reaction vessels in and out of the cavity [5].

It is also important to highlight that single-mode reactors process comparatively small volumes (0.2 to about 150 ml) when compared to multimode reactors (liter scale) and that monomode cavities are especially valuable when small amounts of reagents are used [5,24]. It can be explained because the single-mode instruments produce uniform energy distribution and higher power density that results in more efficient coupling with small samples [8].

The main consequence is that it allows the achievement of a higher reproducibility and predictably of results. Concerning organic or medicinal chemistry for example, yields can therefore be optimized (a difficult task when using traditional microwave oven). Moreover, much higher field strengths can be obtained in single-mode systems, which yields faster heating [4].

Regarding the commercially available monomode reactors, most companies offer a variety of diverse reactor platforms with different degrees of sophistication with respect to automation, database capabilities, safety features, temperature and pressure monitoring, vessel design and prices [5].

MICROWAVES IN CHEMICAL REACTIONS

Since the introduction of MAOS in 1986, shorter times for reactions as well as alteration in product distributions (outcome of the synthesis), compared to those using conventional heating, have led the researchers to discuss the nature of these effects [4,19]. Despite the basic understanding of high-frequency electromagnetic irradiation and microwave-matter interactions, the exact reasons why and how microwaves enhance chemical processes are still not fully understood. Thus, the investigation of microwave effects is an extremely complex subject [3].

A chemical reaction is a process that results in the interconversion of reactants into one or more products. Basically, chemical reactions encompass changes that strictly involve the motion of electrons in the breaking and forming of chemical bonds. Energy is necessary to break chemical bonds in the starting substances and it is released once new bonds are formed [20]. However, it is not necessary to absorb sufficient energy to break chemical bonds in order to have a significant influence on reaction kinetics. Stuerga and Gaillard have correctly pointed out that microwave energy is not large enough to break chemical bonds [21].

In 1889, the Swedish scientist Svante Arrhenius introduced an important equation that describes the rate of a chemical reaction. According to Arrhenius equation ($K = A\,e^{-Ea/RT}$), the reaction rate constant (K) is dependent on two factors: the frequency of collisions between molecules that have the correct geometry for a reaction to occur (A) and fraction of those molecules that have the minimum energy required to overcome the activation energy barrier ($e^{-Ea/RT}$) [8].

Considering this equation, there are basically two ways to increase the rate of a chemical reaction. Some authors have proposed that the pre-exponential factor (A) can be affected by microwave irradiation, once the microwave energy induces an increase in molecular vibrations. However, other authors believe that microwave irradiation produces an alteration in the exponential factor ($e^{-Ea/RT}$) by affecting the free energy of activation [4].

Based on these aspects, there are essentially three different possibilities for rationalizing rate enhancements observed in microwave-assisted chemical reactions: (i) thermal effects (kinetics), (ii) specific microwave effects and (iii) non-thermal (athermal) microwave effects [3].

Today most scientists agree that in most cases the reason for the observed rate enhancements is a purely thermal effect (kinetic) [5]. The high reaction temperature causes greater movement of molecules, which leads to a greater number of energetic collisions. This occurs much faster with microwave energy due to high instantaneous heating of the substance(s), above the normal bulk temperature, and it is the primary factor for observed rate enhancements. In these cases, microwave energy affects the temperature parameter in the Arrhenius equation [8].

Taking into account a general reaction coorditate (Fig. **8**), the reaction begins with reactants (A and B), which have a certain level of energy (E_R). These reactants must collide in the correct geometrical orientation to become activated to a higher-level transition state (E_{TS}) in order to complete the transformation.

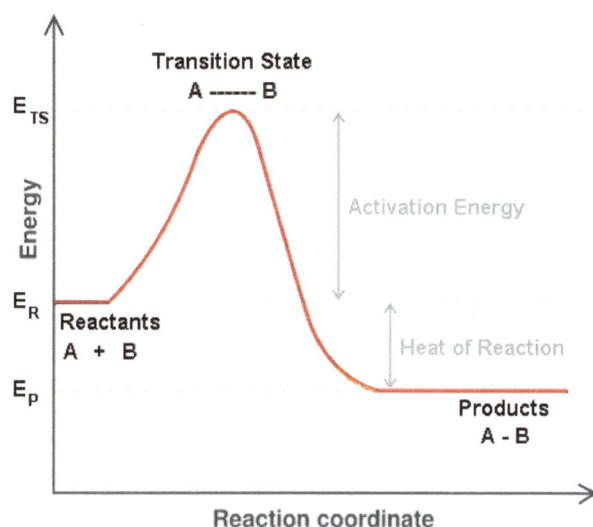

Figure 8: A general reaction coordinate. Figure adapted from Hayes, 2002.

The difference between these energy levels is the activation energy (E_a) required to reach this higher state. Once enough energy is absorbed, the reactants react to give the products (A-B), where the energy state (E_P) is lower than the reactants energy [8].

Microwave irradiation does not affect the activation energy, however it provides the momentum to overcome this barrier. Since the amount of microwave energy being introduced to the system is very large relative to the energy needed to achieve the required activation energy, the reaction is completed more quickly than conventional heating methods.

This is the process that contributes to the increased reaction speeds and higher yields that occurs in microwave chemistry [8].

In addition to the above mentioned thermal effects, microwave effects that are caused by the unique nature of the microwave dielectric heating mechanisms should be termed specific microwave effects. In this category falls: (i) the superheating effect of solvents at atmospheric pressure, (ii) the selective heating of strongly microwave absorbing heterogeneous catalysts or reagents in a less polar reaction medium, (iii) the formation of microscopic hot spots by direct coupling of microwave energy to specific reagents in homogeneous solution and (iv) the elimination of wall effects caused by inverted temperature gradients [5].

The third possibility is related to non-thermal (athermal) microwave effects. These effects have been proposed to result from a direct interaction of the electric field with specific molecules or intermediates in the reaction medium.

It has been argued that the presence of an electric field leads to orientation effects of dipolar molecules and hence changes the pre-exponential factor (A) or the activation energy (E_a) in the Arrhenius equation. However, the area of non-thermal microwave effects is highly controversial [5,17].

DRUG DISCOVERY APPLICATIONS

MAOS have a wide influence in the different phases of the drug discovery process, involving generation of compound libraries, lead discovery and optimization. A major contribution is the reduced time to obtain the desired compounds, making possible a rapid evaluation of the reaction parameters in order to optimize the chemistry involved. As a consequence, the beneficial effects of microwave irradiation are finding an increased role in target discovery, screening, pharmacokinetics and even in the clinical phase, which contributes to expanding the universe of Medicinal Chemistry (Fig. **9**) [13, 17].

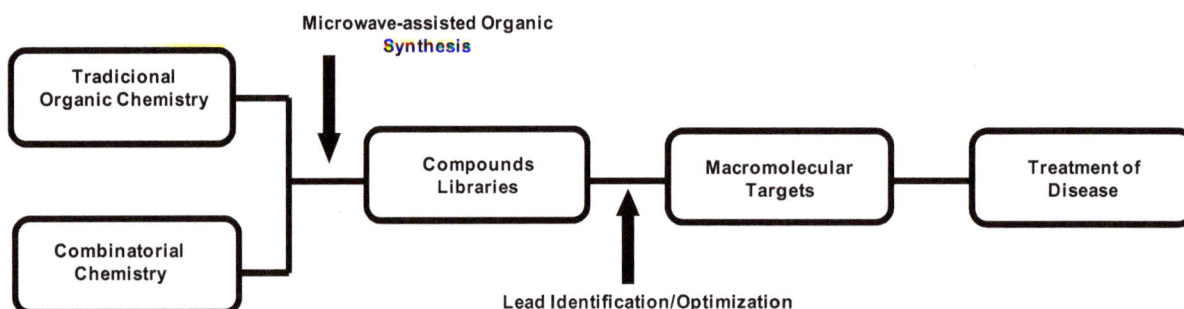

Figure 9: The drug discovery process and the impact of Microwave-Assisted Organic Synthesis on traditional organic/combinatorial chemistry.

Nowadays, many pharmaceutical industrial and academic research groups have adopted MAOS as an excellent alternative for rapid optimization of reactions, for the efficient synthesis of new bioactive chemical entities and generating collections of compounds. In general, the time expended from the design of the compound library to the production stage can be from 15 to 22 weeks (Fig. **10**). In this process, the proof-of-principle stage has the largest proportion, in which many reactions parameters can be evaluated and chemical yields and purities optimized for different strategies [5,17]. Various scientists have published excellent articles/reviews on microwave-assisted rapid organic transformations and their importance and applications in drug discovery process [11, 12, 14, 17, 18, 22, 26, 27, 28].

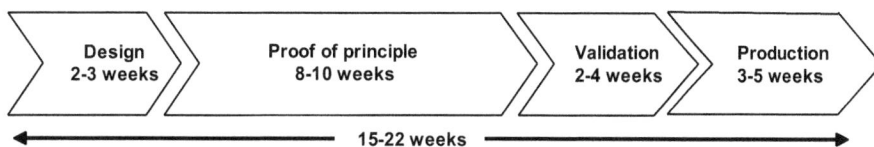

Figure 10: Typical microwave-assisted library synthesis evaluation. Adapted from Kappe and Dallinger, 2006.

The synthesis of several classes of compounds has been reported to be enhanced by microwave irradiation such as quinolines, antibacterial β-lactams, cephalosporins among others. One interesting application of this technique is the preparation of radiopharmaceuticals that contain isotopes with short half-lives (e.g. ^{11}C, ^{122}I and ^{18}F). Some compounds are illustrated in Fig. **11** [13].

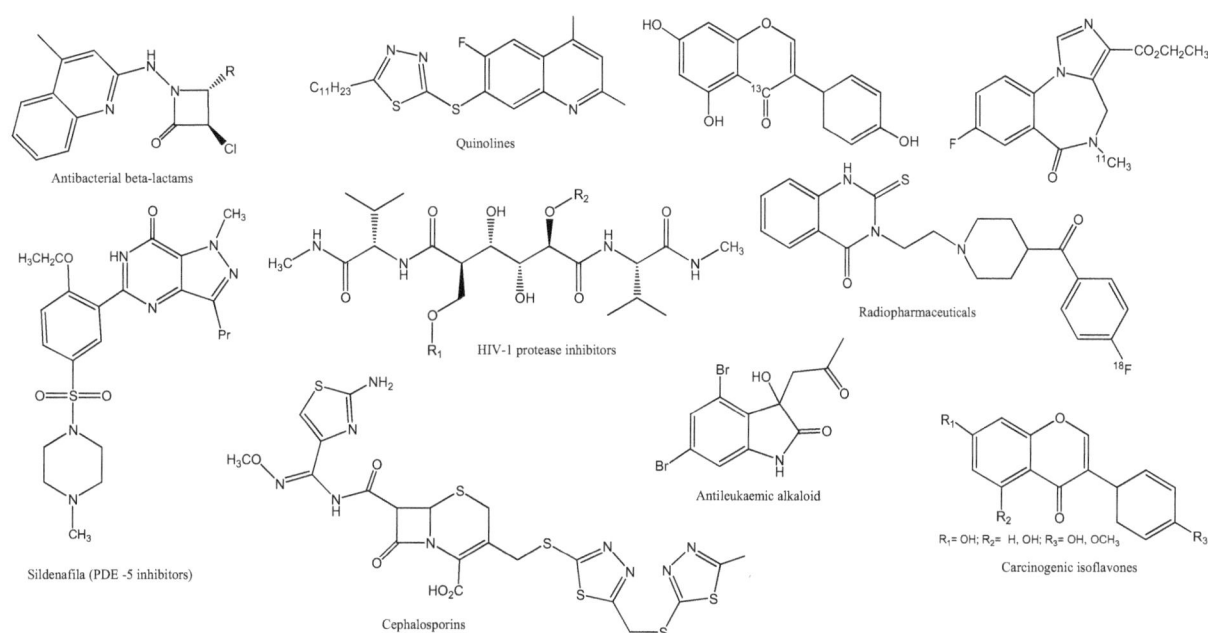

Figure 11: Compounds representing different therapeutic classes.

In fact, combinatorial chemistry and high-throughput screening have contributed to collections of potential lead compounds in a short period of time. In this way, the MAOS have attracted interest from combinatorial/medicinal chemistry researchers due to its increased organic reactions speed and/or improvement in yields for accelerating the discovery of bioactive molecules.

This new technology is able to produce large and diverse libraries by high-throughput, automated, single step, parallel synthesis, especially in the area of multi-component reactions [13].

The high throughput afforded by microwave technology is exemplified by the successful synthesis of a large number of bioactive compounds with great structural diversity. Bagley *et al.* [29] describes a new method for rapid synthesis of pyrimidine libraries (Fig. **12**) for application as ligands for the estrogen receptor, by Bohlmann-Rahtz reaction of alkynones as versatile synthetic intermediates, using microwave dielectric heating.

A series of novel 20-membered macrocycles, selective and potent antagonists at the melanocortin receptor hMC5R, containing an alkylthioaryl bridge within the main ring were synthesized by a tandem combination using solid phase peptide synthesis and microwave-assisted reactions (Fig. **13**) [30].

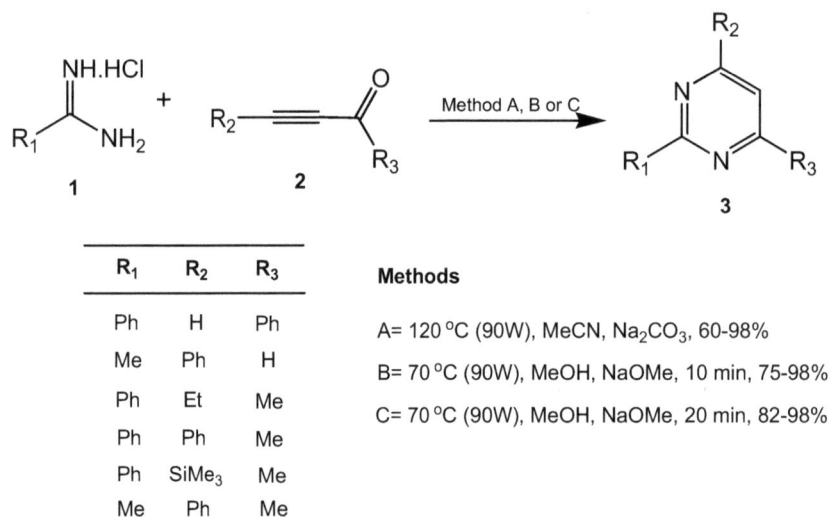

R_1	R_2	R_3
Ph	H	Ph
Me	Ph	H
Ph	Et	Me
Ph	Ph	Me
Ph	SiMe$_3$	Me
Me	Ph	Me

Methods

A= 120 °C (90W), MeCN, Na$_2$CO$_3$, 60-98%

B= 70 °C (90W), MeOH, NaOMe, 10 min, 75-98%

C= 70 °C (90W), MeOH, NaOMe, 20 min, 82-98%

Figure 12: Pyrimidine libraries obtained by MAOS.

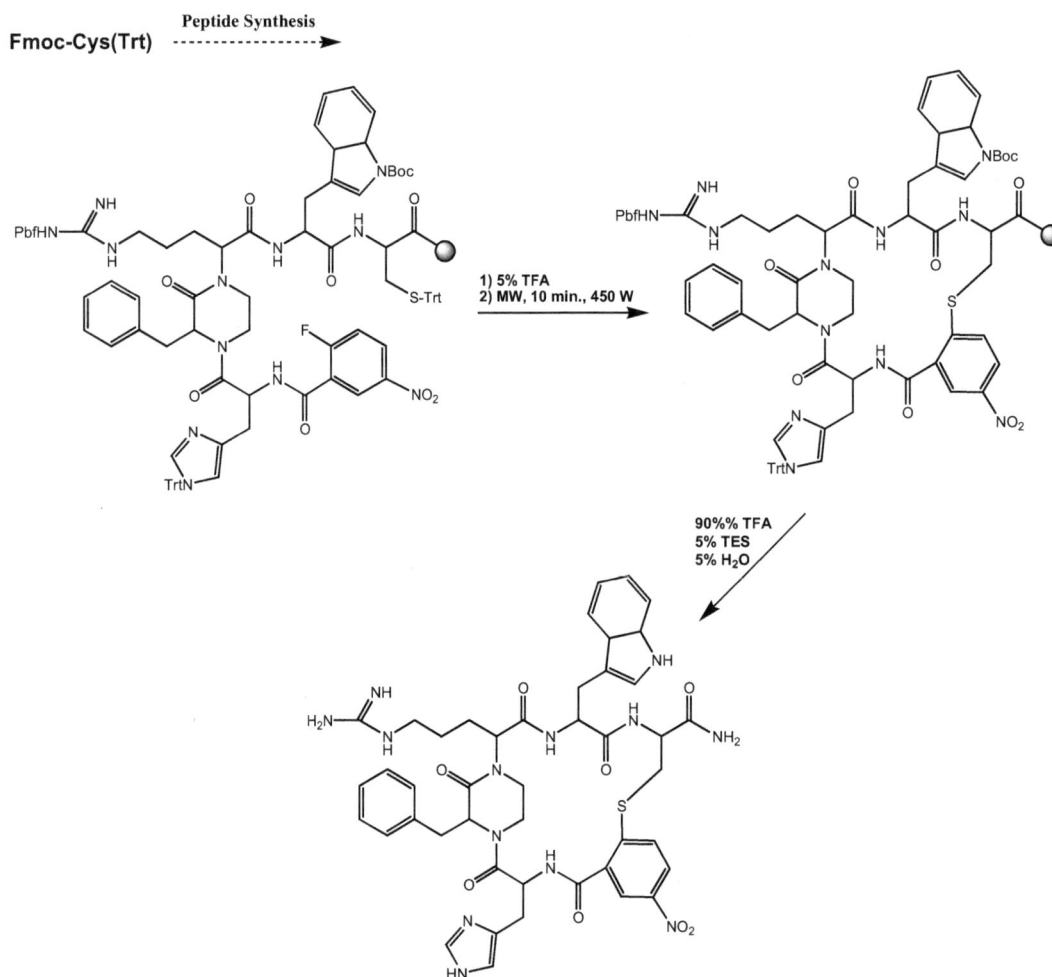

Figure 13: Macrocycles selective and antagonists at the melanocortin receptor hMC5R.

Recently, Awuah and Capretta [31] described a microwave-assisted one-pot method that allows an efficient preparation of flavones, from aryl halides and 2-iodophenol derivatives (Fig. **14**).

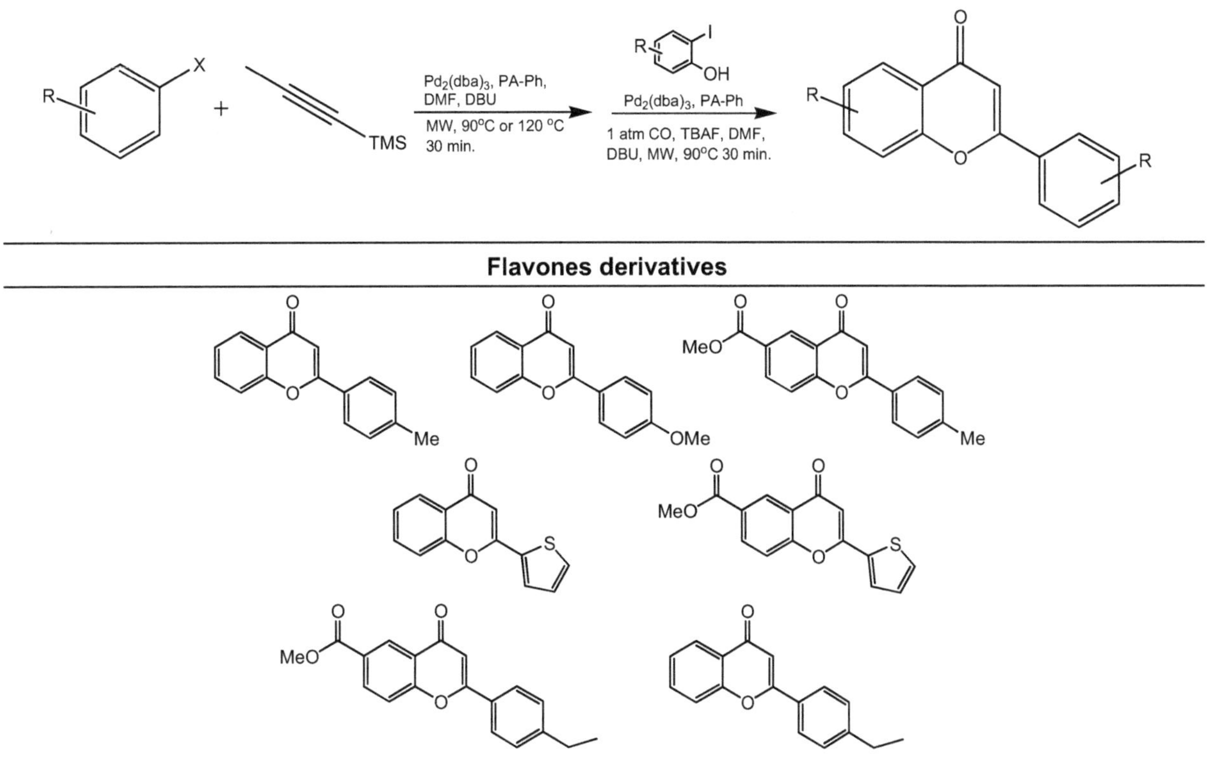

Figure 14: Flavones derivatives obtained via MAOS.

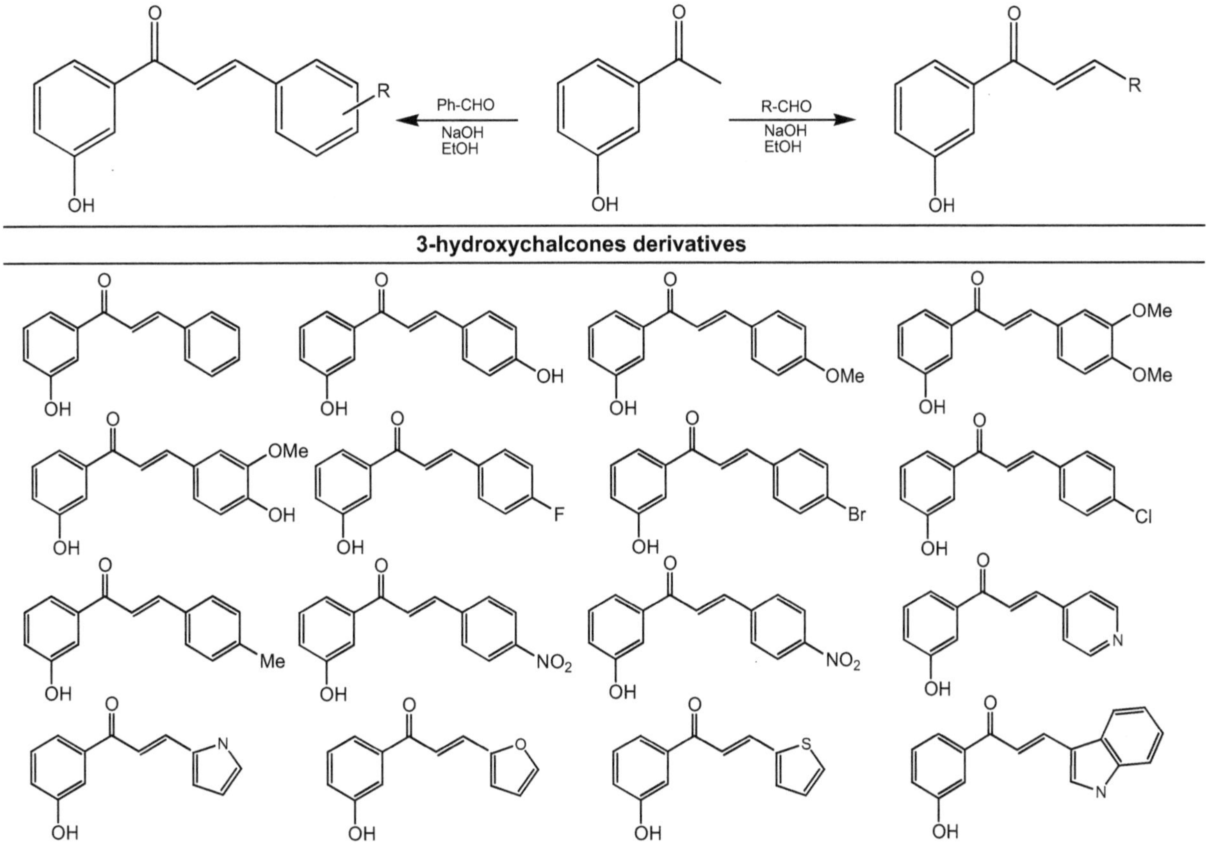

Figure 15: Library of 3-hydroxychalcones derivatives obtained by MAOS, with potential antibacterial activity.

Ansari *et al.* [32a] have developed a microwave synthesis of a 33-membered library of 3-hydroxychalcones by reaction of 3-hydroxyacetophenone with different substituted aryl- and heteroaryl aldehydes under Claisen-Schimidt conditions (Fig. **15**). The reaction time under microwave irradiation had a significant decrease when compared with classical conditions, ranging from 30 seconds to 3 minutes (first method) and from 3 to 5 hours (last method) [32b]. The synthesized chalcones showed potential antibacterial activity, against *B. bronchiseptica* respiratory tract infections.

A series of novel polycyclic-fused isoxazolo[5,4-*b*]pyridines was efficiently synthesized (one pot) under microwave irradiation in water. Isoxazole has been widely used as a key building block for lead compounds which are biologically active.

Its derivatives have diversified pharmacological properties, such as analgesic, anti-inflammatory, anti-HIV, hypoglycemic, anticancer and antibacterial activity (Fig. **16**) [33].

Many 2-pyridone and 2-quinilone analogs display antiulcer, antifungal and antiphlogistic properties and even, some representatives are described as specific non-nucleoside reverse transcriptase inhibitors of human immunodeficiency virus-1 (HIV-1) [34,35].

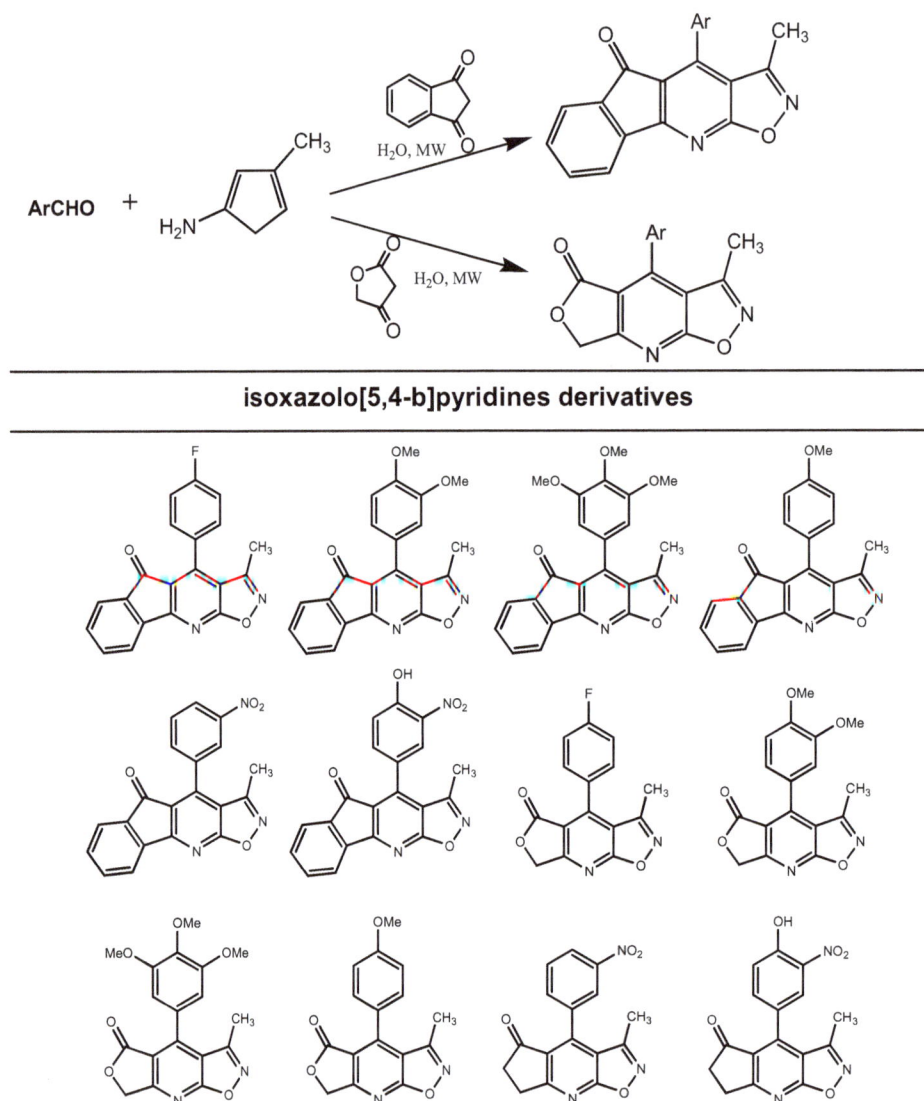

Figure 16: Polycyclic-fused isoxazolo[5,4-*b*]pyridines derivatives synthesized under microwave irradiation in water.

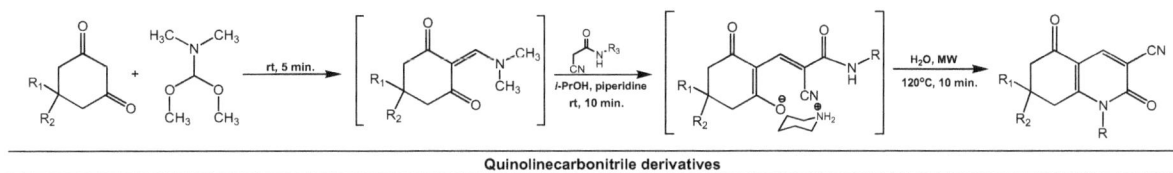

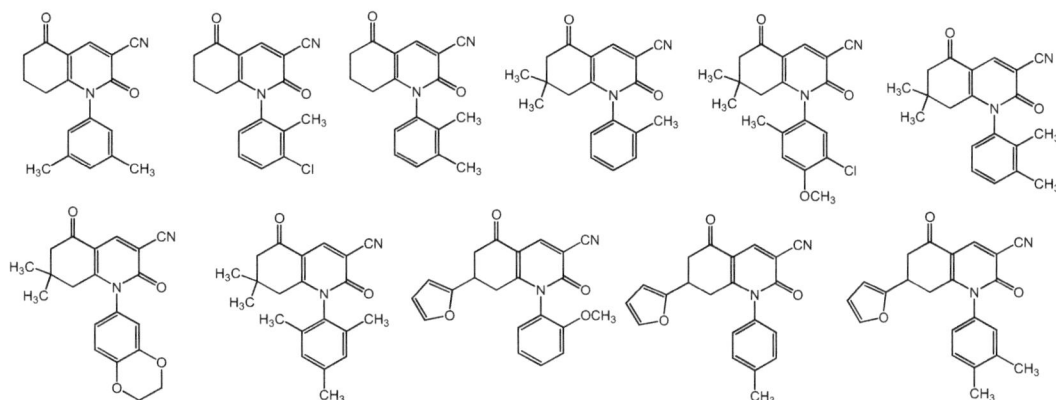

Figure 17: Quinolinecarbonitrile derivatives obtained by MAOS.

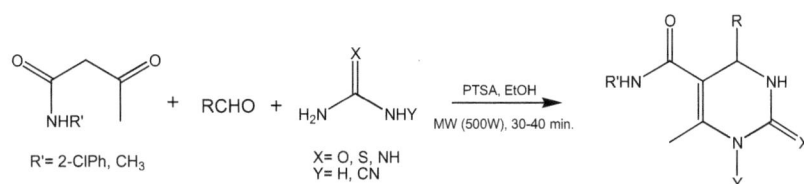

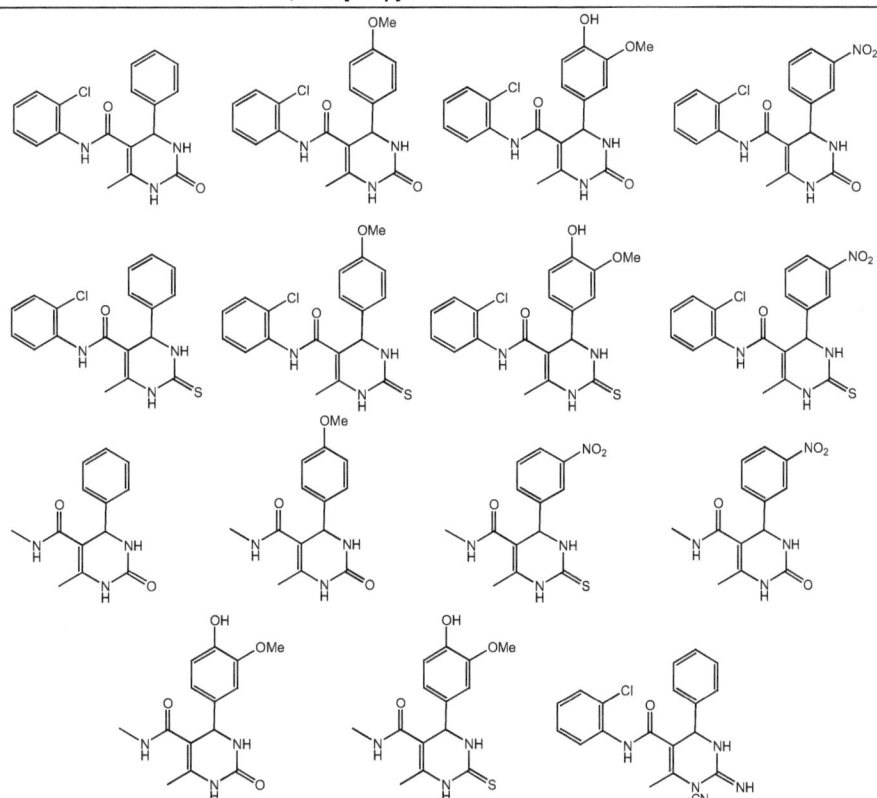

Figure 18: Dihydropyrimidines library with potential anticancer activity.

In this way, Yermolayev, Gorobets and Desenko developed a one-pot three step microwave-assisted method for the synthesis of N1-substituted 2,5-dioxo-1,2,5,6,7,8-hexahydro-3-quinolinecarbonitrile derivatives obtaining 105 compounds library from 1,3-cyclohexanediones, dimethylformamide dimethylacetal and different cyanacetamides (Fig. **17**).

Kumar *et al.* [36] reported the parallel synthesis of some novel dihydropyrimidines from appropriate building blocks using *p*-toluenesulphonic acid as an efficient catalyst and they identified new lead compounds with potential anticancer and antioxidant activity (Fig. **18**).

Some high-yielding MAOS protocols for convenient synthesis of several important heterocyclic derivatives have been widely used as a key building block for pharmaceutical agents, such as 1,2,4-triazines, imidazoles, quinoxalines, pyrazinone, 5-aminooxazoles, pyrazolo[1,5-a]pyrimidines and pyrazolo[3,4-d]pyrimidines.

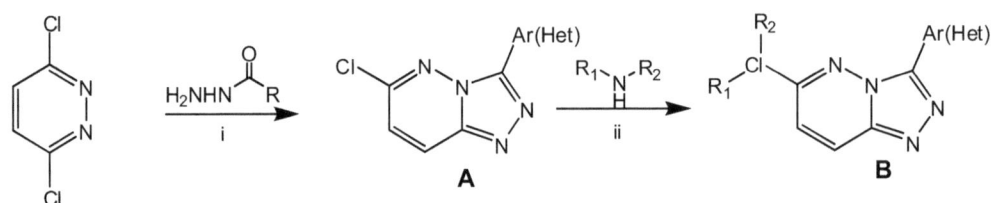

Method 1: (i) 110 °C, 16-60 hours, toluene, yield: < 50%; (ii) 100-140 °C, 8-24 hours, yield: 40-70%.
Method 2: (i) 150 °C, MW, 10 min, 5% H⁺/EtOH, yields: 70-87%; (ii) 180 °C, MW, 15min, DMF, yields: 65-92%.

3-aryl-6-chloro-[1,2,4]triazolo[4,3-*b*]pyridazine derivatives

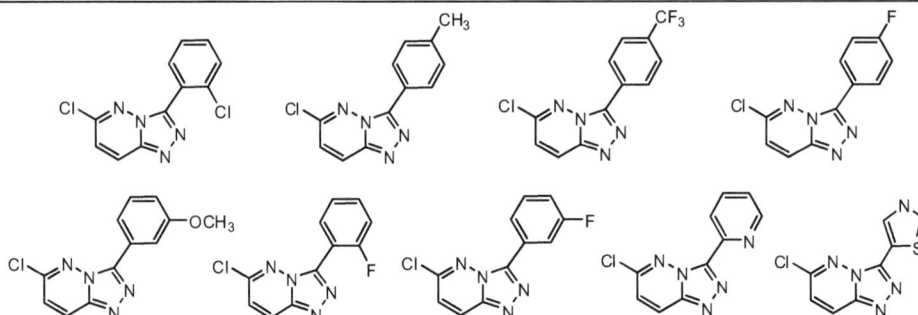

3,6-disubstituted-[1,2,4]triazolo[4,3-b]pyridazine derivatives

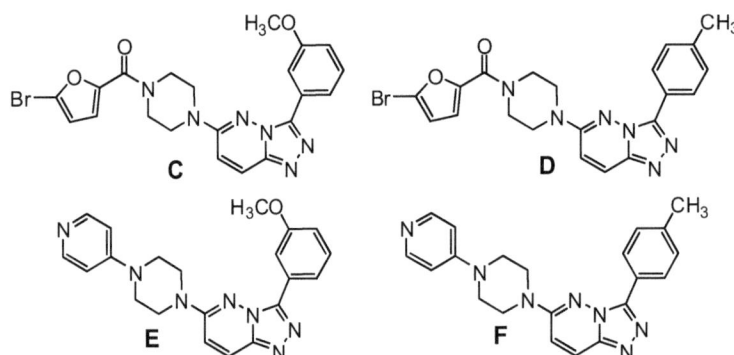

Figure 19: 3,6-disubstituted-[1,2,4]triazolo[4,3-b]pyridazine derivatives and their analogs as leads for potential new therapeutic agents for Parkinson's Disease [31].

Currently, high-yielding and convenient synthesis of the 3,6-disubstituted-[1,2,4]triazolo[4,3-b]pyridazine scaffold **B** analogs have been developed and allowed the identification of new compounds **C**, **D**, **E** and **E** as leads for potential new therapeutic agents for Parkinson's Disease (Fig. **19**) [37a]. In conventional method the scaffold **B** has been synthesized by refluxing for 16-60 hours, to provide the 3-aryl-6-chloro-[1,2,4]triazolo[4,3-b]pyridazine **A** in yields less than 50%. The next step, the introduction of the amino moiety in the 6-position to obtain analogs **B**, occurred at 100-140 °C for 8-30 hours with yields ranging from 40% to 70% [37a, b, c]. The developed general and high-yielding protocols using MAOS allows the reaction time, yields and overall reactions to be dramatically improved. These results can be observed in the reaction scheme shown in Fig. **19** [37a].

Guo *et al.* [38a] reported the optimized synthesis using microwave irradiation and screening of a set of 55 pyridine dicarbonitriles followed by quantitative biological analysis. Previously, these authors described the synthesis of pyridine dicarbonitriles derivatives by conventional heating for 24 hours and yields from 23 to 43% [38b]. When microwave irradiation was used, the reaction time was reduced to 10-120 minutes and the compounds were obtained in 29-51% yield. These compounds were found to be potential prion (infectious agent composed primarily of protein) for disease therapeutics (Fig. **20**).

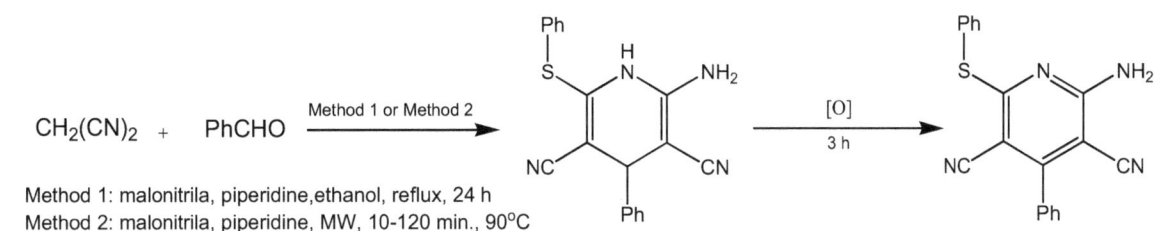

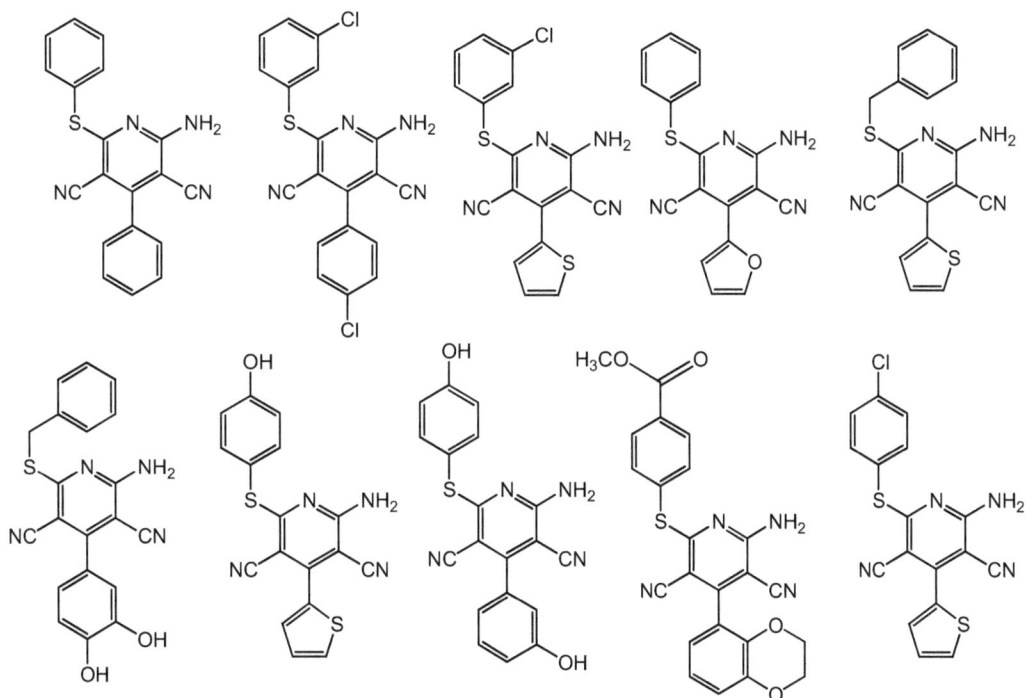

Figure 20: Pyridine dicarbonitriles library obtained by MAOS.

There are many thousands examples of MAOS applications in drug discovery/medicinal chemistry processes reported by both academic and industrial laboratories. It has been contributed in the identification and generation of new compound libraries and lead compounds with different therapeutical applications, such as analgesic, anesthetic, cardiovascular, psychopharmacologic drugs and anti-malarial, respiratory, immunomodulating agents among others (Fig. **21**) [26]. Generally, its most evident improvements are related with considerable reduced time of reaction, with cleaner reactions due to fewer side-reactions, with use of minimal quantities of solvent and the fact that many reactions that previously were not possible can be carried out successfully with microwave irradiation.

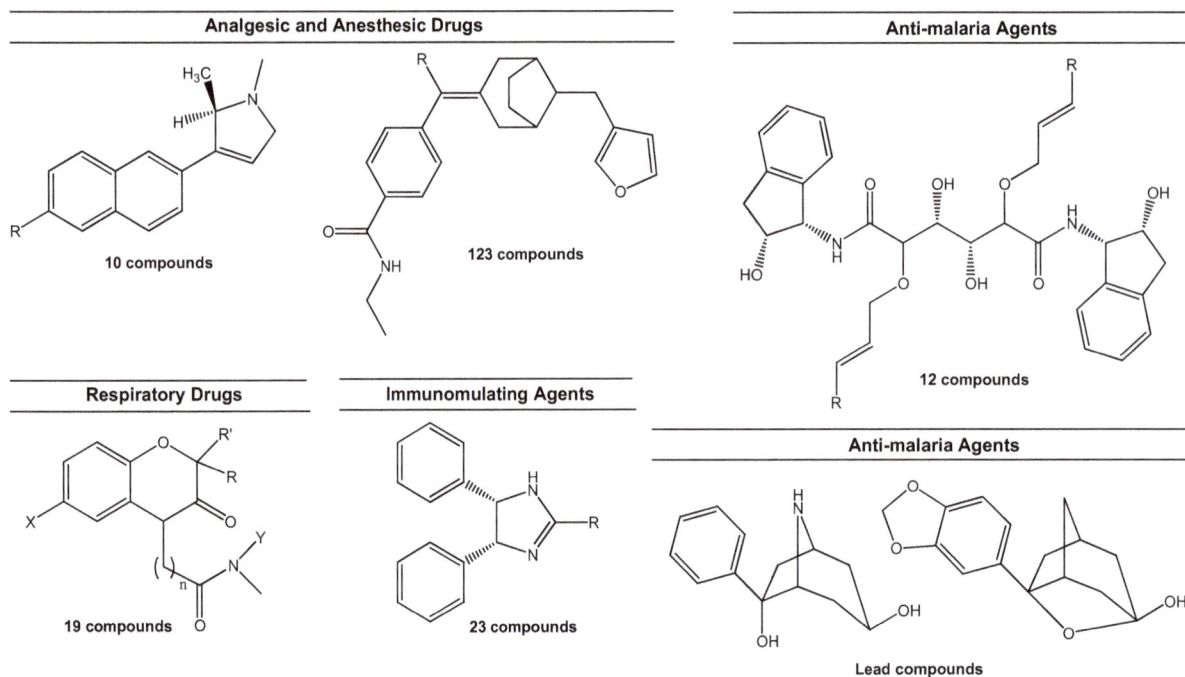

Figure 21: New compound libraries with different therapeutic applications obtained by MAOS.

REFERENCES

[1]   http://www.gallawa.com/microtech/history.html
[2]   http://www.raytheon.com/ourcompany/history/leadership/
[3]   Kappe CO, Stadler A. Weinheim: Microwaves in Organic and Medicinal Chemistry. WILEY-VCH; 2005.
[4]   Lidström P, Tierney J, Wathey B, Westman J. Microwave assisted organic chemistry – a review. Tetrahedron 2001 Aug 29;57:9225-9283.
[5]   Kappe CO. Controlled Microwave Heating in Modern Organic Synthesis. Angew Chem Int Ed 2004;43:6250-6284.
[6]   Gedye R, Smith F, Westaway K *et al.* The Use of Microwave Ovens for Rapid Organic Synthesis. Tetrahedron Lett. 1986, 27(3): 279-282.
[7]   Giguere RJ, Bray TL, Duncan SM, Majetich G. Application of Commercial Microwave ovens to Organic Synthesis. Tetrahedron Letters 1986; 27(41):4945-4948.
[8]   Hayes BL, Microwave Synthesis: Chemistry at the Speed of Light, CEM Publishing, Matthews NC; 2002.
[9]   England R. Microwave Synthesis: A New Wave of Synthetic Organic Chemistry, Personal Chemistry. Chemical Synthesis; 2003
[10]   Larhed M, Hallberg A. Microwave-assisted high-speed chemistry: a new technique in drug discovery. Drug Discovery Today, 2001; 6(8):406-416.
[11]   Shipe WD, Wolkenberg SE, Lindsley CW. Accelerating lead development by microwave-enhanced medicinal chemistry. Drug Discovery Today: Technologies 2005; 2(2):155-161.
[12]   Colombo M, Peretto I. Chemistry strategies in early drug discovery: an overview of recent trends. *Drug Discovery Today* 2008; 13:677-684.
[13]   Wathey B, Tierney J, Lidström P, Westman J. The impact of microwave-assisted organic chemistry on drug discovery. Drug Discovery Today 2002; 7:373-830.
[14]   Mavandadi F, Pilotti A. The impact of microwave-assisted organic synthesis in drug discovery. Drug Discovery Today 2006; 11(3/4), 165-174.
[15]   Gabriel C, Gabriel S, Grant EH, Halstead BSJ, Mingos, DMP. Dielectric parameters relevant to microwave dielectric heating. Chem Soc Rev 1998 Feb 12;27:213-223.
[16]   Mingos DMP, Baghurst D R. Applications of Microwave Dielectric Heating Effects to Synthetic Problems in Chemistry Chemical Society Reviews 1991; 20:1-47.
[17]   Kappe CO, Dallinger D, The impact of microwave synthesis on drug discovery. Nature Reviews Drug Discovery, 2006; 5:51-63.

[18]　Larhed M, Wannberg J, Hallberg A. Controlled Microwave Heating as an Enabling Technology: Expedient Synthesis of Protease Inhibitors in Perspective QSAR Combinatorial Science, 2007; 26:51-68.

[19]　Leadbeater NE, Torenius HM, Tye H. Microwave-assisted Mannich-type three-component reactions Molecular Diversity, 2003; 7:135-144.

[20]　http://www.wikipedia.org/

[21]　Stuerga DAC, Gaillard P. Microwave athermal effects in chemistry: A myth's autopsy.1. Historical background and fundamentals of wave-matter interaction. The Journal of Microwave Power and Electromagnetic Energy, 1996; 31(2):87-100.

[22]　Santagada V, Frecentese F, Perissutti E, Favretto L, Caliendo G. The Application of Microwaves in Combinatorial and High-Throughput Synthesis as New Synthetic Procedure in Drug Discovery. QSAR Combinatorial Science 2004; 23:919-944.

[23]　Lew A, Krutzik PO, Hart ME, Chamberlin AR. Increasing Rates of Reaction: Microwave-Assisted Organic Synthesis for Combinatorial Chemistry. Journal of Combinatorial Chemistry, 2002; 4(2):95-105.

[24]　Kappe C O. High-speed combinatorial synthesis utilizing microwave irradiation. *Current Opinion in Chemical Biology*, 2002; 6: 314-320.

[25]　http://www.milestonesci.com/synth-fund.php

[26]　Alcázar J, Diels G, Schoentjes B. Perspectives of non-nucleoside reverse transcriptase inhibitors (NNRTIs) in the therapy of HIV-1 infection Mini-Reviews in Medicinal Chemistry 2007; 7:345-369.

[27]　Sandoval, W. N.; Pham, V. C.; Lill, J. R. Recent developments in microwave-assisted protein chemistries – can this be integrated into the drug discovery and validation. Drug Discovery Today 2008; 13(23/24):1075-1081.

[28]　Campbell J. and Blackwell H E. Efficient Construction of Diketopiperazine Macroarrays Through a Cyclative-Cleavage Strategy and Their Evaluation as Luminescence Inhibitors in the Bacterial Symbiont *Vibrio fischeri.* Journal of Combinatorial Chemistry 2009; 11:1094-1099.

[29]　Bagley MC, Hughes DD, Lubinu MC, Merritt EA, Taylor PH, Tomkinson NCO. Microwave-Assisted Synthesis of Pyrimidine Libraries. QSAR Combinatorial Science 2004; 23:859-867.

[30]　Grieco P, Cai M, Liu L, Mayorov A, Chandler K, Trivedi D, Lin G, Campiglia P, Novellino E, Hruby VJ. Design and Microwave-Assisted Synthesis of Novel Macrocyclic Peptides Active at Melanocortin Receptors: Discovery of Potent and Selective hMC5R Receptor Antagonists. Journal of Medicinal Chemistry 2008; 51(9):2701-2707.

[31]　Awuah E, Capretta A. Access to Flavones via a Microwave-Assisted, One-Pot Sonogashira-Carbonylation-Annulation Reaction. Organic Letters 2009; 11:3210-3213.

[32]　(a) Ansari FL, Baseer M, Iftikhar F, Kulsoom S, Ullah A, Nazir S, Shaukat A, Haq I, Mirza B. Microwave assisted synthesis, antibacterial activity against *Bordetella bronchiseptica* of a library of 3′-hydroxyaryl and heteroaryl chalcones and molecular descriptors-based SAR. ARKIVOC 2009; (x)318-332. (b) Ansari FL, Umbreen S, Hussain L, Makhmoor T, Nawaz SA, Lodhi MA, Khan SN, Shaheen F, Choudhary MI, Atta-Ur-Rahman, Synthesis and Biological Activities of Chalcones and 1,5-Benzothiazepine Derivatives: promising New Free-radical Scavengers, and Esterase, Urease, and α-Glucosidase Inhibitors. Chem. Biodiv. 2005; *2*:487-496.

[33]　Tu S-J, Zhang X, Han Z, Cao X, Wu S, Yan S, Hao W, Zhang G, Ma N. Synthesis of Isoxazolo[5,4-*b*]pyridines by Microwave-Assisted Multi-Component Reactions in Water Journal of Combinatorial Chemistry 2009; 11(3):42-432.

[34]　Yermolayev SA, Gorobets NY, Desenko SM. Rapid Three-Step One-Pot Microwave-Assisted Synthesis of 2,5-Dioxo-1,2,5,6,7,8-hexahydro-3-quinolinecarbonitrile Library Journal of Combinatorial Chemistry 2009; 11(1):44-46.

[35]　De Clercq E. Perspectives of non-nucleoside reverse transcriptase inhibitors (NNRTIs) in the therapy of HIV-1 infection Farmaco, 1999; 54:26-45.

[36]　Prashantha Kumar BR, Sankar G, Nasir Baig RB, Chandrashekaran S. Novel Biginelli dihydropyrimidines with potential anticancer activity: A parallel synthesis and CoMSIA study European Journal of Medicinal Chemistry 2009; 44:4192-4198.

[37]　(a) Aldrich LN, Lebois EP, Lewis LM, Nalywajko NT, Niswender CM, Weaver CD, Conn PJ, Lindsley CW. MAOS protocols for the general synthesis and lead optimization of 3,6-disubstituted-[1,2,4]triazolo[4,3-b]pyridazines. Tetrahedron Letters 2009; 50:212-215. (b) Cox JM, Harper B, Mastracchio A, Leiting B, Roy RS, Patel RA, Wu JW, Lyons KA, He H, Xu S, Zhu B, Thornberry NA, Weber AE, Edmondson SD. Discovery of 3-aminopiperidines as potent, selective, and orally bioavailable dipeptidyl peptidase IV inhibitors. Bioorg. Med. Chem. Lett. 2007; 17:4579-4583. (c) Carling RW, Moore KW, Street LJ, Wild D, Isted C, Leeson PD, Thomas S, O'Connor D, McKernan RM, Quirk K, Cook SM, Atack JR, Wafford KA, Thompson SA, Dawson GR, Ferris P, Castro JL. 3-Phenyl-6-(2-pyridyl)methyloxy-1,2,4-triazolo[3,4-*a*]phthalazines and Analogues: High-Affinity ç-Aminobutyric Acid-A Benzodiazepine Receptor Ligands with r2, r3, and r5-Subtype Binding Selectivity over r1. J. Med. Chem. 2004; 47(7):1807-1822.

[38] (a) Guo K, Mutter R, Heal W, Reddy TRK, Cope H, Pratt S, Thompson MJ, Chen B. Synthesis and evaluation of a focused library of pyridine dicarbonitriles against prion disease. European Journal of Medicinal Chemistry, 2008; 43:93-106. (b) Reddy TRK, Mutter R, Heal W, Guo K, Gillet VJ, Pratt S, Chen B. Library Design, Synthesis, and Screening: Pyridine Dicarbonitriles as Potential Prion Disease Therapeutics. J. Med. Chem. 2006; 49(2):607-615.

CHAPTER 7

Carbohydrates and Glycoproteins: Cellular Recognition and Drug Design

Vanessa Leiria Campo, Valquiria Aragão-Leoneti, Maristela Braga Martins Teixeira and Ivone Carvalho

School of Pharmaceutical Sciences of Ribeirão Preto, University of São Paulo, Av. do Café, s/n, Monte Alegre, 14040-903, Ribeirão Preto, São Paulo, Brazil

Abstract: The high abundance of carbohydrates in nature and their diverse roles in biological systems validate the increasing interest for their chemical and biological research. Carbohydrates can be found as monomers or oligomers, or as glycoconjugates, which are formed by an oligosaccharide moiety linked to a protein (glycoproteins) or to a lipid moiety (glycolipids). Blood groups determinants (ABH), tumor associated antigens and pathogen binding sites are some of the relevant glycoconjugates found on mammalian cells. It is well known that carbohydrate and glycoconjugate molecules are implicated in many cellular processes, especially in biological recognition events, including cell adhesion, differentiation and growth, signal transduction, protozoa, bacterial and virus infections as well as immune responses. Therefore, the demand for glycans and glycoconjugates for various studies of targets involved in several serious diseases have been continuously growing. In this chapter we will present the design of drugs based on carbohydrate structure for treatment of parasitic diseases (*T. cruzi*) and virus infections (influenza and HIV). In addition, the development of glycoconjugate antitumour vaccines related to the structure of human mucin-associated glycans will also be discussed.

INTRODUCTION

Biological Importance of Carbohydrates and Glycoproteins

In addition to proteins and nucleic acids, carbohydrates constitute the third major class of naturally occurring biopolymers. The peculiar and distinct property of monosaccharides is their polifunctional nature, which provides different positions around the ring that can be connected and allows branching and functionalization.

Moreover, carbohydrate complexity is increased by ring stereocenters and, in contrast to amide or phosphate diester linkages, the formation of each glycosidic linkage creates one new stereogenic center [1, 2].

Therefore, considering only the ten most abundant mammalian monosaccharides (Fig. **1**), more than 100 thousand distinct trisaccharidic structures are theoretically viable, and this number increases significantly with the chain extension.

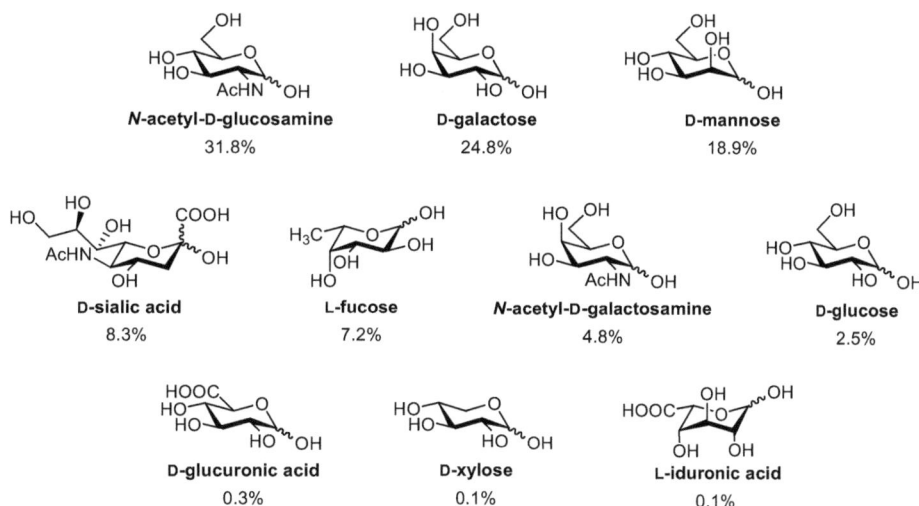

Figure 1: Most frequent mammalian monosaccharides and their respective abundances obtained from GLYCOSCIENCES data base [2].

Carlton A. Taft and Carlos H. T. P. Silva (Eds)

Until 1960s the importance of carbohydrates was restricted to energetic (ex. glucose and glycogen) and structural (ex. chitin in crab shells and cellulose in plants) functions; however, during the last decades carbohydrates have gained more importance considering that they play essential roles as communication molecules in many intercellular and intracellular processes due to their diverse structural arrangements [1, 3].

Carbohydrates can be found as monomers or oligomers, or as glycoconjugates, which are formed by the coupling of glycans to a protein (glycoprotein), to a lipid (glycolipid) or to both lipid and protein (glycosylphosphatidylinositol (GPI)-anchored proteins). The majority of carbohydrates are linked through *O*-glycosidic bonds to the side chains of serine and threonine or through *N*-glycosidic bonds to the side chain of asparagine. The *O*-glycosidic linkages to tyrosine, hydroxylysine and hydroxyproline, as well as *C*-glycosidic attachment to tryptophan, are less common [4]. Blood groups determinants (ABH, etc.), tumor associated antigens (Le$_x$, Le$_y$, etc.) and pathogen binding sites are some of the relevant glycoconjugates found in mammalian cells [5].

It is well known that carbohydrate and glycoproteins expressed in cell surfaces are implicated in many physiological and pathological events, especially in biological recognition processes, including cell adhesion, differentiation and growth, signal transduction, protozoa, bacterial and virus infection as well as immune responses [3-6]. This diversity of activities validate the usage of carbohydrates and glycoproteins for the investigation of biological targets involved in several pathological conditions, such as cancer, auto-immunity, parasitic diseases, virus and bacterial infections, and consequently, for the development of new therapeutic strategies. It is noteworthy that some drugs derived from carbohydrates, either natural or synthetic analogs, were successfully introduced in the market, as is the case of the antiviral oseltamivir phosphate (Tamiflu, Roche®), of the anti-diabetic acarbose (Glucobay, Bayer®), of the antithrombotic heparin and of the aminoglycosidic antibiotics [7].

CELLULAR RECOGNITION

The structure of a specific cell contains codified biological information that other cells can decode. Therefore, as previously mentioned, carbohydrate and glycoconjugate molecules on cell surfaces (Fig. **2**) have been recognized to play crucial roles in many cellular processes involving biological recognition events, binding of toxins, hormones, fertilization and other important roles [8].

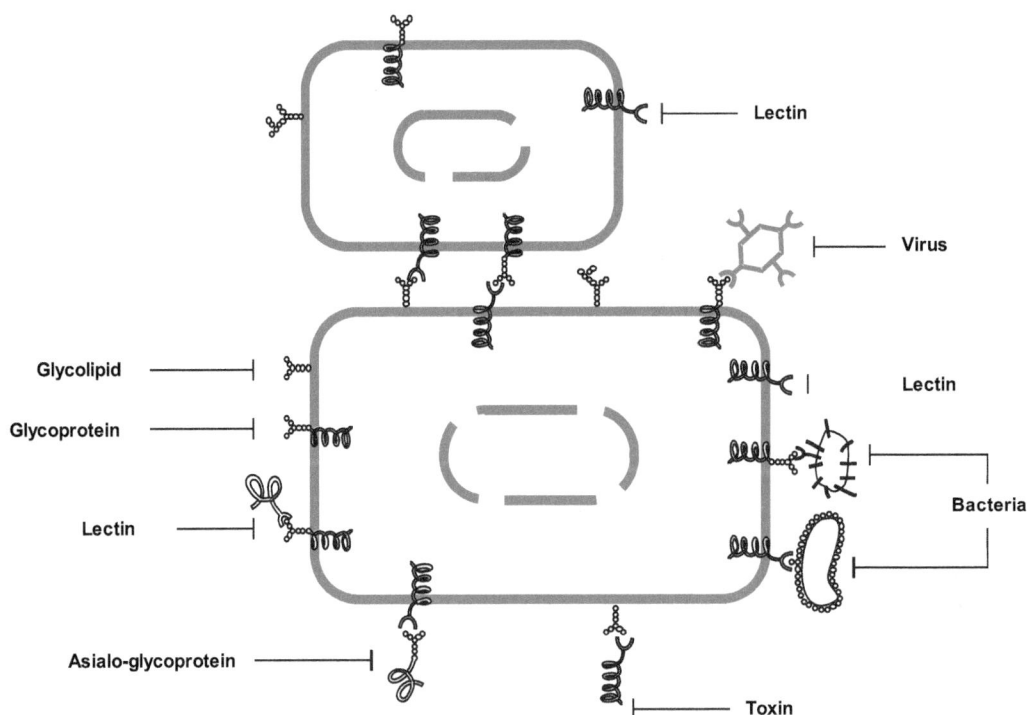

Figure 2: Cell surface lectin-carbohydrate interactions in cellular recognition. Adapted from refs [8] and [9].

Lectins are carbohydrate-specific proteins that function as recognition molecules in several biological systems. They are very important for the investigation of carbohydrates on cell surfaces, especially the alterations that they suffer in malignancy, as well as the isolation and characterization of glycoproteins (Table **1**) [9].

Table 1: Lectin Functions.

Lectin	Role In
Microorganisms	
Amoeba	Infection
Bacteria	Infection
Influenza virus	Infection
Plants	
Various	Defense
Legumes	Symbiosis with nitrogen-fixing bacteria
Animals	
Calnexin, calreticulin, ERGIC-53	Control of glycoprotein biosynthesis
Collectins	Innate immunity
Dectin-1	Innate immunity
Galectins	Regulation of cell growth and apoptosis; regulation of the cell cycle; modulation of cell–cell and cell–substrate interactions
Macrophage mannose receptor	Innate immunity; clearance of sulfated glycoprotein hormones
Man-6-P receptors	Targeting of lysosomal enzymes
L-selectin	Lymphocyte homing
E- and P-selectins	Leukocyte trafficking to sites of inflammation
Siglecs	Cell-cell interactions in the immune and neural system
Spermadhesin	Sperm-egg interaction

Adapted from ref [9].

Thus, the major function of lectins appears to be related to cell recognition by means of carbohydrate-lectin interactions (Table **2**). Each lectin has two or more sugar binding sites and the recognition occurs by molecular interactions between complementary structures on the cell surfaces. This concept represents an extension of the lock-and-key hypothesis introduced by Emil Fischer, yielding the Nobel Prize (chemistry) in 1902, to explain the specificity of interactions between enzymes and their substrates. In the same way that proteins recognize their ligands, lectins can recognize carbohydrates by binding reversibly and with high specificity to mono/oligosaccharides. Nevertheless, they lack catalytic activity and, different to antibodies, are not products of an immune response [10].

Table 2: Carbohydrates and Lectins in Cellular Recognition.

Process	Sugar On	Lectins On
Infection	host cells	microorganisms
Defense	Phagocytes	microorganisms
	Microorganisms	phagocytes
Fertilization	Eggs	(sperm)[a]
leukocyte traffic	Leukocytes	endothelial cells
	endothelial cells	lymphocytes
Metastasis	target organs	malignant cells
	malignant cells	(target organs)[a]
[a] Presumed, no experimental evidence available.		

Adapted from ref [10].

The fundamental role of lectins in cellular recognition has gained remarkable attention by several research groups, which has brought about great advances in this field, with the discovery of myriad functions and applications of lectins [9, 10]. For instance, the investigation of carbohydrate-lectin interactions has allowed the design of drugs based on natural glycan structures with high capacity to interact with specific binding sites, such as those explored for treatment of virus infections and parasitic diseases.

HIV Virus and Drug Design

A crucial feature of the human immunodeficiency virus (HIV) is the presence of complex carbohydrates (glycans) that surround the exposed envelope. However, HIV genome encodes no gene products capable of synthesizing these carbohydrates, being the surface proteins glycosylated by host cellular enzymes. It is well known that this glycosylation process affects significantly the folding of viral glycoproteins, the transmission of the virus and nature of the immune response to infections [11].

The comprehension of the viral life cycle has lead to the identification of targets for drug design. Twenty-five anti-HIV drugs have been formally approved for the treatment of AIDS, which can be divided in seven main categories, as shown in Table **3**. Furthermore, novel anti-HIV drugs are under clinical and preclinical trials related with these viral targets and others, which are involved in viral adsorption processes (mediated by gp 120 glycoprotein), proviral DNA integration or transcription transactivation (Fig. **3**) [12a, 12b].

Table 3: Viral Targets and Approved Anti-HIV Drugs.

Viral Targets	Anti-Hiv Drugs
nucleoside reverse transcriptase inhibitors (**NRTIs**)	zidovudine, didanosine, zalcitabine, stavudine, lamivudine, abacavir, emtricitabine
nucleotide reverse transcriptase inhibitor (**NtRTI**)	tenofovir disoproxil fumarate
non-nucleoside reverse transcriptase inhibitors (**NNRTIs**)	nevirapine, delavirdine, efavirenz, etravirine
protease inhibitors (**PIs**)	saquinavir, ritonavir, indinavir, nelfinavir, amprenavir, lopinavir, atazanavir, fozamprenavir, tipranavir, darunavir
fusion inhibitor (**FI**)	enfuvirtide
co-receptor inhibitor (**CRI**)	maraviroc
integrase inhibitor (**INI**)	raltegravir

The first step in the initiation of infection is the recognition and promoting of cell–virus interactions of a virus particle to a specific receptor on the surface of the target cell. In the HIV and other enveloped viruses, the interaction with the cell receptor is mediated by the envelope glycoprotein. The viral envelope is constituted by a lipid bilayer containing a complex protein denominated *env* that consists of glycoproteins gp41 (transmembrane) and gp120, exposed to the viral surface and anchored (bound non-covalently) to gp41. The receptor for HIV is the CD4 lymphocyte; when the virus approaches the host cell, the gpl20 of HIV binds to CD4. This is the first identified retroviral receptor and also the one most extensively studied [13, 14]. The modulation of the antigenicity of gp120 is dependent on the extension and variability of surface glycosylation and represents an interesting target to be explored in drug design [15].

Carbohydrate-Binding Agents (CBAs)

Taking into account the important role developed by glycans in viral infections, agents that interact with these viral envelope glycans may prevent the efficient entry of the virus into its susceptible target cells. Furthermore, these carbohydrate-binding agents (CBAs) may force the virus to delete part of its surface glycans to escape drug pressure, which can lead to the initiation of an immune response against exposed immunogenic envelope epitopes. Thus, the antiviral mechanisms of the CBAs may comprise direct antiviral activity by binding to glycans of the viral envelope, avoiding virus entrance, and indirect antiviral action from the constant deletions of the envelope glycan shield, triggering the immune system to act against previously hidden immunogenic epitopes of the viral envelope [16].

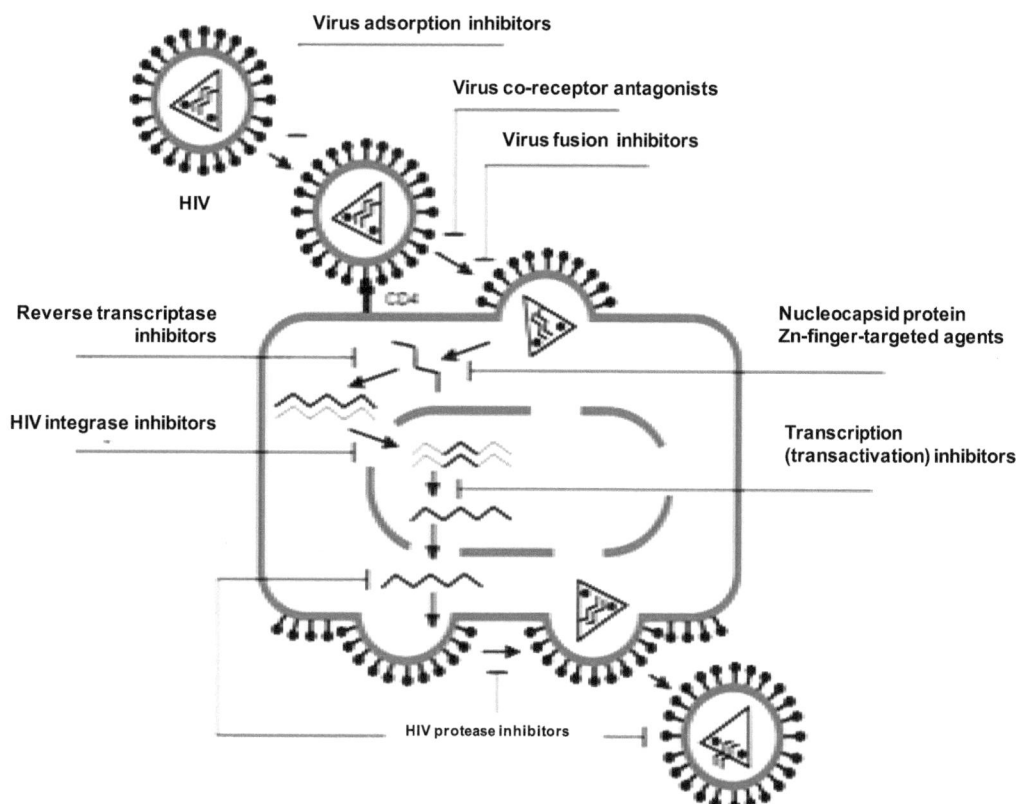

Figure 3: Life cycle of HIV (human immunodeficiency virus) and representation of the targets for anti-HIV drugs. Adapted from ref [12b].

The CBAs can be divided in two categories: lectins that specifically recognize glycan structures, and non-peptidic small-size agents (Fig. **4**) that may have an efficient and often specific affinity for monosaccharide and/or oligosaccharide structures [16]. Besides, various research groups have developed the synthesis and characterization of synthetic CBAs.

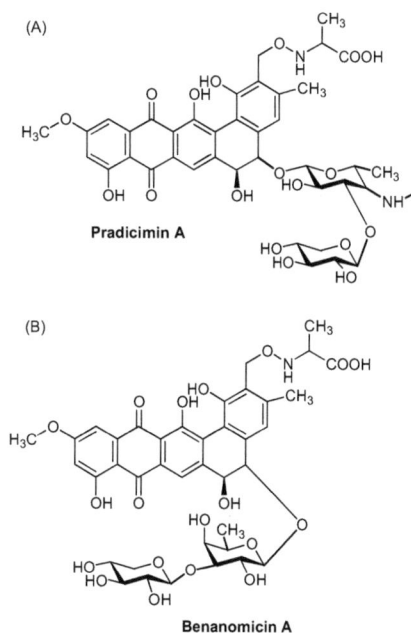

Figure 4: Small-size non-peptidic carbohydrate-binding antigens (CBAs). Pradimicin A (**A**) and benanomicin A (**B**) are produced by *Actinomadura hibiscus* and *Actinomadura spadix*, respectively [16].

Glucosidase Inhibitors

The other class of chemotherapeutics involved in the viral adsorption acts by inhibiting glucosidase, which play a role in glycoprotein biosynthesis. Glucosidases are enzymes that catalyze the cleavage of glycosidic bonds by processing of complex carbohydrates, fundamental in many cellular recognition processes, such as (i) cleavage of diet polysaccharides in monosaccharide, which are metabolically absorbed and used by the organism, (ii) lysosomal glycoconjugate catabolism and glycoprotein processing, and (iii) biosynthesis of oligosaccharides in glycoproteins or glycolipids. Inhibition of these glucosidases can affect quality control, maturation, transport, secretion of glycoproteins, and can alter cell-cell or cell-virus recognition processes [17, 15].

The enzymes glucosidase I and II are involved in key steps during the processing of *N*-linked oligosaccharides by cleaving three terminal glucose residues from the tetradeca-oligosaccharide moiety $Glc_3Man_9GlcNAc_2$ of an important *N*-linked oligosaccharide intermediate (Scheme **1**). Inhibitors of such enzymes affect the formation of these oligosaccharides and have shown remarkable anti-HIV activity, which may lead to unsuccessful completion of gp120 in the viral reproduction [18].

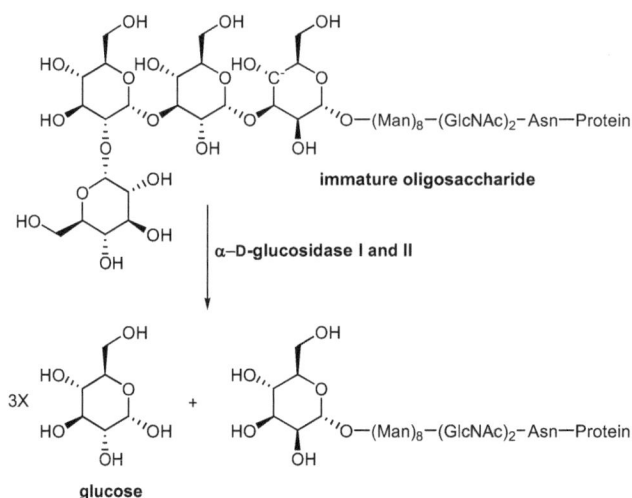

Scheme 1: Processing of *N*-linked oligosaccharides by the action of glucosidase I and II enzymes [15].

The functions of glucosidases in the organism justify the search for potential therapeutic inhibitors to be used in diabetes, obesity, glycosphingolipid lysosomal storage disease, HIV infections, and tumors in general. Some drugs are used as therapeutic agents can be exemplified by acarbose (**1**) (Precose®), miglitol (**2**) (Glyset®), and *N*-butyl-1-deoxynojirimycin (**3**) (Zavesca®) (Fig. **5**). Drugs **1** and **2** are used in the treatment of non-insulin-dependent diabetes, type II, interfering with the digestion of dietary carbohydrates, whilst drug **3** is employed for the control of the metabolic Gaucher's disease [15].

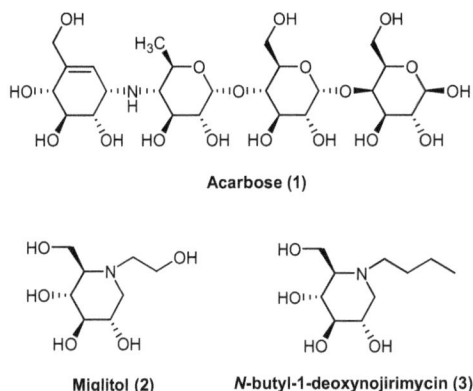

Figure 5: Examples of glucosidase inhibitors available in the therapeutic.

Particularly, treatment with compound **3** leads to structural modifications in gp120 and consequently, expresses viruses that fail to undergo productive post-receptor-binding rearrangements or fusion with the target-cell membrane. However, this drug is moderately tolerated in humans; for antiviral activity, it is necessary to use it in higher concentrations, which causes unwanted inhibition of sucrases in the intestine. Nevertheless, for treatment of glycolipid storage disorders low concentration of this drug is effective [11].

Moreover, glucosidase inhibitors have also been useful for probing biochemical pathways and understanding structure-activity relationships patterns required for mimicking the enzyme transition state. Several types of glucosidase inhibitors have received great attention, such as disaccharides, iminosugars, carbasugars, thiosugars, and non-sugar derivatives [15].

The design of novel compounds with potential glucosidase inhibitory activity requires knowledge of the three-dimensional structures of the human and *Saccharomyces cerevisiae* enzymes, the latter being commercially available and used in biological assays. Considering that these non-solved enzymes are not available in the Protein Data Bank (PDB), a homology model of the *S. cerevisiae* glucosidase was constructed based on a 4-α-glucanotransferase of *Thermotoga maritime* (PDB code 1LWJ), which showed high identity sequence [18, 15].

More recently, the catalytic site of the rat intestinal sucrase was described indicating the sequence identity (84,6%) with human lysosomal α-glucosidase when compared with others homologue proteins, such as the *S. cerevisiae* glucosidase (30% sequence identity). In this study, a 3D model of the rat intestinal sucrase was built, and docking simulations were performed of glucosidase inhibitors as well as pharmacophore modeling and molecular interaction fields studies. It was suggested that the main hydrogen bond interactions of the inhibitor 1-deoxynojirimycin (**4**) with the rat intestinal sucrase model are with residues Asp386, Asp129 and Asp499 (Fig. **6**), in *consensus* with the pharmacophore derived from 17 inhibitors of this enzyme, which are reported from literature. These studies allowed proposal and evaluation of two novel potential α- glucosidase inhibitors as prototypes for design of drugs against HIV virus infection, highlighting the important application of carbohydrate based drugs [19].

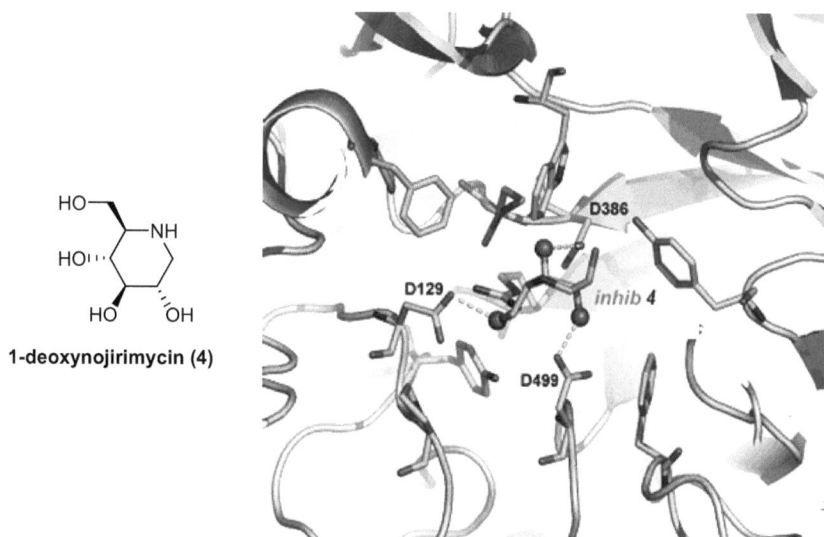

Figure 6: *Ribbons* diagrams of the rat intestinal sucrase model with selected residues of active site. The *consensus* orientation obtained with flexible docking for inhibitor **4**, 1-deoxynojirimycin, is shown in agreement with the pharmacophore modeled, which suggests the hydrogen bonds (dashed lines) with Asp129, Asp386 and Asp499 of the sucrase model as the main interactions of the pharmacophoric groups (hydroxyl groups are represented as spheres) of the α- glucosidase inhibitors –adapted from ref [19].

Design of Influenza Virus Neuraminidase Inhibitors

Influenza is an acute viral infection of the upper respiratory tract that can affect millions of people every year [20], and the emergence of the highly pathogenic avian H5N1 influenza virus, particularly in Asia, highlights the potential impact of influenza virus on humanity, with probability of a human influenza pandemic [21].

Influenza virus (*Myxovirus influenzae*) belongs to the orthomyxoviridae family, which is subdivided into three serologically distinct types: A, B and C. Only influenza virus A and B are of most concern in the human population, with type A considered to be the most likely to cause pandemics. Further classification of influenza virus A is based on the antigenic properties of its surface glycoproteins haemagglutinin (HA) and neuraminidase (NA), which are essential for viral replication, infectivity and the infective cycle of influenza. These glycoproteins are able to recognize the sialic acid *N*-acetylneuraminic acid (Neu5Ac); HA is a lectin that mediates the first contact between the virus and the target host cell through recognition of sialic acid (SA) residues of cell-surface glycoconjugates, while NA is an enzyme that catalyzes the removal of terminal SA linked to glycoproteins and glycolipids, which enables the virus to infect different cells [20, 22].

Neuraminidase plays two critical roles in the life cycle of the virus, including virion progeny release and general mobility of the virus in the respiratory tract. At molecular level, NA promotes the cleavage of the glycosidic bond of glycoproteins and glycolipids, with release of terminal Neu5Ac residues. The enzymatic mechanism involves the formation of a sialosyl cation intermediate (**5**) that adopts a distorted half-chair arrangement. A water molecule then reacts in a stereoselective manner with the sialosyl cation intermediate to afford α-Neu5Ac (**6**) as the first product of release, which then mutarotates to the thermodynamically more favourable β-anomer (**7**) (Scheme **2**) [22, 23].

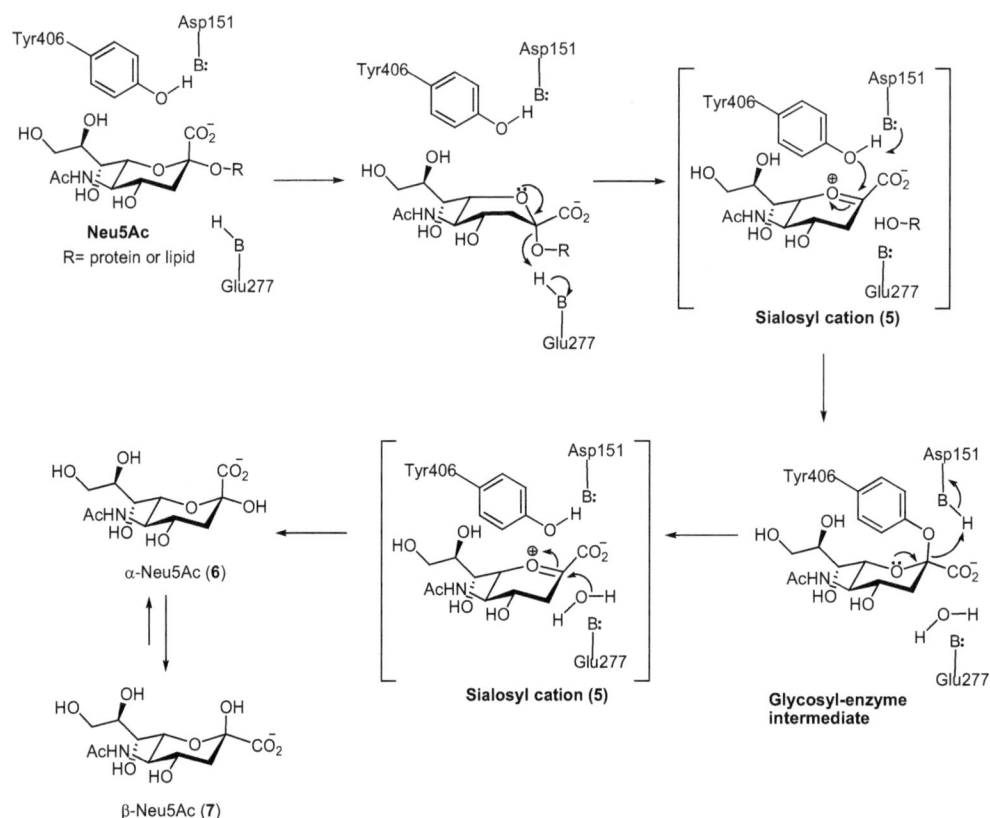

Scheme 2: Enzymatic mechanism of influenza virus neuraminidase.

One of the first inhibitors of neuraminidase was the unsaturated Neu5Ac derivative 2-deoxy-2,3-didehydro-*N*-acetylneuraminic acid (DANA) (**8**) (Fig. **7**), that is an analog of the transition state with a double bond between C-2 and C-3, which makes the ring planar, resembling the sialosyl cation (**5**). The inhibitor DANA (**8**) show a micromolar order inhibition constant ($K_i = 10^{-5}$ to 10^{-6} M) but did not show selectivity for the viral sialidase inhibition and failed in animal models infected with influenza virus. As DANA (**8**), the other designed inhibitors that displayed inhibitory activity contain a double bond in the ring between C-2 and C-3, a carboxylate group at C-2, a positively charged group (in physiological conditions) at C-4 and an *N*- acetamide group at C-5. This is related to the trihydroxylated chain (C7-C9) present in compound (**8**), which can be substituted by a hydrophobic and branching group (Fig. **7**) [23].

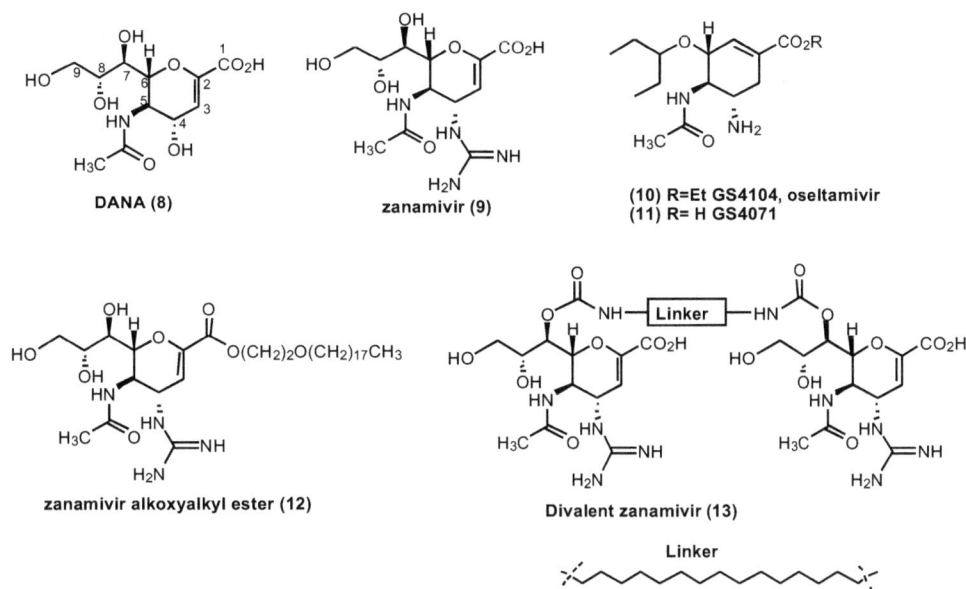

Figure 7: Chemical structures of selected inhibitors of influenza virus neuraminidase.

The determination of the crystal structure of the influenza virus neuraminidase complexed with sialic acid and DANA (**8**) proved to be very useful for the design of new antiinfluenza drugs [22-24]. After analyzing the interactions of (**8**) with the active site of neuraminidase (Fig. 8) it was possible to predict structural modifications that, in principle, could increase the inhibitory effect of this compound.

Thus, the principal modification of (**8**), predicted to significantly improve affinity for the enzyme, was the substitution of the C-4 hydroxyl group with a guanidinyl functionality to provide 4-deoxy-4-guanidino-Neu5Ac2en (**9**) [25].

This improvement in affinity was possible due to interactions between two conserved C-4 binding domain amino acids (Glu119 and Glu227) and the larger basic C-4 guanidinyl moiety (Fig. **8**). Compound (**9**) showed high selectivity for viral sialidase, presenting an inhibition constant of nanomolar order (0.1 to 1 nM), and was selected as the lead drug candidate by Glaxo under the generic name zanamivir.

Considering its limited oral bioavailability (due to its highly polar nature and rapid excretion of the compound), zanamivir was developed in an inhaled form and was approved by FDA in 1999 with the trade name Relenza [22].

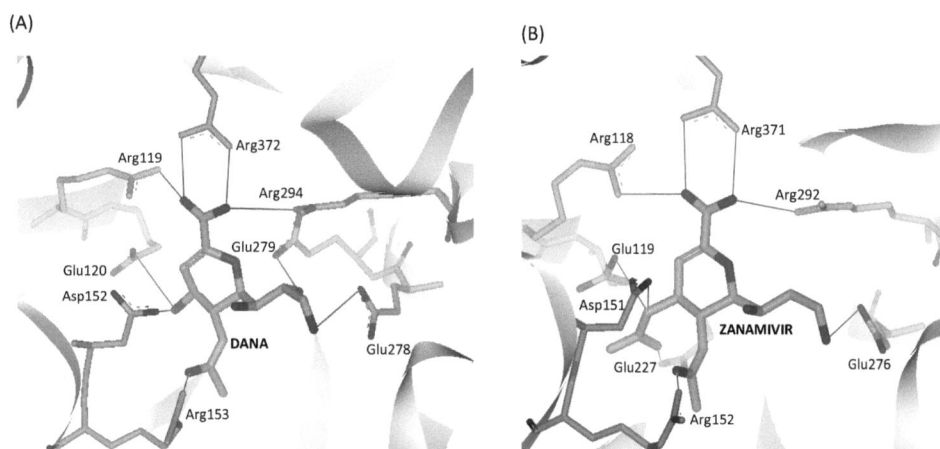

Figure 8: Crystallographic complexes of DANA (**8**) and zanamivir (**9**) with influenza virus neuraminidase (NA). (A) Main interactions of (**8**) with the active site of NA (PDB code 1NNB); (B) Main interactions of (**9**) with the active site of NA (PDB code 2HTQ).

Based on DANA (**8**) and zanamivir (**9**) as prototypes, other neuraminidase inhibitors derived from non-carbohydrate templates were developed in order to facilitate the synthetic process and to increase the bioavailability after oral administration. Among these inhibitors is the cyclohexene derivative oseltamivir (**10**) (GS4104), which is an ethyl ester prodrug of the corresponding active carboxylate (**11**) (GS4071) and is now marketed by Roche under the trade name Tamiflu (Fig. **7**). If the ring structure is not considered, the greater difference between GS4071 (**11**) and zanamivir (**9**) is that (**11**) has a hydrophobic group [3-*O*-(1'-etylpropyl)] replacing the trihydroxylated chain present in zanamivir structure [23, 26, 27]. The crystallographic complex of neuraminidase-GS4071 shows that (**11**) binds in an identical manner to zanamivir (**9**) and other Neu5Ac2en derivatives, but the architecture of the active site is altered upon binding. Specifically, Glu276 reorients outwards from the glycerol side-chain binding domain to interact with Arg224, generating a considerable hydrophobic area within this domain (Fig. **9**) [22].

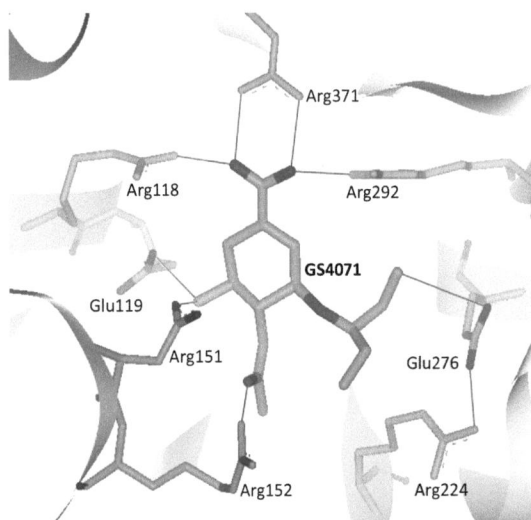

Figure 9: Crystallographic complex of influenza virus neuraminidase-GS4071 (PDB code 2HU4): main interactions of GS4071 (**7**) (active carboxylate) with the active site of neuraminidase.

During the past two years, novel prodrug zanamivir derivatives that may display improved pharmacokinetics compared with zanamivir have been prepared. For example, the alkoxyalkyl ester (**12**) of zanamivir, with long alkyl chains chosen to equilibrate the high hydrophilicity of the molecule, showed protective effects against influenza infection in mice upon oral or intraperitoneal administration. The divalent zanamivir (**13**) containing a linker length of 16-18 atoms displayed *in vitro* and *in vivo* inhibition of influenza, being approximately 100-fold more potent than zanamivir. It also provided protective effects in a mouse model of influenza infection, using a single intranasal dose at considerably lower drug level than for zanamivir. Thus, considering these improved characteristics, this compound is currently being developed by Biota (Australia) and Sankyo (Japan) as a long-acting inhaled sialidase inhibitor [28].

Design of Trypanosoma cruzi trans-Sialidase Inhibitors

Trypanosoma cruzi trans-Sialidase (TcTS) and Mucin Molecules

Chagas' disease, a systemic chronic parasitic infection caused by the protozoan parasite *Trypanosoma cruzi*, is endemic in South and Central America, Mexico and the southern United States, being considered one of the most serious parasite diseases in tropical regions [29, 30]. There are currently 8 to 10 million people infected and a further 28 million, mainly in Latin America, are at risk of infection [31, 32]. Typically, 30-40% of the chagasic individuals show clinical symptoms of the chronic phase associated with neuronal, cardiac and digestive dysfunctions, and at least 12.500 die every year [32]. Thus, there is an urgent need for new therapeutics against this disease.

The parasite *Trypanosoma cruzi* sheds a developmentally regulated enzyme called *trans*-sialidase, which is involved in interactions between host cells and parasite that are crucial for cellular invasion processes and infection. *Trypanosoma cruzi trans*-sialidase (TcTS) belongs to the family of glycoproteins expressed on the surface of the parasite and constitutes one of the few examples of natural surface glycosyltransferases found in eucariotes. *T. cruzi* can not synthesize sialic acid itself and uses a *trans*-sialidase enzyme to scavenge this monosaccharide from host glycoconjugates to sialylate acceptors molecules, such as GPI-anchored mucins that are present in parasite plasma membrane [33]. This enzyme is a *trans*-glycosidase specific to catalyze, preferentially, the transfer of sialic acid from host to mucin glycoproteins, originating α-2,3-linkages with acceptor β-galactose molecules in the parasite surface (Scheme **3**) [34]. However, although it is primarily a transferase, it does have residual hydrolase activity [35]. TcTS behaves as a sialyltransferase *in vivo* and *in vitro* in the presence of suitable sugar acceptor substrates (terminal galactose in glycoconjugates), and different from typical sialyltransferases (E.C. 2.4.99.X), catalyzes the transfer reaction with retention of configuration and does not require sugar-nucleotides (i.e. CMP-sialic acid) as the monosaccharide donor [34].

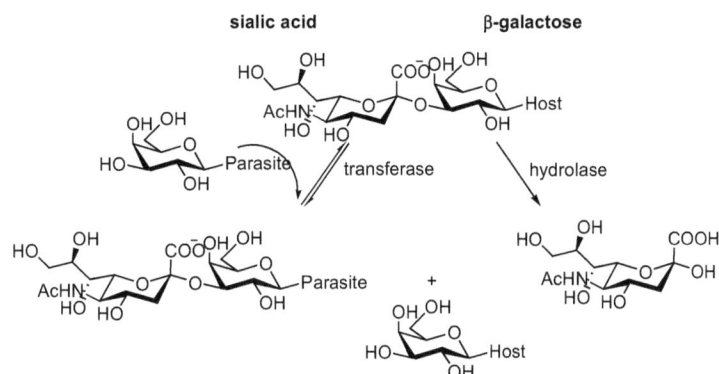

Scheme 3. Transfer of sialic acid by *T. cruzi trans*-sialidase.

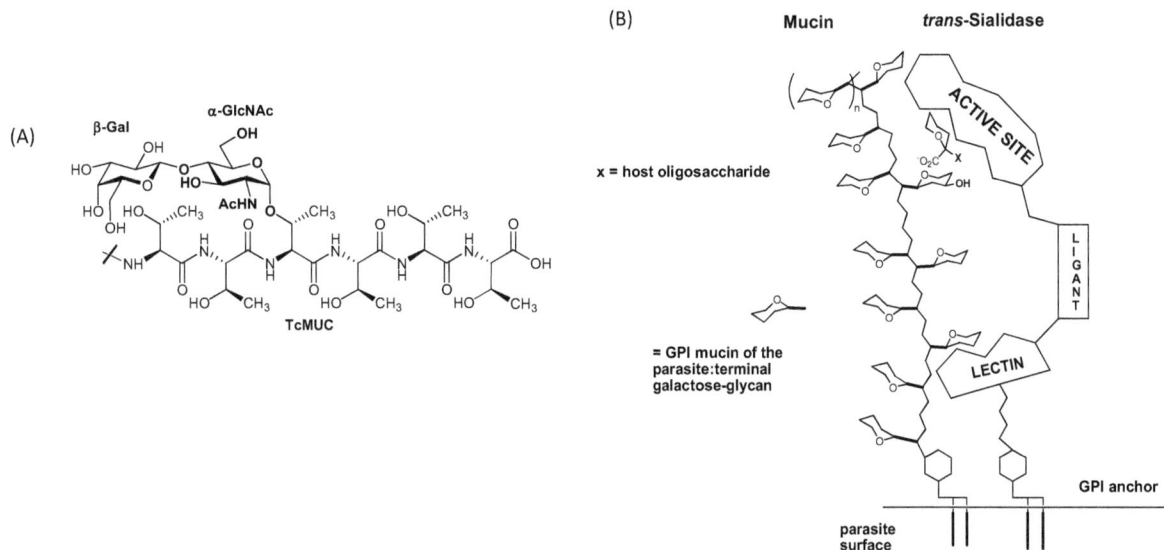

Figure 10: A) Representation of *T. cruzi* mucin molecule (TcMUC). B) Model of recognition and sialylation by TcTS.

T. cruzi mucins (TcMUC) are highly glycosylated (about 60% carbohydrate by weight), polyanionic glycoproteins attached to the membrane by GPI that are rich in Thr, Ser and Pro residues (Thr$_8$LysPro$_2$) [33, 36], but contain few hydrophobic amino acids. The *O*-glycans of *T. cruzi* mucins resemble those of mammalian mucins, although the oligosaccharides are linked to the threonine or serine of the parasite protein via an α-linked *N*-acetyl-glucosamine (GlcNAc) rather than an α-linked *N*-acetyl-galactosamine (GalNAc), as in vertebrate mucins (Fig. **10**) [37]. In general, about 20% of the total *O*-GlcNAc is non-substituted, whereas the remainder can be substituted by one or/up to five galactose residues, in a parasite strain-dependent manner. Most of the Gal residues are present as β-galactopyranose linked as linear and branched side chains to the 4 and 6-positions of the GlcNAc, but in some strains a β-galactofuranose residue can also be linked to the 4-position of the GlcNAc. Besides being involved in the attachment and subsequent penetration of the parasite into host cells, the sialylated mucin molecules also serves to mask the presence of the parasite from the host immune response, conferring resistance to complement and protect against antibody mediated lyses. Therefore, the fundamental role of TcTS in the cellular invasion process parallel to the fact that it is not present in host cells validate this enzyme as an important target for design of antichagasic drugs [38, 39].

TcTS: Mechanism of Action and Design of Inhibitors

Recent determined crystal structure of TcTS [33] showed that it consists of two domains: the *N*-terminal catalytic domains (residues 1-371) connected through a long α helix (residues 372-394) to a *C*-terminal lectin-like domain (residues 395-632), which contains the "shed acute antigen phase" (SAPA), with 12 repeated units of amino acids in tandem, not necessary for the enzymatic activity [34] (Fig. **11A**). The active site of TcTS has several common features with microbial sialidases, for example, an arginine triad (Arg35, Arg245 and Arg314), which interacts with the carboxylate group of sialic acid, besides other important residues essential for stabilization of the transition state (Tyr342, Glu230) and catalysis (Asp59) [35]. A second site, the sialic acid acceptor site, accommodates the β-galactose moiety and contains the amino acids Tyr119 and Trp312 that plays a key role in the *trans*-sialidase activity of TcTS (Fig. **11B**) [40].

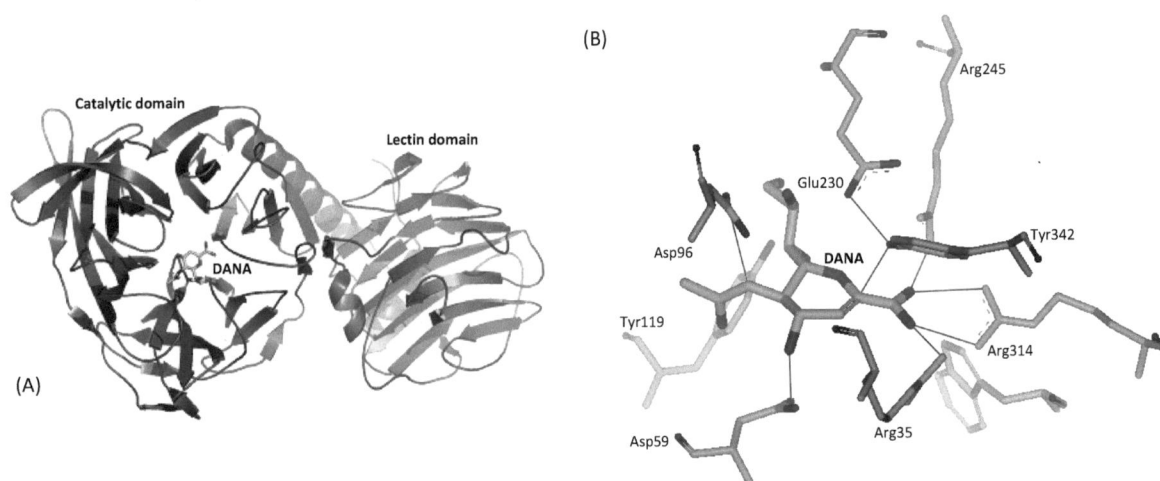

Figure 11: (A) Crystallographic complex of TcTS with DANA (PDB code 1MS8). (B) Main interactions of DANA with the active site of TcTS.

TcTS catalyzes the transglycosylation reaction via a bisubstrate double displacement (ping-pong) mechanism (Scheme **4**), as the binding of lactose to the enzyme active site occurs only after entrance of the sialic acid. After binding of sialic acid donor substrate in the active site, the hydroxyl group of Tyr342, assisted by Glu230 acting as general base, reacts as a nucleophile, with displacement of the protonated group and formation of a covalently bound TcTS-sialoside intermediate. In the next step, the 3-hydroxyl group of the acceptor galactoside, in the presence of Asp59 as a base catalyst, performs a nucleophilic substitution, resulting in the retention of configuration of the sialic acid moiety [41].

Compounds tested as potential TcTS inhibitors can be grouped in two categories, depending on the active site regions they target, namely sialic acid mimetics and sialic acid donor/acceptor substrate mimetics [41]. In the first group, the strategy to mimic sialic acid, as utilized in the development of the influenza neuraminidase inhibitors, has been explored in search of potential TcTS inhibitors. Nevertheless, DANA (**8**) (Fig. **12**), which is a potent inhibitor of influenza neuraminidase, showed a weak inhibition of TcTS (Ki 1.54 mM) despite its favorable interactions in the active site. It shows that key amino acid differences, responsible for the different activity of TcTS, are also responsible for the lower inhibition observed for DANA [35, 42].

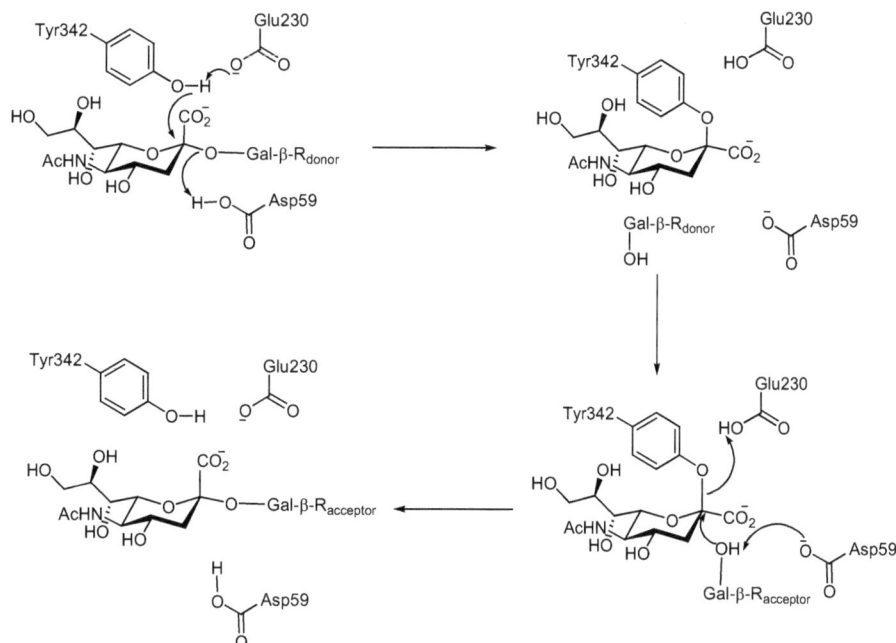

Scheme 4: Mechanism of transglycosylation reaction catalyzed by TcTS.

The fluorinated derivative of sialic acid 2,3-difluorsialic acid (**14**) (Fig. **12**), investigated by Withers in 2003, inhibits TcTS time-dependently by forming a covalent bond with the hydroxyl group of a Tyr 342. However, complete inactivation requires very high concentrations (20 mM) and the enzyme spontaneously recovers activity after removal of excess of the inhibitor and when incubated with the natural acceptor lactose [**15**].

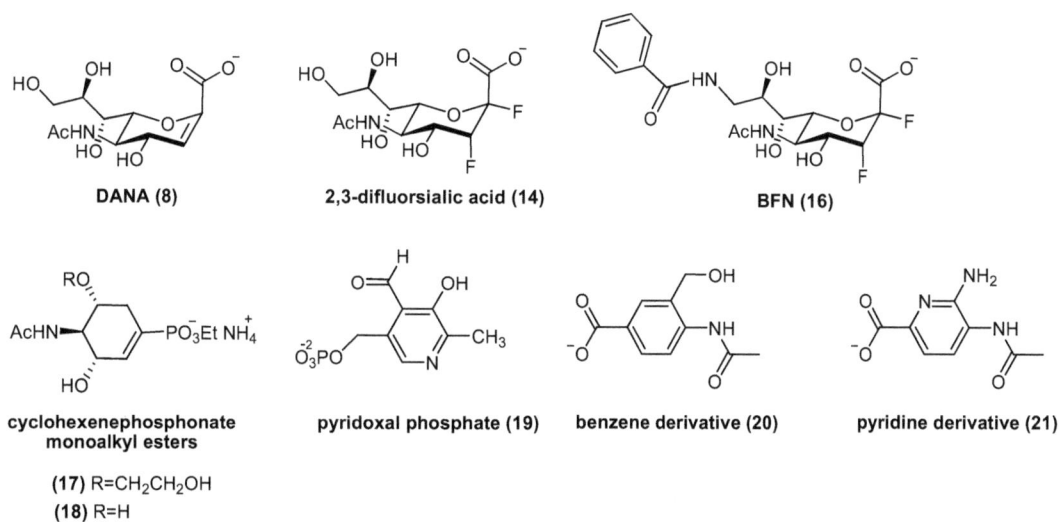

Figure 12: Sialic acid mimetics against TcTS.

More recently, taking into consideration the hydrophobic region around C-9 of sialic acid in the TcTS donor active site, Withers *et al.* developed the synthesis of new derivatives of (**14**), containing aromatic groups at C-9, such as the 9-benzoyl-3-fluoro-*N*-acetyl-neuraminic acid (BFN) (**16**) (Fig. **13**).

Analysis of the covalent intermediate formed between TcTS and BFN (**16**) revealed that the presence of the benzoyl substituent at C-9 induces a reorientation of the whole glycerol side chain compared to the unsubstituted covalent complex (Fig. **13**).

As a consequence, the benzoyl group occupies the space that should accommodate lactoside acceptors, leading to inactivation of transglycosylation by TcTS [43].

The other weak inhibitors of TcTS described are the two cyclohexenephosphonate monoalkyl esters (**17**) (IC_{50} = 4.7 mM) and (**18**) (IC_{50} = 5.7 mM) [45], and the pyridoxal phosphate (**19**) (K*i* 7.3 mM) (Fig. **12**) [46].

Douglas and co-workers have been investigating a synthetic strategy that involves the replacement of the tetrahydropyran ring of sialic acid by simpler cyclic structures such as benzene or pyridine, as exemplified by compounds (**20**) and (**21**) (Fig. **12**) [47], with IC_{50} of 0.54 mM and 0.44 mM, respectively.

Although these structures showed good fit in predicted docked conformation, they did not indicate strong TcTS inhibition.

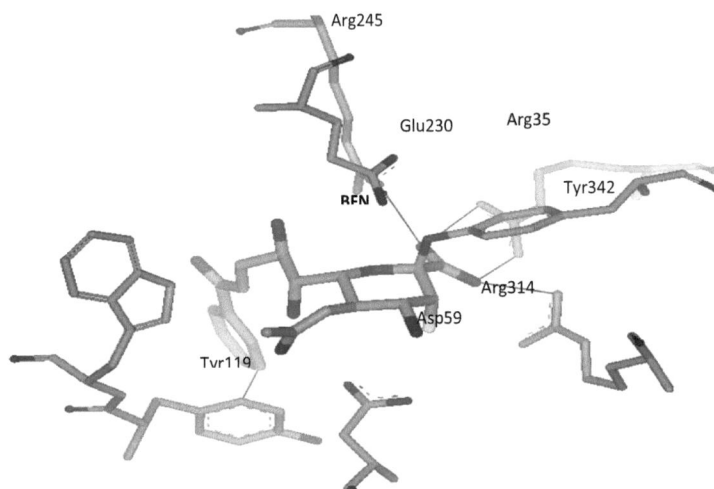

Figure 13: Covalent intermediate formed between TcTS and BFN, and presence of benzoyl group in the acceptor site. (PDB code 3B69).

The sialic acid donor/acceptor substrate mimetics were designed to occupy, simultaneously, the binding sites of the donor substrate (sialic acid) and the acceptor substrate (β-galactose).

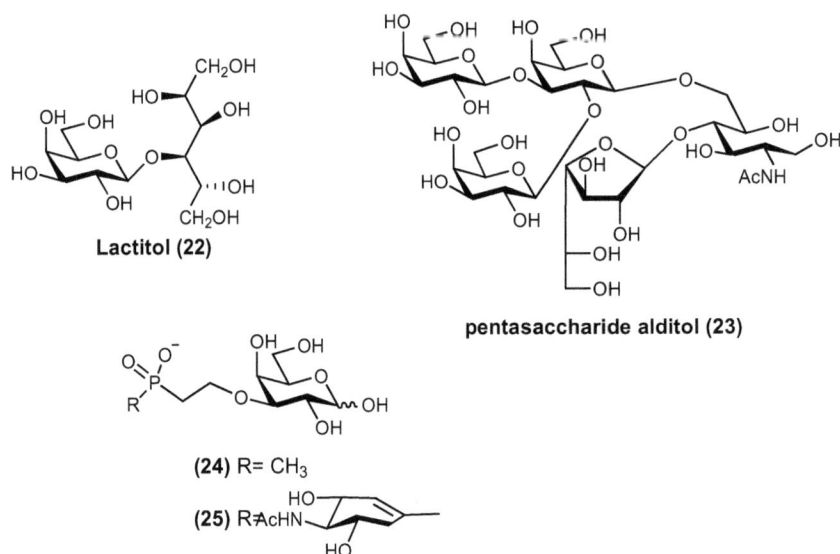

Lactitol (22)

pentasaccharide alditol (23)

(24) R= CH$_3$

(25) R≠AcHN

Figure 14: Sialic acid acceptor substrate mimetics.

Alternatively, other compounds were designed to target essentially the sialic acid acceptor pocket. Lactitol (**22**) (Fig. **14**) is the best lactose analogue discovered so far able to inhibit TcTS reaction toward substrates such as lactose/ *N*-acetyllactosamine, with an IC_{50} of 0.57 mM; It is also verified that it reduced infection of mammalian cells by 20-27% [48].

However, this compound does not inhibit the enzymatic catalytic activity of TcTS, acting as a preferential sialic acid acceptor in comparison with conventional substrates.

Alditol oligosaccharides, such as tetra- and pentasaccharide alditols, containing an external unit of galactofuranose (**23**) (Fig. **14**) were also synthesized by Agusti and co-workers as potential substrates for sialic acid transfer, inhibiting the transfer of sialic acid to the substrate *N*-acetyllactosamine with IC_{50} values in the same order of lactitol, between 0.6 and 4 mM [49].

Galactose-phosphonate derivatives that targeted both the sialic acid and sialic acid acceptor sites have been recently reported, with stronger inhibition being verified for compounds (**24**) (IC_{50} 3 mM) and (**25**), (IC_{50} 1.5 mM) [50] (Fig. **14**).

DEVELOPMENT OF GLYCOCONJUGATE ANTITUMOR VACCINES

For over a century, immunization techniques have noticeably contributed to human health. Although vaccine development proved to be successful, it has been previously based on trial-and-error approaches, through research lacking both comprehension of the immune system molecular functioning and the requirements to produce an effective vaccine.

The ongoing elucidation of the mechanisms driving the immune response has emphasized the relevant role played by chemical synthesis in the rational design and optimization of therapeutic agents able to interfere in such processes [51].

Reverse vaccinology comprises an innovative approach involving the recognition and characterization of key epitopes on selected antigens, which are bound by neutralizing or inhibitory antibodies, later on used for guiding effective vaccine design.

Once the target is established, small and synthetically accessible planned structures may be built mimicking only important epitopic regions, which allows focusing on the immune reaction [51].

Antigen selection from infectious agents is relatively straightforward by searching post-infection immune sera, as such antigens are foreign structures for the human organism and behave immunogenically.

In contrast, due to the self character of cancer cells, natural antibodies against tumor antigens are not generally found in cancer patients.

The choice of targets for cancer vaccine development is complicated and requires more elaborate tools, such as genomics and proteomics [52-54].

Carbohydrate antigens are broad-spectrum markers in that they are found in many surface molecules expressed on a variety of tumor types, acting as signatures associated with malignancy [53].

Amongst tumoral antigens identified so far, carbohydrates are considered the most appropriate and clinically relevant targets for inducing active immunity [52, 54].

Several tumor-associated glycoproteic and glycolipidic antigens, such as the mucin-*O*-linked truncated glycans Tn, sialyl-Tn (STn) and Thomsen-Friedenreich (TF), as well as the lipid tail-containing Globo-H, gangliosides (GM2, GD2, GD3) and Lewis (X, Y) (Fig. **15**), have been adopted as targets [55].

These targets are used for the development of therapeutic vaccines against cancer, since their occurrence in normal tissues is limited [55].

Whilst the overexpression of such antigens on cancer cells surface is often correlated with a poor prognosis for the patient, vaccination based on synthetic tumor-associated epitopes exploits exactly this feature for driving the immune system to produce a tumor-specific response [56, 57].

Antigenic carbohydrates alone trigger a T cell-independent immune response through direct activation of B lymphocytes, resulting in the production of low affinity IgM antibodies.

Application of carbohydrates as vaccines is conditioned to their coupling to immunogenic carrier proteins or peptides, such as bovine serum albumin (BSA), keyhole limpet hemocyanin (KLH) or poliovirus-derived peptide (PV).

Such an approach ensures the stimulation of T lymphocytes, which does not recognize intact antigens but are sensitized by antigenic peptide fragments processed and presented via Major Histocompatibility Complex.

Besides stimulating the carbohydrate-specific response on cytotoxic T-cells, this approach also activates helper T cells that release cytokines promoting isotype switch and affinity maturation of immunoglobulins produced by B cells.

Additional response against carbohydrate antigens is accomplished through co-administration of an immunological adjuvant such as the saponin QS-21, from *Quillaja saponaria* [51, 53, 55, 57, 58].

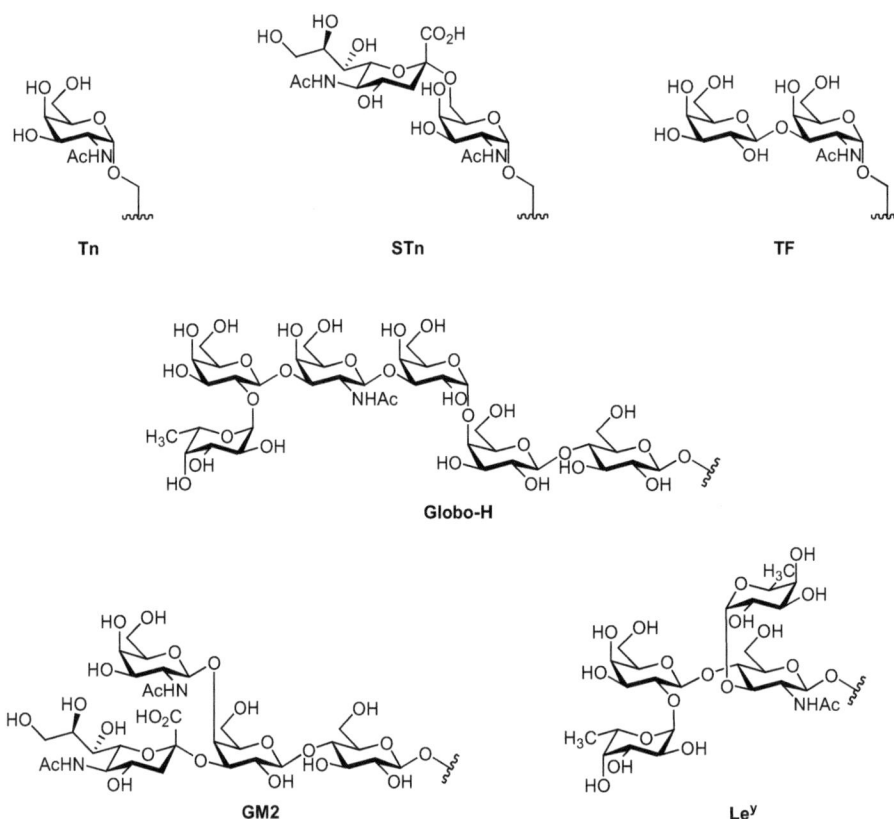

Figure 15: Tumor-associated carbohydrate antigens.

Cytotoxic lymphocytes and antibodies directed against synthetic tumoral antigens are capable of recognizing native epitopes in circulating and metastatic malignant cells, causing their eradication and protecting the organism from tumoral growth and recurrence [51, 55-58]. With the aim of improving immunogenicity, vaccine candidates commonly take advantage of multivalency to mimic more properly the dense display of carbohydrates on cell surfaces. Tumor-associated carbohydrate antigens grouped in dendrimers or clusters are far more efficient in eliciting a protective response than the isolate analog. Cutting-edge research has focused on polyvalent constructs, including up to seven distinct tumoral antigens assembled in a single molecule [52, 53].

Numerous clinical trials ultimately attest the potential of synthetic carbohydrate vaccines for cancer therapy, as promising results were obtained for vaccinations performed with diverse fully synthetic glycoconjugates. A typical example is a phase I clinical trial involving biochemically relapsed prostate cancer patients, who were immunized with a preparation containing Tn clusters (a trimer, specifically) conjugated to KLH carrier protein in the presence of the saponin immunologic adjuvant QS-21 (Fig. **16**). Vaccination safety was established and patients developed good antibody responses against Tn(c), both IgM and IgG, confirming the immunogenicity of the vaccine even at the lowest dose administered (3 μg of Tn(c) per vaccination). Although neither reactivity of sera from immunized patients by flow cytometry nor antibody-dependant cell-mediated cytotoxicity could be demonstrated, overall clinical prognostic was satisfactory. Slope of PSA levels (biochemical marker for prostate cancer) declined for several months after completion of vaccinations, compared to pretreatment period, which may correlate with favorable outcome, possibly delaying cancer radiographic progression [59]. Therefore, in close future active specific immunotherapy is expected to become an alternative or adjuvant approach for cancer treatment [52].

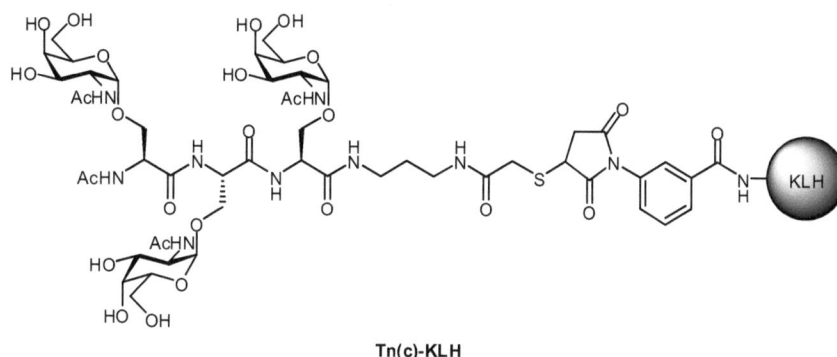

Tn(c)-KLH

Figure 16: Tn cluster conjugated to KLH carrier protein as a vaccine against prostate cancer.

REFERENCES

[1]   Holemann A, Seeberger PH. Carbohydrate diversity: synthesis of glycoconjugates and complex carbohydrates. Curr Opin Biotechnol 2004; 15(6): 615-622.

[2]   Werz DB, Ranzinger R, Herget S *et al.* Exploring the structural diversity of mammalian carbohydrates ("Glycospace") by Statistical Databank Analysis. ACS Chem Biol 2007; 2(10): 685-691.

[3]   Doores KJ, Gamblin DP, Davis BG. Exploring and exploiting the therapeutic potential of glycoconjugates. Chemistry - A European Journal 2006; 12(3): 656-665.

[4]   Sznaidman, M. Bioorganic Chemistry: Carbohydrate*s*. New York: Oxford University Press; 1999.

[5]   Scott AM, Pratt MR, Hruby VJ *et al.* Solid-phase synthesis of *O*-linked glycopeptide analogues of enkephalin. J. Org. Chem 2001 6; 66(7): 2327-2342.

[6]   Davis BG. Synthesis of glycoproteins. Chem. Rev. 2002; 102(2): 579-601.

[7]   Seeberger PH, Werz, DB. Synthesis and medical applications of oligosaccharides. Nature 2007; 446(7139): 1046-1051.

[8]   Kiso M, Ishida H, Ando H. Complex carbohydrate synthesis. Weinheim: Wiley-VCH; 2003.

[9]   Sharon N, Lis H. History of lectins: from hemagglutinins to biological recognition molecules. Glycobiology 2004 30; 14(11): 53R-62R.

[10] Sharon N, Lis H. Lectins: carbohydrate-specific proteins that mediate cellular recognition. Chem Rev 1998 19; 98(2): 637-674.

[11] Scanlan CN, Offer J, Zitzmann N, Dwek, RA. Exploiting the defensive sugars of HIV-1 for drug and vaccine design. Nature 2007 26; 446: 1038-1045.

[12a] De Clerq E. Anti-HIV drugs: 25 compounds approved within 25 years after the discovery of HIV. Int J Antimicrob Agents 2009; 33: 307-320.

[12b] De Clerq E. Antivirals and antiviral strategies. Nat Rev Microbiol 2004; 2: 704-720.

[13] Vaishnav, Y. N.; Wong-Staal, F. The biochemistry of Aids. Annu Rev Biochem 1991; 60: 577-630.

[14] Melo EB, Carvalho I. α e β-Glucosidases como alvos moleculares para desenvolvimento de fármacos. Quím. Nova 2006; 18; 29(4): 840-843.

[15] Melo EB, Gomes, AS, Carvalho I. α- and β-Glucosidase inhibitors: chemical structure and biological activity. Tetrahedron 2006; 7; 62: 10277-10302.

[16] Balzarini J. Targeting the glycans of glycoproteins: a novel paradigm for antiviral therapy. Nat. Rev. Microbiol 2007; 5: 583-597.

[17] Nasi R, Patrick BO, Sim L, Rose DR, Pinto BM. Studies Directed toward the Stereochemical structure determination of the naturally occurring glucosidase inhibitor, kotalanol: synthesis and inhibitory activities against human maltase glucoamylase of seven-Carbon, Chain-Extended Homologues of salacinol. J Org Chem 2008; 24; 73(16): 6172-6181.

[18] Silva CHTP, Carvalho I, Taft CA. Homology modeling and molecular interaction field studies of α-glucosidases as a guide to structure-based design of novel proposed anti-HIV inhibitors. J. Comput.-Aided Mol. Des. 2005; 19: 83-92.

[19] Gomes AS, Silva CHTP, Silva VB, Carvalho I. Structure and ligand-based drug design to propose novel α-glucosidase inhibitors. Current Biactive Compounds 2009; 5: 99-109.

[20] Zhang J, Wang Q, Fang H *et al.* Design, synthesis, inhibitory activity and SAR studies of pyrrolidine derivatives as neuraminidase inhibitors. Bioorg. Med. Chem 2007; 1; 15(7): 2749. 2749-2758.

[21] Itzstein MV. Disease-associated carbohydrate-recognising proteins and structure-based inhibitor design. Curr. Opin. Struct. Biol., 2008; 18: 558-566.

[22] Itzstein MV. The war against influenza: discovery and development of sialidase inhibitors. Nat. Rev. Drug Discov. 2007; 6(12), 967-974.

[23] Fátima A, Baptistella LHB, Pilli RA. Ácidos siálicos-da compreensão do seu envolvimento em processos biológicos ao desenvolvimento de fármacos contra o agente etiológico da gripe. Quim. Nova 2005; 11; 28(2): 306-316.

[24] Colman PM. Influenza virus neuraminidase: structure, antibodies, and inhibitors Protein Sci. 1994; 3: 1687-1696.

[25] Itzstein MV, Dyason JC, Oliver SW *et al.* A study of the active site of influenza virus sialidase: an approach to the rational design of novel anti-influenza drugs. J. Med. Chem. 1996; 39: 388-391.

[26] Hanessian S, Wang J, Montgomery D *et al.* Design, synthesis, and neuraminidase inhibitory activity of GS-4071 analogues that utilize a novel hydrophobic paradigm. Bioorg. Med. Chem. Lett. 2002; 2; 12(23): 3425-3429.

[27] Kim CU, Lew W, Willians MA *et al.* Influenza neuraminidase inhibitors possessing a novel hydrophobic interaction in the enzyme active site: design, synthesis, and structural analysis of carbocyclic sialic acid analogues with potent anti-influenza activity. J. Am. Chem. Soc. 1997; 119: 681-690.

[28] Itzstein MV. Avian influenza vírus, a very sticky situation. Curr. Opin. Chem. Biol. 2008; 12: 102-108.

[29] Linares GEG, Ravaschino EL, Rodriguez JB. Progresses in the field of drug design to combat tropical protozoan parasitic diseases. Curr Med. Chem. 2006; 13(3): 335-360.

[30] Renslo R, Mckerrow JH. Drug discovery and development for neglected parasitic diseases. Nature Chem. Biol 2006; 2: 701-710.

[31] Gascón J, Albajar P, Canãs E *et al.* Diagnosis, management, and treatment of chronic chagas′heart is not endemic.Rev. Esp Cardiol. 2007; 60: 285-293.

[32] Word Health Organization. Reporte del grupo de trabajo científico sobre la enfermedad de Chagas. 2005. Buenos Aires. WHO, 2007.

[33] Previato LM, Previato JO, Jones C *et al.* Structure of *O*-glycosidically linked oligosaccharides from glycoproteins of *Trypanosoma cruzi* CL-Brener strain: evidence for the presence of *O*-linked sialyl-oligosaccharides. J. Biol. Chem. 1995; 270: 7241.

[34] Ribeirão M, Pereira-Chioccola VL, Eichinger D *et al.* Temperature differences for *trans*-glycosylation and hydrolysis reaction reveal an acceptor binding site in the catalytic mechanism of *Trypanosoma cruzi trans*-sialidase. Glycobiology 1997; 7: 1237.

[35] Buschiazzo A, Amaya MF, Cremona ML *et al.* The crystal structure and mode of action of *trans*-sialidase, a key enzyme in *Trypanosoma cruzi* pathogenesis. Molecular Cell 2002; 10(4): 757-768.

[36] Agrellos OA, Jones C, Todeschini AR *et al.* A novel sialylated and galactofuranose-containing *O*-linked glycan, Neu5Acα2→3Galpβ1→6(Galfβ1→4)GlcNAc, is expressed on the sialoglycoprotein of *Trypanosoma cruzi* Dm28c. Mol. Biochem. Parasit. 2003; 126: 93-96.

[37] Buscaglia CA, Campo VA, Frasch ACC *et al. Trypanosoma cruzi* surface mucins: host-dependent coat diversity. Nat Rev Microbiol 2006; 4(3): 229-236.

[38] Corey WT, Lima MF, Villalta F. *Trypanosoma cruzi* uses a 45-KDa mucin for adhesion to mammalian cells. Biochem Biophys Res Commun. 2002; 290: 29-34.

[39] Pereira VL, Serrano A, Almeida IC *et al.* Mucin-like molecules form a negatively charged coat that protects *Trypanosoma cruzi* trypomastigotes from killing by human anti-α-galactosyl antibodies. Journal of Cell Science 2000; 113(7): 1299-1307.

[40] Amaya MF, Watts AG, Damager I *et al.* Structural insights into the catalytic mechanism of *Trypanosoma cruzi trans*-sialidase. Structure 2004; 12: 775-784.

[41] Neres J, Bryce RA, Douglas KT. Rational drug design in parasitology: *trans*-sialidase as a case study for Chagas' disease. Drug Discovery Today 2008; 13(3): 110-117.

[42] Paris G, Ratier L, Amaya MF *et al.* A sialidase mutant displaying *trans*-sialidase activity. J. Mol. Biol 2005; 345: 923-934.

[43] Watts AG, Damager I, Amaya ML *et al. Trypanosoma cruzi trans*-sialidase operates through a covalent sialyl-enzyme intermediate: tyrosine is the catalytic nucleophile. J. Am. Chem. Soc. 2003; 25; 125(25): 7532-7533.

[44] Buchini S, Buschiazzo A, Withers SG. A new generation of specific *Trypanosoma cruzi trans*-sialidase inhibitors. Angew. Chem. Int. Ed. 2008 Feb 25; 47(14): 2700-2703.

[45] Streicher H, Busse H. Building a successful structural motif into sialylmimetics-cyclohexenephosphonate monoesters as pseudo-sialosides with promising inhibitory properties. Bioorg. Med. Chem. 2006 Feb 15; 14(4): 1047-1057.

[46] Ferrero-Garcia MA, Sanches DO, Frasch AC *et al.* The effect of pyridoxal 5'-phosphate and related compounds on *Trypanosoma cruzi trans*-sialidase. J. An. Asoc. Quim. Arg 1993; 81: 127-132.

[47] Neres J, Bonnet P, Edwards PN, *et al.* Benzoic acid and pyridine derivatives as inhibitors of *Trypanosoma cruzi trans*-sialidase. Bioorg. Med. Chem. 2007 Mar 1; 15(5): 2106-2119.

[48] Agusti R, Paris G, Ratier L *et al.* Lactose derivatives are inhibitors of *Trypanosoma cruzi trans*-sialidase activity toward conventional substrates *in vitro* and in vivo. Glycobiology 2004; 14: 659-670.

[49] Agusti R, Giorgi ME, Mendoza VM *et al.* Comparative rates of sialylation by recombinant *trans*-sialidase and inhibitor properties of synthetic oligosaccharides from *Trypanosoma cruzi* mucins-containing galactofuranose and galactopyranose. Bioorg. Med. Chem. 2007; 1; 15(7): 2611-2616.

[50] Busse H, Hakoda M, Stanley M *et al.* Galactose-phosphonates as mimetics of the sialyltransfer by trypanosomal sialidases. J. Carbohydr. Chem. 2007; 26(3): 159-194.

[51] Robinson JA. Horizons in chemical immunology: approaches to synthetic vaccine design. Chimia 2007, 61(3): 84-92.

[52] Slovin SF, Keding SJ, Ragupathi G. Carbohydrate vaccines as immunotherapy for cancer. Immunol Cell Biol 2005, 83(4): 418-428.

[53] Cunto-Amesty G, Monzavi-Karbassi B, Luo P *et al.* Strategies in cancer vaccines development. Int J Parasitol 2003, 33(5-6): 597-613.

[54] Keding SJ, Endo A, Danishefsky SJ. Synthesis of non-natural glycosylamino acids containing tumor-associated carbohydrate antigens. Tetrahedron 2003, 59(35): 7023-7031.

[55] Vichier-Guerre S, Lo-Man R, Huteau V *et al.* Synthesis and immunological evaluation of an antitumor neoglycopeptide vaccine bearing a novel homoserine Tn antigen. Bioorg Med Chem Lett 2004, 14(13): 3567-3570.

[56] Galonic DP, Gin, DY. Chemical glycosylation in the synthesis of glycoconjugate antitumor vaccines. Nature 2007, 446(7139): 1000-1007.

[57] Brocke C, Kunz H. Synthesis of tumor-associated glycopeptide antigens. Bioorg Med Chem 2002, 10(10): 3085-3112.

[58] Meinjohanns E, Meldal M, Jensen T *et al.* Versatile solid-phase thiolytic reduction of azido and N-Dts groups in the synthesis of hemoglobin (67-76) O-glycopeptides and photoaffinity labeled analogs to study glycan T-cell specificity. J. Chem. Soc., Perkin Trans. 1 1997, (6): 871-884.

[59] Slovin SF, Ragupathi G, Musselli C *et al.* Fully synthetic carbohydrate-based vaccines in biochemically relapsed prostate cancer: clinical trial results with α-N-acetylgalactosamine-O-serine/threonine conjugate vaccine. J Clin Oncol 2003, 21(23): 4292-4298.

Subject Index

www.ingramcontent.com/pod-product-compliance
Lightning Source LLC
Chambersburg PA
CBHW041710210326
41598CB00007B/598